The Role of Foods and Nutritional and Botanical Supplements for the Enhancement of Human Health and Performance

The Role of Foods and Nutritional and Botanical Supplements for the Enhancement of Human Health and Performance

Guest Editor

Robert M. Hackman

MDPI

Basel • Beijing • Wuhan • Barcelona • Belgrade • Novi Sad • Cluj • Manchester

Guest Editor
Robert M. Hackman
Department of Nutrition
University of California Davis
Davis, CA
USA

Editorial Office
MDPI AG
Grosspeteranlage 5
4052 Basel, Switzerland

This is a reprint of the Special Issue, published open access by the journal *Nutrients* (ISSN 2072-6643), freely accessible at: https://www.mdpi.com/journal/nutrients/special_issues/H5D478S07X.

For citation purposes, cite each article independently as indicated on the article page online and as indicated below:

Lastname, A.A.; Lastname, B.B. Article Title. *Journal Name* **Year**, *Volume Number*, Page Range.

ISBN 978-3-7258-7454-5 (Hbk)
ISBN 978-3-7258-7455-2 (PDF)
https://doi.org/10.3390/books978-3-7258-7455-2

Contents

About the Editor

Robert M. Hackman

Robert M. Hackman is a nutritionist in the Department of Nutrition at the University of California, Davis. His research addresses the role of foods and nutritional and botanical supplements for enhancement of human health and performance. His work on dietary supplements includes a focus on medicinal mushroom mycelia, and the authentication of botanical extracts. Prof. Hackman's research on foods includes the role of fruits, nuts, wine and berries on vascular function, inflammation, skin aging and eye health.

nutrients

MDPI

Article

Monoterpenoids from the Roots of *Liquidambar formosana* (Formosan Sweet Gum) Exhibit Senomorphic Activity Against Cellular Senescence

Minh Thi Tuyet Le †, Quang Huy Vu †, Van-Hieu Mai, Jorge Eduardo Ponce-Zea, Seri Choi, Jin-Pyo An and Won-Keun Oh *

Research Institute of Pharmaceutical Sciences, College of Pharmacy, Seoul National University, Seoul 08826, Republic of Korea; lethituyetminh19289@gmail.com (M.T.T.L.); 2023-23730@snu.ac.kr (Q.H.V.); maihieu@snu.ac.kr (V.-H.M.); jepz210689@snu.ac.kr (J.E.P.-Z.); loyalmintt2@naver.com (S.C.); ntopjp77@gmail.com (J.-P.A.)

* Correspondence: wkoh1@snu.ac.kr; Tel.: +82-2-880-7872

† These authors contributed equally to this work.

Abstract: Background/objectives: Cellular senescence is a hallmark of aging that contributes to tissue dysfunction and age-related diseases. This process is characterized by the activation of the cyclin-dependent kinase inhibitor p16^{INK4A} and the secretion of pro-inflammatory factors collectively known as the senescence-associated secretory phenotype (SASP). In this study, we used human lung-derived cells, including A549 and IMR90 fibroblasts, to identify bioactive compounds from the roots of *Liquidambar formosana* that suppress p16^{INK4A} activity and attenuate SASP expression. Methods: Bioactivity-guided isolation was performed to obtain target compounds. The structures of the new compounds were elucidated using extensive 1D and 2D NMR spectroscopic analyses as well as high-resolution mass spectrometry. All isolated compounds were evaluated for their ability to inhibit p16^{INK4A}, a key regulator of the cell cycle and an important tumor suppressor protein. Results: Two previously undescribed monoterpenoids (**1** and **2**), characterized as cinnamic acid esters with a monoterpene-derived core, were isolated from the roots of *L. formosana*, along with six known compounds (**3–8**). Notably, compound **3** exhibited promising inhibition of p16^{INK4A} with an IC_{50} value of 3.9 μM. Furthermore, this compound attenuated the senescence phenotype, as demonstrated by β-galactosidase staining and RT-qPCR analysis. This represents the first report identifying bioactive monoterpenoids from *L. formosana* that inhibit aging-related biomarkers such as p16^{INK4A}. Conclusions: These results suggest that cinnamic acid-conjugated monoterpenoids may serve as interesting lead structures for the development of agents targeting the p16^{INK4A} pathway for the treatment of aging-associated diseases. Further studies will be required to clarify the mechanisms of action of this compound and to evaluate its in vivo efficacy.

Keywords: *Liquidambar formosana*; cellular senescence; monoterpenoids; senomorphic effects; SASP inhibition

1. Introduction

The genus *Liquidambar*, commonly known as sweet gum, belongs to the family Altingiaceae and comprises approximately 15 species of deciduous trees widely distributed across East Asia, North America, and the Mediterranean region. Among these, *Liquidambar styraciflua* (American sweet gum) is the most widely recognized species, primarily found in North America [1]. Another important species is *Liquidambar formosana* (Formosan sweet gum), which is native to East Asia and has been traditionally used in folk medicine [2]. Recent studies have revealed several biological activities associated with *L. formosana*. The balsam of this species exhibits antifungal activity, with compounds such as 3α,25-dihydroxyolean-12-en-28-oic acid and bornyl cinnamate showing inhibitory effects against wood-decaying fungi, including *Lenzites betulina* and *Laetiporus sulphureus* [3]. In addition, the ethyl acetate fraction of *L. formosana* leaf extract has demonstrated antioxidant, hypoglycemic, anti-glycation, and antidiabetic properties [4]. Yao Zhu et al. further reported the chemical composition and antimicrobial activities of *L. formosana* oleoresins, identifying 15 pentacyclic triterpenoids, predominantly of the lupane and oleanane types, suggesting potential applications in the treatment of pathological angiogenesis [5].

Aging is a progressive pathophysiological process that leads to an irreversible decline in organ function. Numerous studies have shown that aging increases the risk of various common chronic diseases [6], including diabetes, neurodegenerative disease, cardiovascular disease, chronic obstructive pulmonary disease (COPD), and idiopathic pulmonary fibrosis (IPF). Cellular senescence, one of the hallmarks of aging, is a state of stable cell cycle arrest induced by diverse stressors such as DNA damage, oxidative stress, oncogene activation, and telomere shortening [7]. Although senescent cells lose their proliferative capacity, they remain metabolically active and acquire a pro-inflammatory phenotype known as the senescence-associated secretory phenotype (SASP), characterized by the secretion of cytokines, chemokines, proteases, and growth factors. While senescence plays beneficial roles in tumor suppression and tissue repair, its age-related accumulation promotes chronic inflammation and contributes to pathologies such as cancer, fibrosis, and neurodegeneration [8].

Consequently, targeting senescent cells has emerged as a promising therapeutic approach for age-associated diseases. Two main pharmacological strategies are currently under investigation: senolytics, which selectively eliminate senescent cells, and senomorphics, which modulate the senescent phenotype without inducing cell death, often by suppressing SASP factors or restoring cellular function [9]. Among the key biomarkers of cellular senescence, $p16^{INK4A}$, a cyclin-dependent kinase inhibitor encoded by the CDKN2A gene, plays a critical role [10]. $p16^{INK4A}$ functions as a tumor suppressor by inhibiting cyclin-dependent kinases CDK4 and CDK6, thereby blocking the phosphorylation of the retinoblastoma protein (pRB) and inducing cell cycle arrest in the G1 phase [11]. While $p16^{INK4A}$ is essential for maintaining cellular homeostasis, its aberrant overexpression has been implicated in aging and age-related diseases. Elevated levels of $p16^{INK4A}$ are frequently observed in aged tissues, where it promotes the accumulation of senescent cells and the activation of SASP secretion. Recent studies have further revealed that $p16^{INK4A}$ functions not only as a biomarker of cellular senescence but also as an active driver of aging-related pathologies by impairing tissue regeneration and promoting degenerative processes.

Therefore, modulation of $p16^{INK4A}$ expression using natural products or herbal medicines has emerged as a promising therapeutic strategy to delay senescence and promote healthy aging. Among the potential candidates, bakuchiol, a phenolic monoterpene isolated from *Psoralea corylifolia*, has been reported to exert a broad range of pharmacological activities, including significant anti-aging effects [12]. The roots of *L. formosana*, rich in phenolic monoterpenoids, represent another potential source of senescence-modulating agents. However, the anti-senescence potential of these compounds remains largely unexplored.

2. Materials and Methods

2.1. General Experimental Procedures

A JASCO P-2000 polarimeter (JASCO International Co. Ltd., Tokyo, Japan) was used to determine optical rotations and a Chirascan-Plus spectrometer (Applied Photophysics Ltd.,

Surrey, UK) was employed to record UV and electronic circular dichroism (ECD) spectra. IR spectra were measured using a Nicolet 6700 Fourier transform infrared spectrometer (Thermo Fisher Scientific, Waltham, MA, USA). 1D and 2D NMR spectra were acquired on a JEOL 400 MHz spectrometer, and data processing and assignments were performed with MestReNova 14.2 (Mestrelab Research, Santiago de Compostela, Spain). High-resolution electrospray ionization mass spectrometry (HR-ESI-MS) was performed on an Agilent Infinity UHPLC 1290 system equipped with an Agilent qTOF mass spectrometer 6530 (Agilent Technologies, Santa Clara, CA, USA). Compound purification was performed using a Gilson HPLC system with UV detection at 210 and 254 nm (Gilson Inc., Middleton, WI, USA), using a C18 column (10 × 250 mm, 10 μm particle size). Column chromatography (CC) was carried out with silica gel (particle size: 63–200 μm, Zeochem AG, Rüti, Switzerland), RP-C18 (particle size: 75 μm, Nacalai Tesque, Kyoto, Japan), and Sephadex LH-20 (GE Healthcare, Little Chalfont, UK). Thin-layer chromatography (TLC) was conducted using silica gel 60 F254 and RP-18 F254S plates (Merck, Darmstadt, Germany). All solvents were purchased from Daejung Chemical (Siheung, Republic of Korea).

2.2. Plant Material

The roots of *Liquidambar formosana* were collected in 2022 from the Gwangyang branch of the Seoul National University Forests (35°2′3.336″ N, 127°36′16.056″ E), Republic of Korea. Voucher specimen (SNU-2022-07) was deposited in the Herbarium of the College of Pharmacy, Seoul National University, Seoul, Republic of Korea. The plant was authenticated through integrated morphological and anatomical analyses by Hak-Ki Park from the Gwangyang branch of the Seoul National University Forests.

2.3. HR-ESI-MS/MS and Molecular Networking

HR-ESI-MS/MS analyses were performed on an Agilent 6530 Q-TOF mass spectrometer (Agilent Technologies, Santa Clara, CA, USA) interfaced with an Agilent 1260 Infinity UPLC and fitted with an ACQUITY UPLC BEH C18 column (2.1 × 100 mm i.d., 1.7 μm). The mobile phase gradient employed H_2O with 0.1% formic acid (A) and MeCN (B), programmed from 10% B to 90% B over 20 min at 0.3 mL/min, maintained at 100% B for 4 min at 0.5 mL/min, returned to 10% B in 0.1 min, and equilibrated for 2 min at 0.3 mL/min. Nitrogen was used as both the drying and collision gas in the ESI source. The electrospray ionization parameters were optimized as follows: drying gas flow rate, 10 L/min; capillary temperature, 350 °C; sheath gas temperature, 350 °C; sheath gas flow, 12 L/min; nebulizer pressure, 30 psi. Additional source parameters included a capillary voltage (VCap) of 4000 V, fragmentor voltage of 180 V, skimmer voltage of 60 V, and an octopole RF peak voltage of 750 V. Data acquisition was performed in both positive and negative ionization modes with MS scanning from m/z 100–1000. Auto-MS/MS data were acquired in data-dependent mode with a fixed collision energy of 50 eV. ProteoWizard was employed to transform raw data files into mzML (Version 3.0, Palo Alto, CA, USA). Data processing was performed using MZmine software (version 4.0.3) through a workflow: mzML file import, peak threshold setting, chromatogram building, deconvolution, isotope grouping, join alignment, and gap filling. The processed data were exported as mgf-clustered spectral files and corresponding CSV metadata files (containing retention times, peak areas, and molecular formula assignments) using the integrated "Export for GNPS" and "Export to CSV file" functions. Molecular networking analysis was performed using the spectral/molecular networking module in MZmine. Library matching against the Global Natural Products Social Molecular Networking (GNPS) spectral databases required a minimum cosine score of 0.7 and at least four matched fragment ions. Network visualization and analysis were accomplished using Cytoscape software (version 3.10.3) (Figure S1).

2.4. Extraction and Isolation

The ground roots (3 kg) of *Liquidambar formosana* were extracted three times with 70% EtOH (5 L, 99 min each; Powersonic 420 ultrasonic cleaner, Hwashin Tech, Seoul, Republic of Korea) at room temperature to obtain a crude extract, which was then dried under reduced pressure. The dried crude root extract was partitioned between n-hexane, ethyl acetate, n-butanol, and water to obtain four respective fractions. The hexane fraction was chromatographed using an MPLC system (Biotage, Uppsala, Sweden) equipped with an RP-C18 column (40–60 μm particle size, MeOH/H_2O = 10/90 to 100/0), yielding three fractions (M1 to M3). Fraction M2 (2 g) was subjected to MPLC on a normal-phase (NP) column and eluted with n-hexane/EtOAc (85/15 to 100/0), yielding three subfractions. Fraction M2.1 (1.5 g) was further chromatographed on an RP column (40–60 μm particle size; MeOH/H_2O = 80/20 to 100/0) to obtain three subfractions. Fraction M2.1.3 (500 mg) was purified by semi-preparative HPLC (MeCN/H_2O, isocratic 90%) to yield compound **7** (100 mg, 23 min), compound **6** (32 mg, 21.5 min), compound **3** (30 mg, 17 min), compound **4** (4 mg, 15 min), compound **5** (7 mg, 12.5 min), compound **2** (8 mg, 16.5 min), compound **1** (4 mg, 20.5 min), and compound **8** (2 mg, 13.5 min).

β-Pinenyl cinnamate (**1**): Pale yellow amorphous powder; $[\alpha]_D^{25}$ + 99.6 (*c* 0.1, MeOH); IR (KBr) ν_{max} 3898, 3730, 3564, 2930, 2353, 1711, 1636, 1513, 1452, 1278, 1166, 981, 769, 684; ^1H and ^{13}C NMR; see Table 1 and Figures S2–S10 in Supplementary Materials; HRESIMS m/z 283.1707 $[M + H]^+$ (calcd for $C_{19}H_{23}O_2$ at 283.1693, m/z error 4.9 ppm).

Table 1. ^1H- and ^{13}C-NMR spectroscopic data of compounds **1** and **2** in $CDCl_3$ [a].

Position	**1** [b]		**2**	
	δ_H (*J* in Hz)	δ_C	δ_H (*J* in Hz)	δ_C
1	7.37 (m)	129.0	7.37 (m)	129.0
2	7.38 (m)	130.3	7.38 (m)	130.4
3	7.37 (m)	129.0	7.37 (m)	129.0
4	7.52 (m)	128.2	7.53 (m)	128.2
5		134.6		134.5
6	7.52 (m)	128.2	7.53 (m)	128.2
7	7.68 (d, 16.0)	144.6	7.70, (d, 16.0)	144.9
8	6.45 (d, 16.0)	119.0	6.47, (d, 16.0)	118.2
9		166.7		167.0
12	5.70 (d, 8.0)	68.8	4.60 (2H, s)	70.3
13		150.5		129.3
14	2.56 (t, 5.45)	50.9	7.38 (m)	130.7
15		40.7	2.26 (2H, br s)	26.5
16	2.02 (m)	39.7	2.28 (2H, br s)	30.9
17	1.88 (m), 2.45 (m)	33.5		145.8
18	4.93 (br s), 5.11 (br s)	114.4	6.38, (dd, 17.6, 10.8)	138.9
19	1.58 (m), 1.69 (m)	28.1	5.07 (d, 10.8), 5.24 (d, 17.6)	116.1
20	0.73 (3H, s)	22.1	1.71 (3H, s)	14.2
21	1.31 (3H, s)	26.0	5.02 (d, 12.3)	113.3

[a] Assignments were based on COSY, HSQC, and HMBC experiments. [b] ^1H and ^{13}C NMR spectra were acquired at 400 and 100 MHz, respectively.

Myrcenyl cinnamate (**2**): Pale yellow amorphous powder; $[\alpha]_D^{25}$ + 107.8 (*c* 0.1, MeOH); UV (MeOH) λ_{max} (log ε) 252 (−1.95), 350 (−1.85); IR (KBr) ν_{max} 3898, 3730, 3564, 2930, 2353, 1711, 1636, 1513, 1452, 1278, 1166, 981, 769, 684; ^1H and ^{13}C NMR; see Table 1 and Figures S11–S17; HRESIMS found m/z 283.1694 $[M + H]^+$ (calcd for $C_{19}H_{23}O_2$ at 283.1693, m/z error 0.3 ppm)

Limonenyl cinnamate (**3**): Pale yellow amorphous powder; ^{1}H NMR (400 MHz, $CDCl_3$) δ_H 7.68 (dd, *J* = 16.0, 4.5 Hz, 1H), 7.58–7.48 (m, 2H), 7.44–7.34 (m, 3H), 6.46 (dd, *J* = 16.0, 11.6 Hz, 1H), 5.62 (tp, *J* = 2.8, 1.4 Hz, 1H), 4.59 (s, 2H), 2.43 (dt, *J* = 8.6, 5.6 Hz, 1H), 2.31 (dt, *J* = 15.2, 1.6 Hz, 1H), 2.18 (td, *J* = 5.6, 1.5 Hz, 1H), 2.12 (dqd, *J* = 5.9, 2.9, 1.2 Hz, 1H), 1.30 (s, 3H), 1.22 (d, *J* = 8.7 Hz, 1H), 0.86 (s, 3H); ^{13}C NMR (100 MHz, $CDCl_3$) δ_C 167.0, 144.8, 143.2, 134.6, 130.4, 128.2, 128.2, 121.6, 118.3, 67.2, 43.7, 40.8, 38.2, 31.6, 31.4, 29.8, 26.2, 21.2.; HRESIMS *m/z* 283.1706 $[M + H]^+$ (calcd for $C_{19}H_{23}O_2$ at 283.1693, *m/z* error 4.6 ppm).

4-Isopropylbenzyl cinnamate (**4**): Pale yellow amorphous powder; ^{1}H NMR (400 MHz, $CDCl_3$) δ_H δ 7.72 (d, *J* = 16.0 Hz, 1H), 7.55–7.48 (m, 2H), 7.41–7.32 (m, 5H), 7.25 (d, *J* = 5.2 Hz, 2H), 6.48 (d, *J* = 16.0 Hz, 1H), 5.22 (s, 2H), 1.29–1.22 (m, 6H); ^{13}C NMR (100 MHz, $CDCl_3$) δ_C 167.0, 149.3, 145.2, 133.5, 130.5, 129.0, 128.7, 128.2, 126.8, 118.1, 66.5, 34.1, 24.1; HRESIMS *m/z* 281.1556 $[M + H]^+$ (calcd for $C_{19}H_{23}O_2$ at 281.1536, *m/z* error 7.11 ppm).

Cinnamyl cinnamate (**5**): Pale yellow amorphous powder; ^{1}H NMR (400 MHz, $CDCl_3$) δ_H 7.74 (d, *J* = 16.0 Hz, 1H), 7.54 (dt, *J* = 6.3, 3.8 Hz, 3H), 7.45–7.35 (m, 6H), 7.34–7.31 (m, 2H), 6.53–6.43 (m, 1H), 4.88 (dd, *J* = 6.4, 1.3 Hz, 2H); ^{13}C NMR (100 MHz, $CDCl_3$) δ_C 166.9, 145.3, 134.5, 134.4, 130.5, 129.1, 128.8, 128.3, 128.2, 126.8, 123.4, 118.1, 65.3, 29.9.

Myrthenyl cinnamate (**6**): Pale yellow amorphous powder; ^{1}H NMR (400 MHz, $CDCl_3$) δ_H 7.68 (d, *J* = 16.0 Hz, 1H), 7.54 (dq, *J* = 5.7, 3.2 Hz, 2H), 7.41–7.36 (m, 3H), 6.48 (d, *J* = 16.0 Hz, 1H), 5.02 (ddd, *J* = 10.0, 3.5, 2.1 Hz, 1H), 2.42 (ddt, *J* = 13.9, 10.0, 4.0 Hz, 1H), 2.05 (ddd, *J* = 12.7, 9.1, 4.4 Hz, 1H), 1.85–1.68 (m, 2H), 1.42–1.23 (m, 3H), 1.06 (dd, *J* = 13.8, 3.5 Hz, 1H), 0.95 (s, 3H), 0.90 (s, 3H), 0.89 (s, 3H); ^{13}C NMR (100 MHz, $CDCl_3$) δ_C 167.1, 144.9, 143.2, 134.6, 130.4, 129.0, 128.2, 128.2, 121.7, 118.3, 67.3, 43.8, 40.9, 38.2, 31.6, 31.4, 29.8, 26.3, 21.2; HRESIMS *m/z* 283.1691 $[M + H]^+$ (calcd for $C_{19}H_{23}O_2$ at 283.1693, *m/z* error −0.71 ppm).

Bornyl cinnamate (**7**): Pale yellow amorphous powder; ^{1}H NMR (400 MHz, $CDCl_3$) δ_H 7.68 (d, *J* = 16.0 Hz, 1H), 7.54 (dq, *J* = 5.7, 3.2 Hz, 2H), 7.41–7.36 (m, 3H), 6.48 (d, *J* = 16.0 Hz, 1H), 5.02 (ddd, *J* = 10.0, 3.5, 2.1 Hz, 1H), 2.42 (ddt, *J* = 13.9, 10.0, 4.0 Hz, 1H), 2.05 (ddd, *J* = 12.7, 9.1, 4.4 Hz, 1H), 1.85–1.68 (m, 2H), 1.42–1.23 (m, 3H), 1.06 (dd, *J* = 13.8, 3.5 Hz, 1H), 0.95 (s, 3H), 0.90 (s, 3H), 0.89 (s, 3H); ^{13}C NMR (100 MHz, $CDCl_3$) δ_C 167.5, 144.4, 134.7, 130.3, 129.0, 128.2, 119.0, 80.1, 49.1, 48.0, 45.1, 37.0, 29.8, 28.2, 27.4, 19.9, 19.0, 13.7; HRESIMS *m/z* 285.1846 $[M + H]^+$ (calcd for $C_{19}H_{25}O_2$ at 285.1849, *m/z* error −1.07 ppm).

3-Phenylpropyl cinnamate (**8**): Pale yellow amorphous powder; ^{1}H NMR (400 MHz, $CDCl_3$) δ_H 7.68 (d, *J* = 16.0 Hz, 1H), 7.57–7.51 (m, 2H), 7.40 (dt, *J* = 4.6, 2.7 Hz, 3H), 7.33–7.27 (m, 2H), 7.24–7.17 (m, 3H), 6.45 (d, *J* = 16.0 Hz, 1H), 4.24 (t, *J* = 6.5 Hz, 2H), 2.75 (dd, *J* = 8.6, 6.8 Hz, 2H), 2.13–1.99 (m, 2H); ^{13}C NMR (100 MHz, $CDCl_3$) δ_C 167.2, 144.9, 141.4, 134.6, 130.4, 129.0, 128.6, 128.2, 126.2, 118.3, 64.1, 32.4, 30.5.; HRESIMS *m/z* 267.1375 $[M + H]^+$ (calcd for $C_{19}H_{23}O_2$ at 267.1380, *m/z* error −1.87 ppm).

2.5. ECD Calculation

A conformational search was performed using the GMMX extension in Gaussian View 9 with MMFF94s molecular force-field calculations and an energy cutoff of 3.5 kcal/mol. Conformers with populations greater than 1% were selected and then subjected to DFT optimization followed by frequency calculations at the B3LYP/6-31G(d) level of theory in the gas phase using Gaussian 16. Upon completion, Gibbs free energies were extracted, and Boltzmann populations were calculated. Conformers with a Boltzmann population greater than 1% were selected for ECD simulation using time-dependent DFT (TD-DFT) at the B3LYP/6-31G(d) level of theory in MeOH (IEFPCM solvent model), considering up to the first 20 excitation states (compound **1**). The Boltzmann-averaged spectra were visualized using SpecDis 1.70 software, with a half-bandwidth correction of 0.2–0.3 eV and a UV shift correction of 0–20 nm.

2.6. Cell Culture

The lung cancer cell line A549 was obtained from the Korean Cell Line Bank. A549 cells were cultured in Roswell Park Memorial Institute (RPMI) 1640 medium (Welgene, Daegu, Republic of Korea) supplemented with 10% fetal bovine serum (FBS) (Gibco, Waltham, MA, USA) and 1% penicillin-streptomycin (P/S; Gibco) under a humidified atmosphere containing 5% CO_2 at 37 °C. IMR90 human lung fibroblasts (American Type Culture Collection, ATCC, CCL-186) were maintained in Minimum Essential Medium (MEM) supplied with 10% FBS (Gibco) and 1% P/S at 37 °C with 5% CO_2. Cells were subcultured every 48 hr.

2.7. $p16^{INK4A}$ Promoter Activity-Related Luciferase Reporter Assay

A549 cells were seeded at a density of 80,000 cells/mL in 96-well plates. After 24 hr of incubation, they were washed with phosphate-buffered saline (PBS) and transfected with a plasmid mixture and Lipofectamine 2000 (Invitrogen, Carlsbad, CA, USA) for 7 hr in Opti-MEM. The plasmid mixture contained 0.07 μg pGL3_$p16^{INK4A}$ plasmid encoding the human $p16^{INK4A}$ promoter (GenBank accession no. NM_000077.4) and firefly luciferase, and 0.03 μg pSV-beta-galactosidase plasmid (Promega, Madison, WI, USA) as an internal standard. The following day, cells were treated with compounds and navitoclax (as a positive control) for 20 h, followed by lysis with cell culture lysis buffer (Promega). Luciferase activity was measured using a firefly luciferase assay kit (Promega) and normalized to β-galactosidase activity.

2.8. MTT Assay

Cell viability was assessed by the (3-(4,5-dimethyl-2-thiazolyl)-2,5-diphenyl-2H-tetrazolium bromide (MTT; Sigma, St. Louis, MO, USA) assay. A volume of 20 μL of the 2 mg/mL MTT solution was added to each well in a 96-well plate, and the plates were incubated at 37 °C in the dark for 4 h. After incubation, the supernatant was removed, and the formazan crystals were dissolved in 100 μL of DMSO. The absorbance was obtained at 540 nm using a microplate reader (VersaMax™, Molecular Devices, San Jose, CA, USA).

2.9. Senescence-Associated β-Galactosidase Staining

IMR90 cells were seeded at 50,000 cells/mL in 24-well plates and incubated for 24 h. Bleomycin (40 μg/mL; Tokyo Chemical Industry, Tokyo, Japan) was added to all wells except the untreated control. After 48 h, the test compounds were introduced and cells were further incubated for 48 h. Cells were stained using a senescence-associated β-galactosidase (SA-β-gal) staining kit (Cell Signaling Technology, Danvers, MA, USA) according to the manufacturer's instructions. The stained cells were observed under a microscope (Olympus Corporation, Tokyo, Japan). All reactions were independently performed in triplicate. The expression level of X-gal was normalized to that of the control group.

2.10. RNA Extraction and Quantitative Real-Time Polymerase Chain Reaction (qRT-PCR)

IMR90 cells were seeded as described above and treated with bleomycin (40 μg/mL) for 48 h, followed by exposure to the test compounds for an additional 48 h. Total RNA was extracted using NucleoZOL (Macherey-Nagel, Düren, Germany) after 48 h of compound treatment. One μg of total RNA was used for cDNA synthesis with the Thermo cDNA Synthesis Kit (Thermo Fisher Scientific). Real-time qPCR was performed by the AccuPower 2X GreenStarTM qPCR Master Mix (Bioneer, Daejeon, Republic of Korea). All reactions were performed in independent triplicates. The expression levels of all markers were normalized to 18s ribosomal RNA.

2.11. Statistical Analyses

The data were analyzed using GraphPad PRISM 10.4.1 software (GraphPad Software, Inc., La Jolla, San Diego, CA, USA) and are expressed as the mean ± standard error of the mean (SEM) from three independent experiments. To compare group means, analysis of variance (ANOVA) was performed, followed by Dunn's multiple comparison test for post hoc analysis. Statistical significance was established at * $p < 0.05$, ** $p < 0.01$, *** $p < 0.001$, and **** $p < 0.0001$.

3. Results

3.1. Feature-Based Molecular Networking of the Liquidambar formosana Root Extract

The GNPS molecular network highlighted six noteworthy clusters, including coumarins, gallotannins, monoterpenoids, fatty acids, triterpenoids, and flavonoids. In the triterpenoid cluster, four compounds were annotated using the GNPS platform against the online GNPS database, namely, betulonic acid, sumaresinolic acid, ursolic acid, and oleanolic acid. The largest cluster displayed the presence of numerous compound classes, including monoterpenoids such as (−)-carveol (m/z: 135.1170) and α-pinene (m/z: 137.1320), along with coumarins and fatty acids.

To enhance the annotation of metabolites from *L. formosana* roots, a local database was established by searching Reaxys for compounds previously isolated from *L. formosana*. This local database was then imported into MZmine to calculate the possible adducts and annotate features by matching with the corresponding m/z values. The result showed that many nodes were annotated, including a monoterpene cluster [linalool (m/z 137.1320)]; a gallotannin cluster [3,4,5-trimethoxyphenyl-6-O-syringoyl-D-glucopyranoside (m/z 527.1729) and 2,4,6-tri-O-galloyl-D-glucose (m/z 619.0930)]; and a triterpene cluster [melliferone (m/z 435.3257) and 28-diepoxyoleanane-3-one (m/z 437.3414)]. Catechin (m/z 273.0757) and gallocatechin (m/z 289.0707) were also putatively identified. However, a significant number of molecular features remained unannotated, which represents a well-known challenge in metabolomic analysis, where many detected chemical signals cannot be identified using standard library matching. To address this bottleneck, we applied the Structural similarity Network Annotation Platform for Mass Spectrometry (SNAP-MS). This tool is designed to annotate molecular networking subnetworks without relying on experimental MS^2 spectral libraries, instead leveraging the principle that the distribution of molecular formulae within a natural product family is often highly diagnostic. For each subnetwork, SNAP-MS searches each parent mass against a comprehensive reference database, in this instance, the COCONUT database, which contains over 600,000 compounds from natural sources. It retrieves all potential candidate structures for each mass and then groups them into compound families based on structural similarity. These families are scored and ranked according to their coverage, defined as the number of distinct masses from the original subnetwork represented within that family. This approach enables more accurate prediction of a compound family for an entire subnetwork, even when individual members are absent from spectral libraries [13].

Results from SNAP-MS suggested six clusters with top candidates, including xanthones, monoterpenoids, diarylheptanoids, stilbenoids, coumarins, and cinnamic acid-conjugated monoterpenoids (Figure S18). Among them, the cluster of cinnamic acid-conjugated monoterpenoids is described in Figure 1B. MS/MS analysis revealed a characteristic fragment at m/z 131.05. This fragment corresponds to the protonated cinnamic acid moiety, providing strong experimental evidence for the presence of a cinnamate substructure across the molecular family. Using this ion as a marker, we extracted the ion chromatogram (± 0.05 Da) of the enriched fraction and observed several peaks whose MS^2 spectra contained m/z 131.05. The corresponding precursor ions were m/z 265, 267, 281,

283, and 285, consistent with multiple monoterpene–cinnamate conjugates. This combination of computational prediction from SNAP-MS and direct experimental evidence from the MS/MS data provided valuable guidance for the subsequent targeted isolation of these novel compounds.

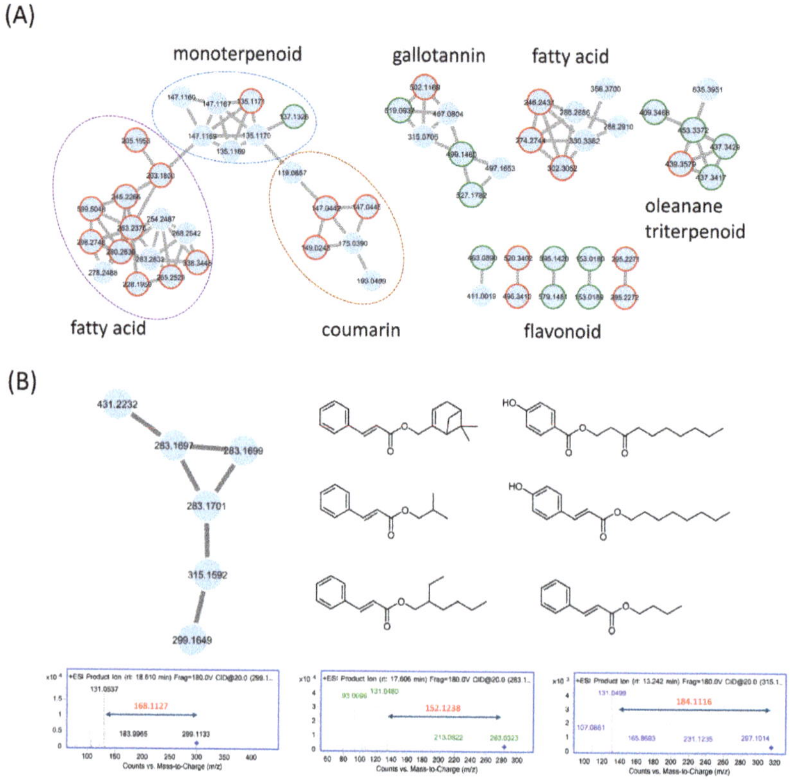

Figure 1. (**A**) Clusters of interest from molecular networking of the crude extract from the roots of *L. formosana* using UPLC qTOF-MS/MS data acquired in the positive mode. Nodes were grouped into chemical classes, and clusters were circled as follows: blue for monoterpenoids, purple for fatty acids, and orange for coumarins. Individual nodes annotated by GNPS are highlighted with a red ring, while nodes putatively identified from the literature (via a Reaxys search for compounds previously reported from *L. formosana*) are marked with a green ring. (**B**) The target cluster for isolation (left) and suggested structures for cluster (right), as revealed by SNAP-MS and tandem MS analyses, show cinnamic acid derivatives bearing possible monoterpene moieties.

3.2. *Isolation and Structural Elucidation of New Compounds* **1** *and* **2**

The structure of compound **1** was deduced using ^{1}H and ^{13}C NMR, one- and two-dimensional spectroscopy, as well as IR and MS analyses (Figure 2). *UPLC* qTOF-MS/MS analysis of **1** yielded a protonated molecular ion $[M + H]^+$ at m/z 283.1710 (calcd for $C_{19}H_{23}O_2$, 283.1693), consistent with a molecular formula of $C_{19}H_{22}O_2$, indicating nine degrees of unsaturation. The ^{1}H NMR spectrum exhibited characteristic signals of a trans-disubstituted double bond at δ_H 7.68 and 6.45 (each d, J = 16.0 Hz), an oxygenated methine at δ_H 5.70, two protons of an exomethylene group (δ_H 5.11, 4.93), and a vinyl methyl group at δ_H 0.73 and 1.31 (each s). The ^{13}C NMR data, in conjunction with DEPT experiments, revealed 19 resonances attributable to one carbonyl (δ_C 166.7), six aromatic carbons (δ_C 128.2, 128.2, 129.0, 129.0, 130.3, 134.6), four olefinic carbons (δ_C 144.6, 119.04, 150.5, 114.4), two quaternary sp3 carbons (δ_C 40.7, 150.5), two methylenes (δ_C 28.1, 33.5) including one exomethylene (δ_C 114.4), and two methyl carbons (δ_C 22.1, 26.0). COSY, HSQC, and HMBC spectral data provided additional evidence to confirm the structure of compound **1**. The COSY spectrum of compound **1** displayed connectivities between H-16 (δ_H 2.02, m) and H-17 (δ_H 1.88, 2.45, each m), H-16 and H-19 (δ_H 1.58, 1.69, each m), H-19 and H-14 (δ_H 2.56, t, J = 5.4 Hz), and H-17 and H-12 (δ_H 5.70, d, J = 8.0 Hz) (Figure 3A). The HMBC spectrum of compound **1** showed significant correlations from the exomethylene protons (δ_H 4.93, 5.11, each br s, H-18) to C-13 (δ_C 150.5), C-12 (δ_C 68.8), and C-14 (δ_C 50.9). The signals for H-19 correlated with C-13, C-14, C-15 (δ_C 40.7), C-16 (δ_C 39.7), and C-17 (δ_C 33.5), whereas H-20 (δ_H 0.73) and H-21 (δ_H 1.31) showed correlations with C-15 and C-21 (δ_C 26.0). In addition, the correlations of H-7 (δ_H 7.68, d, J = 16.0 Hz) with C-5 (δ_C 134.6), C-6 (δ_C 128.2), and C-4 (δ_C 128.2), as well as the correlation of H-8 (δ_H 6.45, d, J = 16.0 Hz) with C-5, supported the proposed structure as a cinnamic acid conjugated with β-pinene. The relative configuration of **1** was determined based on diagnostic NOE correlations (Figure 3B). NOE correlations between Me-20 and H-14, and between Me-20 and H-16, revealed an α-orientation, whereas the NOE correlation between Me-21 and H-12 indicated a β-orientation. Based on the relative configuration, the absolute configuration of **1** was assigned as 14S,12R,16S by ECD calculations (Figure 3C). Therefore, compound **1** was characterized as β-pinenyl cinnamate.

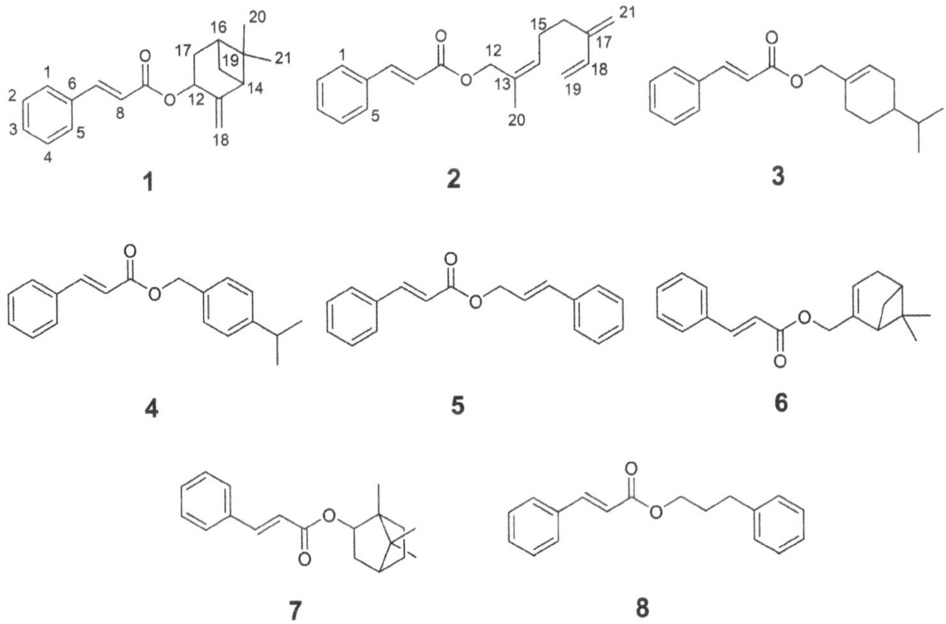

Figure 2. Chemical structures of eight compounds isolated from the roots of *L. formosana*. Using a bioactivity-guided isolation strategy, the 70% EtOH root extract was partitioned with n-hexane, followed by MPLC and HPLC. The chemical structures of each compound were elucidated based on 1D and 2D NMR, IR, and high-resolution mass spectrometry. Compounds **1** and **2** were identified as newly discovered natural products.

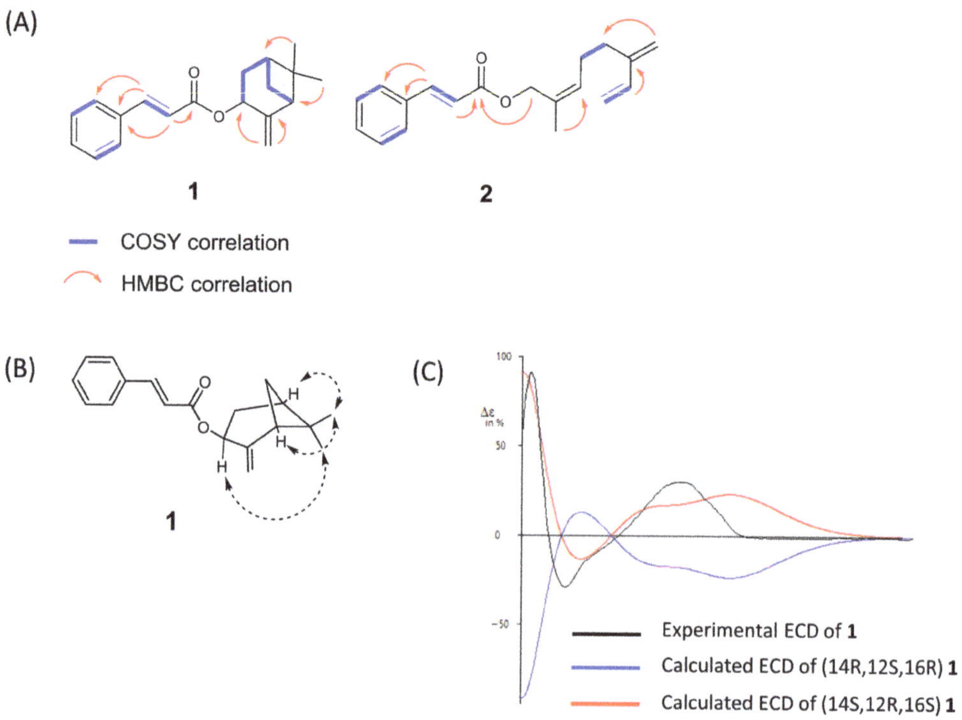

Figure 3. (**A**) Key COSY (blue bold lines) and HMBC (red arrows) correlations for compounds **1** and **2**. (**B**) Key NOE correlations for compound **1** (dashed-double-headed arrows), with the relative configuration assigned based on NOE data. (**C**) Experimental and calculated ECD spectra of **1**. Conformers with populations greater than 1% were optimized and frequency-verified by DFT [B3LYP/6-31G(d), gas phase; Gaussian 16]. The experimental ECD (black) was in good agreement with the calculated spectrum (red), establishing the absolute configuration as 14S,12R,16S.

The structure of compound **2** was elucidated through comprehensive analysis of ^{1}H and ^{13}C NMR, one and two-dimensional spectroscopic techniques, as well as IR and MS data. HR-ESI-MS analysis of **2** showed a protonated molecular ion $[M + H]^+$ at m/z 283.1715, consistent with the molecular formula of $C_{19}H_{22}O_2$ (calcd m/z 283.1693), indicating nine degrees of unsaturation. The ^{1}H NMR spectrum exhibited characteristic signals of a trans-disubstituted double bond at δ_H 7.70 and 6.47 (each d, J = 16.0 Hz), an oxygenated methylene at δ_H 4.60 (s, 2H), and a vinyl methyl group at δ_H 1.71 (s). The ^{13}C NMR spectrum, in conjunction with DEPT experiments, revealed 19 resonances, corresponding to one carbonyl carbon (δ_C 167.0), six aromatic carbons (δ_C 129.0, 129.0, 128.2, 128.2, 130.4, 134.5), eight olefinic carbons (δ_C 145.8, 144.9, 138.9, 130.7, 129.3, 118.2, 116.1, 113.3), three methylenes (δ_C 26.5, 30.9, 70.3), two exomethylenes (δ_C 113.3, 116.1), and one methyl carbon (δ_C 14.2). The COSY spectrum of **2** revealed key connectivities between H-19 [(δ_H 5.07, d, J = 10.8 Hz), (δ_H 5.24, d, J = 17.6 Hz)] and H-18 (δ_H 6.38, dd, J = 17.6, 10.8 Hz), and H-16 (δ_H 2.28, br s) with H-15 (δ_H 2.26, br s) and H-14 (δ_H 7.38, m), confirming the presence of a myrcene moiety (Figure 3A). HMBC correlations from H-7 (δ_H 7.70, d, J = 16.0 Hz) to C-5 (δ_C 134.5), C-6 (δ_C 128.2), and C-4 (δ_C 128.2), as well as from H-8 (δ_H 6.47, d, J = 16.0 Hz) to C-5 (δ_C 134.5), supported the cinnamic acid substructure. In addition, HMBC correlations from the oxymethylene protons (δ_H 4.60, H-12) to the carbonyl carbon (δ_C 167.0, C-9) established the ester linkage between the cinnamic acid and myrcene unit. Therefore, compound **2** was characterized as myrcenyl cinnamate.

Comparison with previously reported literature allowed us to identify compounds **3–8** as limonenyl cinnamate (**3**) [14], 4-isopropylbenzyl cinnamate (**4**) [15], cinnamyl cinnamate (**5**) [16], myrthenyl cinnamate (**6**) [17], bornyl cinnamate (**7**) [18], and 3-phenylpropyl cinnamate (**8**) [19].

3.3. *Bioactivity of Isolated Compounds from Liquidambar formosana*

Cellular senescence, as described by the Hayflick limit, was first demonstrated by the cessation of cell growth after several passages in cell culture [20]. A key regulator of this process is $p16^{INK4A}$, which initiates and maintains senescence by binding to CDK4/6, thereby inhibiting its kinase activity and preventing phosphorylation of Rb during the G1-to-S transition in order to regulate the cell cycle [21]. Several studies have revealed that $p16^{INK4A}$ expression is significantly increased in senescent cells during natural aging and in age-related diseases [22]. Recent studies have highlighted phenolic compounds, such as cinnamic acid derivatives, for their anti-senescence potential. Kanlayavattanakul et al. showed that hydroxycinnamic acids can alleviate aging in dermal cells [23]. Caffeic acid (3,4-dihydroxycinnamic acid), a plant-derived phenolic antioxidant, has been reported to inhibit skin aging in human keratinocytes (HaCaT cells) [24] and in skin cancer xenograft mouse models [25]. Along with cinnamic acid, numerous studies on the senomorphic effects of monoterpenes have demonstrated their ability to inhibit SASP by modulating key signaling pathways such as NF-κB, mTOR, and JAK/STAT [26]. β-myrcene has been reported to exhibit senomorphic activity, particularly through the direct suppression of IL-6 secretion in human dermal fibroblast cells [27]. Recently, the phenolic monoterpene bakuchiol has been gaining attention for its anti-aging effects [24]. However, few other phenolic monoterpenes or cinnamic acid-conjugated monoterpenes have been identified as anti-aging agents.

In this study, eight isolated compounds (**1–8**) from the ethyl acetate fraction of *L. formosana* were assessed for cytotoxicity. All compounds exhibited over 70% cell viability at a concentration of 10 μM in an MTT cell viability assay (Figure 4A). To evaluate their effect on $p16^{INK4A}$ expression, human lung carcinoma A549 cells, which have a homozygous deletion of $p16^{INK4A}$ gene, were used [28]. A549 cells were co-transfected with $p16^{INK4A}$ promoter-driven luciferase construct and β-galactosidase as an internal standard. Since the expression of $p16^{INK4A}$ is regulated by its promoter, quantifying its transcriptional activity provides a suitable model for assessing this key aging biomarker. As a result of compound treatment at 10 μM, compound **3** significantly reduced luciferase activity driven by the $p16^{INK4A}$ promoter, with an IC_{50} value of 3.9 μM. (Figure 4B–D). Navitoclax, a known senolytic agent, was used as a positive control to determine the downregulation of $p16^{INK4A}$, with normalization by β–galactosidase.

SASP, or senescence-messaging secretome (SMS), includes cytokines such as IL-6, IL-8, IL-1α, and IL-1β, which are characteristic features of senescent cells [29]. These cytokines not only serve as biomarkers but also play functional roles in reinforcing the senescent state and affecting surrounding tissues. For instance, interleukin-6 (IL-6) can induce premature senescence through activation of signal transducer and activator of transcription 3 (STAT3) signaling [30]. IL-8 is similarly overexpressed in senescent fibroblasts via autocrine signaling through the IL-8 pathway [31]. Besides IL-6 and IL-8, IL-1 family members, including membrane-bound IL-1α and soluble IL-1β, have also been studied as markers of senescence. Given this, we employed the bleomycin-induced senescence model in IMR90 fibroblasts, a well-established system for cellular aging studies, which leads to changes in the mRNA levels of SASP factors [32–34]. In this experiment, senescence was induced in IMR90 fibroblasts by a 2-day bleomycin pretreatment, followed by exposure to compound **3** for 48 h. The expression of four major SASP-associated genes (IL-6, IL-8, IL-1α, and IL-1β) was reduced in a dose-dependent manner upon treatment with compound **3** (Figure 5). At 10 μM, compound **3** markedly suppressed the expression of all four cytokines compared with the bleomycin-only control, with reductions of 68.55% for IL-6, 52.75% for IL-8, 57.18% for IL-1α, and 75.83% for IL-1β. At 5 μM, partial reductions were observed for IL-1α and IL-1β, whereas IL-6 and IL-8 remained largely unchanged. In contrast, treatment with 2.5 μM compound **3** did not produce significant effects on any of the tested markers. These findings indicate that compound **3** exerts the most robust and consistent inhibitory effects on SASP gene expression at 10 μM.

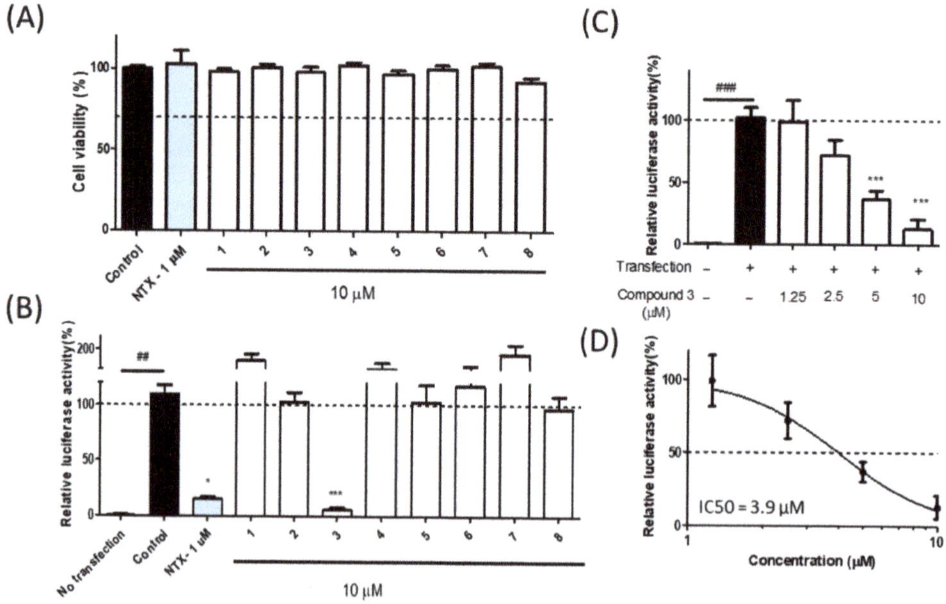

Figure 4. Effect of compounds on inhibition of the p16^{INK4A} promoter activity. (**A**) Cell viability of compounds **1–8** from *L. formosana* was measured using an MTT assay. Cell viability results are expressed as relative values compared with the untreated group (set at 100%). Bar colors indicate groups: black, control; blue, navitoclax treated control; white, experimental. (**B**) Inhibitory effects of compounds **1–8** on p16^{INK4A} promoter activity. Bar colors indicate groups as in panel (**A**). (**C**,**D**) Inhibitory effect of compound **3** in a dose-dependent manner (1.25, 2.5, 5, and 10 μM). (**C**) Compound **3** reduced p16^{INK4A} promoter activity (black, control; white, treated. (**D**) Dose–response curve of compound **3** based on data from panel (**C**). Data were normalized to β-galactosidase activity and are presented as mean ± SEM (n = 3). Statistical analysis was performed using one-way ANOVA followed by Dunn's multiple comparisons test (* $p < 0.05$, *** $p < 0.001$ vs. control; ## $p < 0.01$, ### $p < 0.001$ vs. no transfection control).

Senescence cell morphology typically displays an enlarged, flattened shape, together with molecular features such as increased p16^{INK4A} expression and reduced Rb phosphorylation. SA-β-gal is a well-established biomarker for the detection of the senescent phenotype. SA-β-gal staining is based on the detection of lysosomal β-galactosidase, which cleaves X-gal to produce a visible blue precipitate at pH 6.0 [12]. To validate the senomorphic activity of compound **3**, SA-β-gal staining was performed on bleomycin-induced senescent IMR90 fibroblasts. As shown in Figure 6A, cells exposed to bleomycin for 4 days displayed a pronounced increase in SA-β-gal-positive staining, characterized by enlarged and flattened morphology with extensive blue precipitates, compared with the untreated control group. In contrast, treatment with compound **3** for 48 h following bleomycin pretreatment markedly reduced the proportion of SA-β-gal-positive cells in a concentration-dependent manner. At 10 μM, treatment of compound **3** led to a marked reduction in SA-β-gal staining, whereas cells treated with 5 μM and 2.5 μM showed a moderate decrease compared with the bleomycin-only group. Quantitative analysis confirmed these observations (Figure 6B). Bleomycin pretreatment increased the proportion of SA-β-gal-positive area to nearly 100% relative to the control, whereas subsequent treatment with compound **3** reduced this value to 41.82 ± 26.72% at 10 μM, 43.07 ± 12.36% at 5 μM, and 46.84 ± 10.87% at 2.5 μM. These results demonstrate that compound **3** significantly attenuates bleomycin-induced cellular senescence, with the strongest inhibitory effect observed at the highest tested concentration (10 μM).

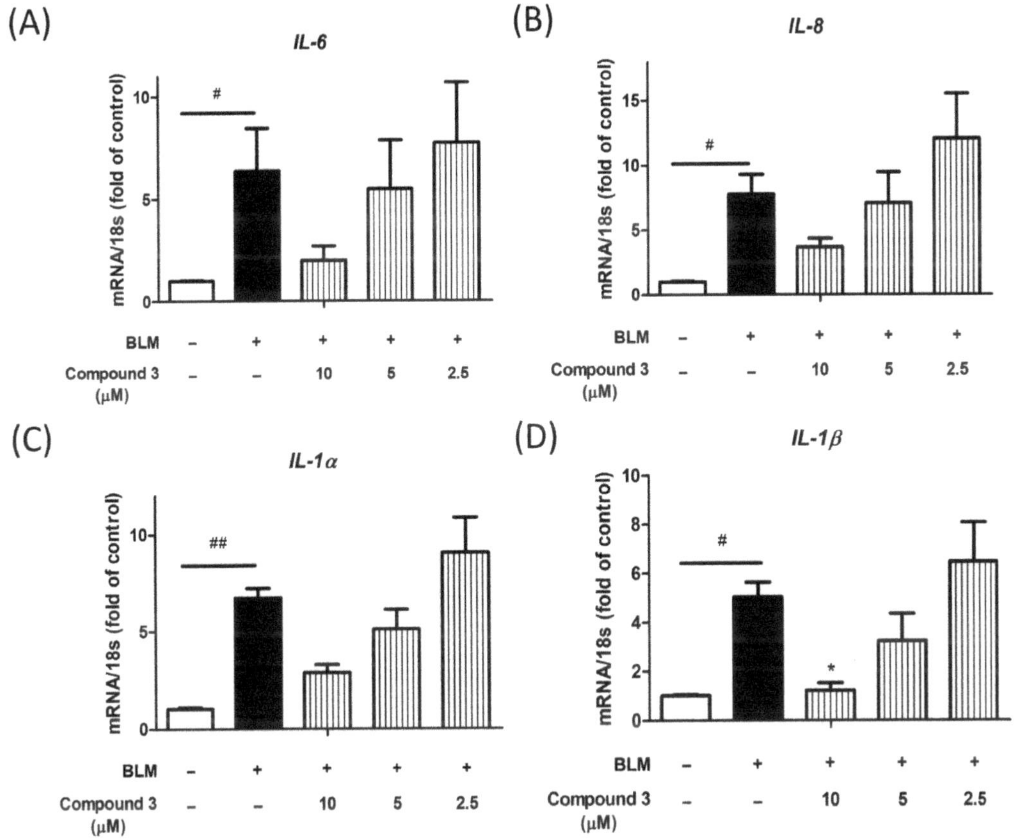

Figure 5. Senomorphic effects of compound **3** on rescuing replicative senescence and inhibiting SASP mRNA expression. IMR90 cells were exposed to bleomycin (BLM, 40 μg/mL) for 2 days and subsequently treated with the indicated compounds for an additional 2 days, after which total RNA was extracted for analysis. Compound **3** was tested in a dose-dependent manner (2.5, 5, and 10 μM) for its effects on SASP markers IL-6 (**A**), IL-8 (**B**), IL-1α (**C**), and IL-1β (**D**). Data are expressed as mean ± SEM (n = 3). Bar shading and pattern denote the following groups: white (control), black (bleomycin-only control), and striped (experimental). Statistical analysis was performed using one-way ANOVA followed by Dunn's multiple comparisons test (* $p < 0.05$ vs. BLM-treated group for 2 days; # $p < 0.05$, ## $p < 0.01$ vs. control).

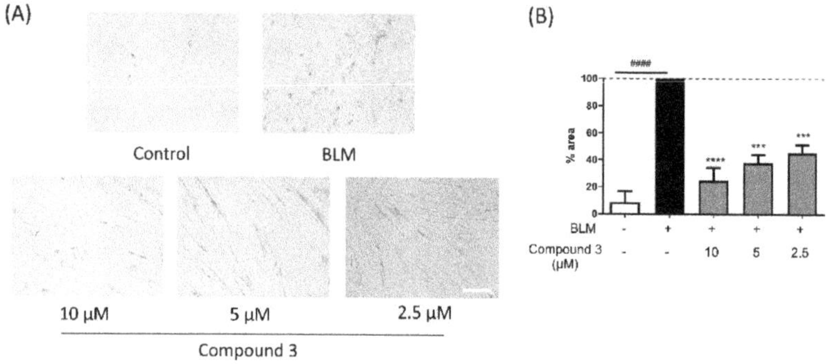

Figure 6. Results of the senescence-associated β-galactosidase (SA-β-gal) staining (**A**) and quantification. Bar shading denotes the following groups: white (control), black (bleomycin-only control), and gray (experimental). (**B**). IMR90 cells were exposed to bleomycin (BLM, 40 μg/mL) for 2 days and subsequently treated with the indicated compounds for an additional 2 days. Cells were then analyzed by SA-β-gal staining. Compound **3** was tested in a dose-dependent manner (2.5, 5, and 10 μM). The proportion of SA-β-gal-positive cells was significantly reduced in the compound **3**-treated groups compared with the bleomycin-only control. Data are presented as mean ± SEM (n = 3). Statistical analysis was determined using one-way ANOVA followed by Dunn's multiple comparisons test (*** $p < 0.001$, **** $p < 0.0001$ vs. 2-day BLM-treated group; #### $p < 0.0001$ vs. control). Scale bars = 200 μm.

4. Discussion

In this study, two new compounds (**1** and **2**), along with six known compounds, were isolated from the root of *L. formosana* based on a bioactivity-guided isolation approach (Supplementary Figure S20). With the increasing use of high-resolution mass spectrometry, FBMN has been proven to be an efficient and reliable method for dereplication and chemical profiling of natural products due to the availability of ever-growing public databases. By using this method, two new compounds were isolated, thereby enhancing the chemical diversity of this plant.

Since its discovery, $p16^{INK4A}$ has been shown to have a strong correlation with aging and cellular senescence [35]. Previous studies have demonstrated that ionizing radiation can induce senescence via the ROS-mediated $p16^{INK4A}$ pathway in human vascular smooth muscle cells [36] and mouse hippocampus cells [37]. In this study, we initially performed a $p16^{INK4A}$ promoter activity inhibition screening assay to identify bioactive compounds that inhibit $p16^{INK4A}$ expression, a major biomarker of senescence. Using A549 cells, which have a homozygous deletion of the $p16^{INK4A}$ gene [28], and co-transfected with the $p16^{INK4A}$ gene and β-galactosidase as an internal standard, compound **3** was identified as a potent $p16^{INK4A}$ inhibitor with an IC_{50} of 3.9 μM. SASP expression is regulated through multiple transcriptional and signaling pathways, with NF-κB identified as a master regulator [38]. In senescent cells, damaged DNA released into the cytoplasm forms cytoplasmic chromatin fragments (CCFs) that activate the cGAS–STING–NF-κB pathway, leading to the secretion of pro-inflammatory cytokines such as IL-6, IL-8, IL-1α, and IL-1β [39,40]. Other regulatory factors of the SASP include C/EBPß, GATA4, p38 MAP-kinase, mTOR, JAK/STAT, and Notch pathway [41]. Additionally, several studies have suggested that senomorphic compounds may regulate epigenetic mechanisms that control SASP transcription [42,43]. IL-6 plays a central role in the SASP network [44], IL-8 serves as a chemoattractant cytokine [45], and IL-1 (α and β) initiates signaling cascades that induce IL-6 and IL-8 expression [46]. Hence, suppressing SASP cytokines offers a strategic approach to mitigating the harmful effects of senescence. In this study, compound **3** isolated from the root of *L. formosana* significantly reduced SASP markers (IL-6, IL-8, IL-1α, and IL-1β). These results demonstrate that our compound exerts SASP marker-reducing effects at much lower concentrations than previously reported compounds. Lim et al. reported that avenanthramide C, a compound extracted from oats, suppressed IL-6 and IL-8 expression in senescent human dermal fibroblasts (HDFs) at 120 μM [47]. Other well-studied senomorphic candidates, such as fisetin and quercetin, typically require concentrations above 20 μM to achieve comparable effects [48,49]. Collectively, these benchmarks highlight the superior potency of compound **3** and support its potential as a lead scaffold for the development of senescence-modulating therapeutics.

To further confirm the senescence phenotype, SA-β-gal staining was performed. This histochemical assay uses the chromogenic substrate X-gal, detectable at pH 6.0, which yields an insoluble blue compound when cleaved by β-galactosidase [50]. The results demonstrated that compound **3** exhibits the most promising SASP-inhibitory activity among the isolated compounds. According to our data, compound **3** exhibits superior SA-β-gal inhibition at relatively lower concentrations compared to previously reported compounds or extracts. Previous studies showed that ginsenosides from heat-processed ginseng at 120 °C, when administered to endothelial progenitor cells at 200 μg/mL, reduced SA-β-gal positivity from 93.8% to 62.5% [36]. Extracts from *Silybum marianum* flowers demonstrated senotherapeutic-like effects, significantly decreasing the proportion of SA-β-gal-positive senescent HDFs by 33.2% at 200 μg/mL [37]. Kaempferol-type compounds from *Nephelium lappaceum* were also reported to reduce the proportion of SA-β-gal-positive cells by approximately 50% [38]. Although compound **3** was not evaluated for activity using the same cell system as the previously reported compounds, these results support the potential of compound **3** as a novel senomorphic agent for the treatment of aging-associated diseases by targeting $p16^{INK4A}$ expression, SASP modulation, and morphological features of cellular senescence.

This study has several limitations that should be acknowledged. Our findings were primarily obtained from continuous cell lines, including A549 lung carcinoma cells and IMR90 fibroblasts, which may not fully recapitulate the complexity of primary human tissues or patient-derived senescent cells. Although these models are well established for senescence research, the translational relevance of our results remains to be validated in more physiologically relevant systems. While we demonstrated that compound **3** effectively reduced $p16^{INK4A}$ promoter activity, SASP cytokine expression, and SA-β-gal positivity, its precise molecular targets and upstream regulatory pathways remain undefined (Supplementary Figure S21). Further studies using primary cells, patient-derived models, and in vivo systems will therefore be necessary to confirm the senomorphic activity of compound **3** and to elucidate its mechanism of action. These investigations will not only validate the therapeutic potential of compound **3** but also provide broader insights into the role of monoterpenoids in modulating cellular senescence. Future work should further address the heterogeneity of senescence by testing compound **3** across diverse senescence inducers to better clarify its global molecular effects.

5. Conclusions

In this study, by using FBMN powered by the GNPS database, the chemical profile of *L. formosana* was established, revealing the presence of flavonoid glycosides, amides, and triterpenoids. Eight meroterpenoids were further identified by integrating SNAP-MS. Two undescribed compounds (**1** and **2**) were isolated, and their structures were characterized by NMR and other spectroscopic techniques. Evaluation of these compounds demonstrated their ability to inhibit senescence markers, including $p16^{INK4A}$, SASP, and SA-β-gal staining, with compound **3** emerging as the most potent inhibitor. To our knowledge, this is the first report to identify a cinnamic acid-conjugated monoterpennoid from *L. formosana* that targets aging-related biomarkers. These findings highlight the potential as promising therapeutic candidates for aging-associated diseases through the modulation of cellular senescence.

Supplementary Materials: The following supporting information can be downloaded at https://www.mdpi.com/article/10.3390/nu17213321/s1. Figure S1: The feature based molecular networking of the total extract from the root of *L. formosana*; Figure S2: IR(KBr) spectrum of compound **1**; Figure S3: UV spectrum of compound **1**; Figure S4: ECD spectrum of compound **1**; Figure S5: ^{1}H NMR spectrum of compound **1**; Figure S6: ^{13}C NMR spectrum of compound **1**; Figure S7: eHSQC spectrum of compound **1**; Figure S8: HMBC spectrum of compound **1**; Figure S9: COSY spectrum of compound **1**; Figure S10: NOESY spectrum of compound **1**; Figure S11: IR(KBr) spectrum of compound **2**; Figure S12: UV spectrum of compound **2**; Figure S13: ^{1}H NMR spectrum of compound **2**; Figure S14: ^{13}C NMR spectrum of compound **2**; Figure S15: eHSQC spectrum of compound **2**; Figure S16: HMBC spectrum of compound **2**; Figure S17: COSY spectrum of compound **2**; Figure S18: High-confidence subnetwork (component index 5) and representative compounds predicted by SNAP-MS; Figure S19: Conformers of compound **1**; Figure S20: Bioactivity-guided isolation workflow targeting cellular senescence modulators; Figure S21: Cell viability of bleomycin-treated IMR90 fibroblasts in response to compound **3**; Figure S22: Proposed mechanism of compound **3** action in the p16INK4A pathway; Table S1: Energies and atomic Cartesian coordinates of geometry-optimized conformers of compound **1** at B3LYP/6-31g(d) in methanol. Table S2: Calculated excited state transition wavelengths, oscillator strengths and rotatory strengths for geometry-optimized conformers of compound **1** at B3LYP/6-31g(d) in methanol.

Author Contributions: Conceptualization, M.T.T.L. and W.-K.O.; methodology, Q.H.V. and V.-H.M.; formal analysis, V.-H.M., S.C. and J.E.P.-Z.; investigation, M.T.T.L. and J.-P.A.; resources, Q.H.V.; writing—original draft preparation, M.T.T.L. and Q.H.V.; writing—review and editing, W.-K.O.; supervision, W.-K.O.; project administration, W.-K.O.; funding acquisition, W.-K.O. All authors have read and agreed to the published version of the manuscript.

Funding: This research was supported by grants from the Basic Science Research Programs (RS-2022-NR070150) and (RS-2023-00218616) through the National Research Foundation of Korea (NRF) funded by the Ministry of Science and ICT in Korea.

Institutional Review Board Statement: Not applicable.

Informed Consent Statement: Not applicable.

Data Availability Statement: The data that support the findings of this study are available from the corresponding author upon reasonable request.

Conflicts of Interest: The authors declare no conflicts of interest.

Abbreviations

The following abbreviations are used in this manuscript:

CCFs	Cytoplasmic chromatin fragments
ECD	Electronic circular dichroism
GNPS	Global natural products social molecular networking
HMBC	Heteronuclear multi-bond correlation
HPLC	High-performance liquid chromatography
HRESIMS	High-resolution electrospray ionization mass spectrometry
HSQC	Heteronuclear single quantum coherence
LC-MS	Liquid chromatography–mass spectrometry
NMR	Nuclear magnetic resonance
SASP	Senescence-associated secretory phenotype
STAT3	Signal transducer and activator of transcription 3

References

1. Ma, Y.; Ding, S.; Qiu, Y. Chromosome-level genome assembly of American sweetgum (*Liquidambar styraciflua*, Altingiaceae). *Sci. Data* **2024**, *11*, 1078. [CrossRef]
2. Ouyang, X.L.; Yi, S.; Lu, H.; Wu, S.; Zhao, H. *Liquidambar formosana* Hance: A mini-review of chemical constituents and pharmacology. *Eur. J. Med. Plants* **2016**, *17*, 1–11. [CrossRef]
3. Chien, S.-C.; Xiao, J.-H.; Tseng, Y.-H.; Kuo, Y.-H.; Wang, S.-Y. Composition and antifungal activity of balsam from *Liquidambar formosana* Hance. *Holzforschung* **2013**, *67*, 345–351. [CrossRef]
4. Zhang, L.; Zhu, M.F.; Tu, Z.C.; Zhao, Y.; Wang, H.; Li, G.J.; Sha, X.M. a-Glucosidase inhibition, anti-glycation and antioxidant activities of *Liquidambar formosana* Hance leaf, and identification of phytochemical profile. *S. Afr. J. Bot.* **2017**, *113*, 239–247. [CrossRef]
5. Zhu, Y.; Guan, Y.-J.; Chen, Q.-Z.; Yuan, L.-H.; Xu, Q.-Q.; Zhou, M.-L.; Liu, H.; Lin, W.; Zhang, Z.-D.; Zhou, Z.-L. Pentacyclic Triterpenes from the resin of *Liquidambar formosana* have anti-angiogenic properties. *Phytochemistry* **2021**, *184*, 112676. [CrossRef]
6. Niccoli, T.; Partridge, L. Ageing as a risk factor for disease. *Curr. Biol.* **2012**, *22*, R741–R752. [CrossRef] [PubMed]
7. Kumari, R.; Jat, P. Mechanisms of cellular senescence: Cell cycle arrest and senescence associated secretory phenotype. *Front. Cell Dev. Biol.* **2021**, *9*, 645593. [CrossRef]
8. Saito, Y.; Yamamoto, S.; Chikenji, T.S. Role of cellular senescence in inflammation and regeneration. *Inflamm. Regen.* **2024**, *44*, 28. [CrossRef]
9. Zhang, L.; Pitcher, L.E.; Prahalad, V.; Niedernhofer, L.J.; Robbins, P.D. Targeting cellular senescence with senotherapeutics: Senolytics and senomorphics. *FEBS J.* **2023**, *290*, 1362–1383. [CrossRef] [PubMed]
10. Koh, J.; Enders, G.H.; David Dynlacht, B.; Harlow, E.D. Tumour-derived p16 alleles encoding proteins defective in cell-cycle inhibition. *Nature* **1995**, *375*, 506–510. [CrossRef]
11. McConnell, B.B.; Gregory, F.J.; Stott, F.J.; Hara, E.; Peters, G. Induced expression of p16 INK4a inhibits both CDK4-and CDK2-associated kinase activity by reassortment of cyclin-CDK-inhibitor complexes. *Mol. Cell. Biol.* **1999**, *19*, 1981–1989. [CrossRef] [PubMed]
12. Xin, Z.; Wu, X.; Ji, T.; Xu, B.; Han, Y.; Sun, M.; Jiang, S.; Li, T.; Hu, W.; Deng, C.; et al. Bakuchiol: A newly discovered warrior against organ damage. *Pharmacol. Res.* **2019**, *141*, 208–213. [CrossRef] [PubMed]
13. Morehouse, N.J.; Clark, T.N.; McMann, E.J.; van Santen, J.A.; Haeckl, F.J.; Gray, C.A.; Linington, R.G. Annotation of natural product compound families using molecular networking topology and structural similarity fingerprinting. *Nat. Commun.* **2023**, *14*, 308. [CrossRef] [PubMed]
14. Pu, X.Y.; Tian, K.; Sun, J.X.; Wang, W.; Liu, H.C.; Yang, J.; Jiang, M.Y.; Huang, X.Z. Anti-inflammatory monoterpene esters from the stems of Illigera aromatica. *Nat. Prod. Res.* **2021**, *35*, 960–966. [CrossRef]
15. do Vale, J.A.; Rodrigues, M.P.; Lima, Â.M.A.; Santiago, S.S.; de Almeida Lima, G.D.; Almeida, A.A.; de Oliveira, L.L.; Bressan, G.C.; Teixeira, R.R.; Machado-Neves, M. Synthesis of cinnamic acid ester derivatives with antiproliferative and antimetastatic activities on murine melanoma cells. *Biomed. Pharmacother.* **2022**, *148*, 112689. [CrossRef]
16. Shang, X.F.; Xiao, L.; Su, J.T.; Wei, S.Y.; Wang, Y.S.; Yang, J.H. Chemical constituents of *Litsea euosma*. *Chem. Nat. Compd.* **2019**, *55*, 1138–1140. [CrossRef]
17. Bohlmann, F.; Zdero, C. Stevisalicinone (X), a new diterpene type, and other constituents from Stevia species. *Chem. Inform.* **1986**, *17*, 1974–1983.
18. Hayashi, H.; Yasukochi, S.; Sakamoto, T.; Hatano, M.; Ishihara, K. Insight into the mechanism of the acylation of alcohols with acid anhydrides catalyzed by phosphoric acid derivatives. *J. Org. Chem.* **2021**, *86*, 5197–5212. [CrossRef]
19. Funasaka, S.; Mukaiyama, T. A versatile, practical, and inexpensive reagent, pyridine-3-carboxylic anhydride (3-PCA), for condensation reactions. *Bull. Chem. Soc. Jpn.* **2008**, *81*, 148–159. [CrossRef]
20. Hayflick, L. The limited in vitro lifetime of human diploid cell strains. *Exp. Cell Res.* **1965**, *37*, 614–636. [CrossRef]
21. Rayess, H.; Wang, M.B.; Srivatsan, E.S. Cellular senescence and tumor suppressor gene p16. *Int. J. Cancer* **2012**, *130*, 1715–1725. [CrossRef]
22. Baker, D.J.; Wijshake, T.; Tchkonia, T.; LeBrasseur, N.K.; Childs, B.G.; Van De Sluis, B.; Kirkland, J.L.; Van Deursen, J.M. Clearance of p16Ink4a-positive senescent cells delays ageing-associated disorders. *Nature* **2011**, *479*, 232–236. [CrossRef] [PubMed]
23. Kanlayavattanakul, M.; Khongkow, M.; Iempridee, T.; Lourith, N. Food hydroxycinnamic acids alleviate ageing in dermal cells. *Food Prod. Process. Nutr.* **2024**, *6*, 86. [CrossRef]
24. Pluemsamran, T.; Onkoksoong, T.; Panich, U. Caffeic acid and ferulic acid inhibit UVA-induced matrix metalloproteinase-1 through regulation of antioxidant defense system in keratinocyte HaCaT cells. *Photochem. Photobiol.* **2012**, *88*, 961–968. [CrossRef] [PubMed]
25. Yang, G.; Fu, Y.; Malakhova, M.; Kurinov, I.; Zhu, F.; Yao, K.; Li, H.; Chen, H.; Li, W.; Lim, D.Y. Caffeic acid directly targets ERK1/2 to attenuate solar UV-induced skin carcinogenesis. *Cancer Prev. Res.* **2014**, *7*, 1056–1066. [CrossRef] [PubMed]

26. Lagoumtzi, S.M.; Chondrogianni, N. Senolytics and senomorphics: Natural and synthetic therapeutics in the treatment of aging and chronic diseases. *Free Radic. Biol. Med.* **2021**, *171*, 169–190. [CrossRef] [PubMed]
27. Rao, V.S.N.; Menezes, A.M.S.; Viana, G.S.B. Effect of myrcene on nociception in mice. *J. Pharm. Pharmacol.* **1990**, *42*, 877–878. [CrossRef] [PubMed]
28. Adachi, J.; Kohno, T.; Baeg, G.; Akiyama, T.; Yokota, J. Growth suppression of non-small cell lung carcinoma cells by the introduction of the p16 (INK4A) gene. *Int. J. Oncol.* **1997**, *10*, 33–39. [CrossRef]
29. He, S.; Sharpless, N.E. Senescence in health and disease. *Cell* **2017**, *169*, 1000–1011. [CrossRef]
30. Kojima, H.; Inoue, T.; Kunimoto, H.; Nakajima, K. IL-6-STAT3 signaling and premature senescence. *Jak-Stat* **2013**, *2*, e25763. [CrossRef]
31. Wang, T.; Notta, F.; Navab, R.; Joseph, J.; Ibrahimov, E.; Xu, J.; Zhu, C.-Q.; Borgida, A.; Gallinger, S.; Tsao, M.-S. Senescent carcinoma-associated fibroblasts upregulate IL8 to enhance prometastatic phenotypes. *Mol. Cancer Res.* **2017**, *15*, 3–14. [CrossRef]
32. Zhang, X.; Dong, Y.; Li, W.-c.; Tang, B.-x.; Li, J.; Zang, Y. Roxithromycin attenuates bleomycin-induced pulmonary fibrosis by targeting senescent cells. *Acta Pharmacol. Sin.* **2021**, *42*, 2058–2068. [CrossRef]
33. Lim, H.; Park, H.; Kim, H.P. Effects of flavonoids on senescence-associated secretory phenotype formation from bleomycin-induced senescence in BJ fibroblasts. *Biochem. Pharmacol.* **2015**, *96*, 337–348. [CrossRef] [PubMed]
34. Aoshiba, K.; Tsuji, T.; Kameyama, S.; Itoh, M.; Semba, S.; Yamaguchi, K.; Nakamura, H. Senescence-associated secretory phenotype in a mouse model of bleomycin-induced lung injury. *Exp. Toxicol. Pathol.* **2013**, *65*, 1053–1062. [CrossRef]
35. Krishnamurthy, J.; Torrice, C.; Ramsey, M.R.; Kovalev, G.I.; Al-Regaiey, K.; Su, L.; Sharpless, N.E. Ink4a/Arf expression is a biomarker of aging. *J. Clin. Investig.* **2004**, *114*, 1299–1307. [CrossRef] [PubMed]
36. Zheng, X.; Liu, Z.; Bin, Y.; Wang, J.; Rao, X.; Wu, G.; Dong, X.; Tong, F. Ionizing radiation induces vascular smooth muscle cell senescence through activating NF-κB/CTCF/p16 pathway. *Biochim. Biophys. Acta (BBA)-Mol. Basis Dis.* **2024**, *1870*, 166994. [CrossRef] [PubMed]
37. Cheng, Z.; Zheng, Y.Z.; Li, Y.-Q.; Wong, C.S. Cellular senescence in mouse hippocampus after irradiation and the role of p53 and p21. *J. Neuropathol. Exp. Neurol.* **2017**, *76*, 260–269. [CrossRef]
38. Chien, Y.; Scuoppo, C.; Wang, X.; Fang, X.; Balgley, B.; Bolden, J.E.; Premsrirut, P.; Luo, W.; Chicas, A.; Lee, C.S. Control of the senescence-associated secretory phenotype by NF-κB promotes senescence and enhances chemosensitivity. *Genes Dev.* **2011**, *25*, 2125–2136. [CrossRef]
39. Ivanov, A.; Pawlikowski, J.; Manoharan, I.; van Tuyn, J.; Nelson, D.M.; Rai, T.S.; Shah, P.P.; Hewitt, G.; Korolchuk, V.I.; Passos, J.F. Lysosome-mediated processing of chromatin in senescence. *J. Cell Biol.* **2013**, *202*, 129–143. [CrossRef]
40. Dou, Z.; Ghosh, K.; Vizioli, M.G.; Zhu, J.; Sen, P.; Wangensteen, K.J.; Simithy, J.; Lan, Y.; Lin, Y.; Zhou, Z. Cytoplasmic chromatin triggers inflammation in senescence and cancer. *Nature* **2017**, *550*, 402–406. [CrossRef]
41. Fraga, M.F.; Agrelo, R.; Esteller, M. Cross-talk between aging and cancer: The epigenetic language. *Ann. N. Y. Acad. Sci.* **2007**, *1100*, 60–74. [CrossRef] [PubMed]
42. Liu, H.; Xu, Q.; Wufuer, H.; Li, Z.; Sun, R.; Jiang, Z.; Dou, X.; Fu, Q.; Campisi, J.; Sun, Y. Rutin is a potent senomorphic agent to target senescent cells and can improve chemotherapeutic efficacy. *Aging Cell* **2024**, *23*, 13921. [CrossRef]
43. Cuollo, L.; Antonangeli, F.; Santoni, A.; Soriani, A. The senescence-associated secretory phenotype (SASP) in the challenging future of cancer therapy and age-related diseases. *Biology* **2020**, *9*, 485. [CrossRef]
44. Rolt, A.; Nair, A.; Cox, L.S. Optimisation of a screening platform for determining IL-6 inflammatory signalling in the senescence-associated secretory phenotype (SASP). *Biogerontology* **2019**, *20*, 359–371. [CrossRef]
45. Matsushima, K.; Yang, D.; Oppenheim, J.J. Interleukin-8: An evolving chemokine. *Cytokine* **2022**, *153*, 155828. [CrossRef]
46. Schmitz, M.L.; Weber, A.; Roxlau, T.; Gaestel, M.; Kracht, M. Signal integration, crosstalk mechanisms and networks in the function of inflammatory cytokines. *Biochim. Biophys. Acta (BBA)-Mol. Cell Res.* **2011**, *1813*, 2165–2175. [CrossRef]
47. Lim, J.S.; Kim, H.S.; Park, S.C.; Park, J.T.; Kim, H.S.; Oh, W.K. Identification of a novel senomorphic agent, avenanthramide C, via the suppression of the senescence-associated secretory phenotype. *Mech. Ageing Dev.* **2020**, *192*, 111355. [CrossRef]
48. Imb, M.; Véghelyi, Z.; Maurer, M.; Kühnel, H. Exploring senolytic and senomorphic properties of medicinal plants for anti-aging therapies. *Int. J. Mol. Sci.* **2024**, *25*, 10419. [CrossRef] [PubMed]
49. Zhang, L.; Tong, X.; Huang, J.; Wu, M.; Zhang, S.; Wang, D.; Liu, S.; Fan, H. Fisetin alleviated bleomycin-induced pulmonary fibrosis partly by rescuing alveolar epithelial cells from senescence. *Front. Pharmacol.* **2020**, *11*, 553690. [CrossRef]
50. Dimri, G.P.; Lee, X.; Basile, G.; Acosta, M.; Scott, G.; Roskelley, C.; Medrano, E.E.; Linskens, M.; Rubelj, I.; Pereira-Smith, O. A biomarker that identifies senescent human cells in culture and in aging skin in vivo. *Proc. Natl. Acad. Sci. USA* **1995**, *92*, 9363–9367. [CrossRef] [PubMed]

nutrients

MDPI

Article

One-Week Elderberry Juice Intervention Promotes Metabolic Flexibility in the Transcriptome of Overweight Adults During a Meal Challenge

Christy Teets [1], Andrea J. Etter [2] and Patrick M. Solverson [1,*]

[1] Department of Nutrition and Exercise Physiology, Elson S. Floyd College of Medicine, Washington State University, Spokane, WA 99202, USA; christy.teets@wsu.edu
[2] Department of Nutrition and Food Science, University of Vermont, Burlington, VT 05405, USA; andrea.etter@uvm.edu
* Correspondence: patrick.solverson@wsu.edu; Tel.: +1-509-358-7967

Abstract: Background: Metabolic flexibility, the ability to efficiently switch between fuel sources in response to changing nutrient availability and energy demands, is recognized as a key determinant of metabolic health. In a recent randomized controlled human feeding trial, overweight individuals receiving American black elderberry juice (EBJ) demonstrated improvements in multiple clinical indices of metabolic flexibility, but the mechanisms of action were unexplored. The objective of this study was to utilize RNA sequencing to examine how EBJ modulates the transcriptional response to fasting and feeding, focusing on pathways related to metabolic flexibility. Methods: Overweight or obese adults (BMI > 25 kg/m^2) without chronic illnesses were randomized to a 5-week crossover study protocol with two 1-week periods of twice-daily EBJ or placebo (PL) separated by a washout period. RNA sequencing was performed on peripheral blood mononuclear cells from 10 participants to assess transcriptomic responses collected at fasting (pre-meal) and post-prandial (120 min post-meal) states during a meal-challenge test. Results: The fasted-to-fed transition for EBJ showed 234 differentially expressed genes following EBJ consumption compared to 59 genes following PL, with 44 genes shared between interventions. EBJ supplementation showed significantly higher enrichment of several metabolic pathways including insulin, FoxO, and PI3K–Akt signaling. KEGG pathway analysis showed 27 significant pathways related to metabolic flexibility compared to 7 for PL. Conclusions: Our findings indicate that short-term elderberry juice consumption may promote metabolic flexibility in overweight adults.

Keywords: elderberry juice; transcriptome; metabolic flexibility; berry anthocyanins; functional foods; meal tolerance test; obesity; PBMC

1. Introduction

Metabolic flexibility, the ability to efficiently switch between fuel sources in response to changing nutrient availability and energy demands, is recognized as one key determinant of metabolic health. This adaptive capacity enables healthy individuals to preferentially utilize glucose in the fed state and shift toward fatty acid oxidation during fasting. The maintenance of this flexibility is fundamental, as it supports optimal energy balance and cellular resilience across physiological conditions [1–4].

Loss of metabolic flexibility is a driver of metabolic disorders. Metabolic inflexibility precedes and contributes to the development of chronic conditions such as type 2 diabetes,

https://doi.org/10.3390/nu17193142

obesity, hepatic steatosis, and cardiovascular disease [3,4]. Rather than viewing insulin resistance and related comorbidities as triggers of inflexibility, empirical evidence emphasizes that the impaired substrate switching itself initiates a cascade of complications—disrupting insulin action, energy homeostasis, mitochondrial function, and inflammatory control [3,5]. This paradigm shift places the restoration of metabolic flexibility at the center of preventive and therapeutic strategies for metabolic disease [2].

Anthocyanins, the predominant polyphenolic pigments found in berries, are increasingly studied for their role in improving metabolic flexibility. Under certain conditions, anthocyanins modulate insulin signaling, mitochondrial function, inflammation, and nutrient-sensing pathways (e.g., AMPK, PPARs), which restore or enhance fuel switching in obesity or insulin-resistant states [6–8].

American black elderberries (*Sambucus nigra* spp. *canadensis*) have the highest anthocyanin concentrations compared to commonly consumed fruits and exhibit the ability to improve metabolic health in some studies [9]. In our recent randomized controlled human feeding trial involving overweight adults [10], individuals receiving American black elderberry juice (EBJ) demonstrated improvements in multiple indices of metabolic flexibility. These improvements were marked by reduced postprandial glucose and insulin levels, and a decline in respiratory quotient (RQ) in the fasted-to-fed transition, relative to placebo (PL). This suggested enhanced metabolic flexibility without changes in caloric intake or body weight. These findings indicated that EBJ may support dynamic fuel switching while enhancing physiological responses critical for overall well-being. Yet, the underlying molecular mechanisms that drive the effect remain unclear.

Building upon our prior work, our study objective is to investigate these molecular mechanisms by analyzing gene expression profiles from peripheral blood mononuclear cells (PBMCs) collected from participants during a meal tolerance test from the previous clinical study. Using RNA sequencing, we examined how EBJ modulates the transcriptional response to fasting and feeding, focusing particularly on pathways related to metabolic flexibility.

2. Materials and Methods

2.1. Human Clinical Trial

Details of the human clinical trial (NCT 06626373) were previously published [10]. Briefly, 18 overweight and obese adults (15 female) completed a 7-day randomized, diet- and placebo-controlled, crossover trial comparing twice-daily consumption of 355 g of 100% EBJ containing 720 mg/day cyanidin-3-glucoside equivalents (C3GE) or a matched placebo beverage. Each arm included four days of a 100% fully investigator-controlled diet, followed by a three-week washout before crossover. Participants maintained habitual physical activity, completed daily compliance questionnaires, and returned empty food and beverage containers. A 3 h meal tolerance test (MTT) was administered on the morning of day 8 of each arm. The MTT included a high-carbohydrate breakfast (~60 g sugar from waffles and syrup) plus a full daily dose of either EBJ or PL. Serum was collected every 30 min for 3 h. The study was approved by the Washington State University IRB (WSU-IRB 18597) and conducted in accordance with the Declaration of Helsinki, and written informed consent was obtained from all participants.

2.2. RNA Sequencing

RNA sequencing was performed on PBMCs from 10 participants to assess transcriptomic responses. Fasting (pre-meal) and postprandial (120 min post-meal) samples were collected into PAXgene Blood RNA Tubes (Qiagen, Valencia, CA, USA), yielding 40 libraries across fasted and fed states in both treatment arms. RNA was extracted using the

PAXgene Blood RNA Kit (Qiagen, Hilden, Germany). Quality control and sequencing were completed by Novogene (Sacramento, CA, USA). All samples had RNA integrity numbers (RIN) above 7.8 (mean = 8.6). Globin mRNA was depleted using the QIAseq FastSelect-Globin Kit, followed by poly (A) selection. Libraries were prepared with the NEBNext Ultra II Directional RNA Library Prep Kit (New England Biolabs, Ipswich, MA, USA) and sequenced on an Illumina NovaSeq 6000 S1 platform (2 $\times$ 150 bp paired-end reads), targeting approximately 20 million read pairs per sample.

2.3. Read Processing and Alignment

RNA-seq data were processed using Galaxy (v23.1.5dev0) [11]. Quality assessment was performed with FastQC to check read integrity, GC content, and adapter contamination. Trimmomatic removed low-quality bases, adapters, and short or degraded reads [12]. Ribosomal RNA was filtered using SortMeRNA (v2.1), removing 2–5% of reads per sample to focus on mRNA [13]. Cleaned reads were aligned to the GRCh38 human genome using HISAT2 [14], with alignment rates between 87.9% and 98.1%, indicating high mapping quality. Gene-level quantification was performed using featureCounts (v2.0.1) [15] with paired-end, strand-specific settings and Ensembl GRCh38.113 annotations. Multimapping and ambiguous reads were excluded for specificity.

2.4. Differential Gene Expression Analysis

Differential gene expression was analyzed in R (v4.4.1) using DESeq2 and lmerSeq. Genes with fewer than 10 reads in at least four samples were excluded. The variance-stabilizing transformation (VST) was applied with DESeq2 [16] and Ensembl gene IDs were mapped to gene symbols using org.Hs.eg.db [17]. Due to the 2 $\times$ 2 crossover design and repeated sampling, linear mixed-effects models were fit using lmerSeq, with the following model:

$$\sim\text{Treatment} * \text{State} + \text{Sequence} + (1 \mid \text{Participant})$$

where Treatment refers to EBJ vs. PL and State refers to fasted vs. fed. To evaluate potential carryover effects inherent to 2 $\times$ 2 crossovers, we included Sequence (EBJ $\rightarrow$ PL vs. PL $\rightarrow$ EBJ) as a fixed effect, consistent with recommended practice for crossover designs [18]. Sequence tests were adjusted using Benjamini–Hochberg procedures. A random intercept for Participant modeled within-subject correlations. This model aligns with recent recommendations emphasizing the importance of modeling interaction effects and repeated measures in RNA-seq studies [19,20]. Because contrasts are on the VST scale, effect estimates approximate log2 fold-changes. Genes with BH-adjusted $p < 0.05$ and $|\text{log2FC}| > 0.25$ (~19%) were considered differentially expressed. This aims to balance sensitivity and error control for PBMC datasets, where nutritionally induced responses are often present as small per-gene shifts [21,22]. The analysis included the main effects of treatment and metabolic state, their interaction, and pairwise contrasts (e.g., EBJ vs. PL in the fed state). This model-based approach enabled robust detection of expression changes while accounting for inter-individual variability and study design.

2.5. Pathway-Based Filtering of Differentially Expressed Genes

To identify gene expression changes relevant to metabolic regulation, we applied a curated, pathway-driven filtering strategy based on Kyoto Encyclopedia of Genes and Genomes (KEGG) and literature-defined metabolic functions. First, differentially expressed genes (DEGs) with adjusted *p*-value (padj) <0.05 and absolute $\log_2$ fold-change > 0.25 were retained. A custom metabolic flexibility gene whitelist was constructed by aggregating all human genes from 38 KEGG pathways associated with energy metabolism, nutrient sensing, redox regulation, and mitochondrial function (e.g., glycolysis, TCA cycle, insulin signaling, AMPK, autophagy) (Supplementary Table S1). Pathways were queried via KEGG's REST API, and gene symbols, descriptions, and annotations were extracted.

In addition, 74 literature-curated regulators of metabolic flexibility—representing core nodes in pathways such as glucose uptake, fatty acid oxidation, mitochondrial biogenesis, and immunometabolism—were manually added to ensure inclusion of biologically important genes not annotated in KEGG [23–25]. These genes were cross-referenced against the KEGG-derived whitelist, and only those not already represented were retained to avoid duplication. Genes were then filtered by presence in this expanded, non-redundant whitelist.

Filtered DEGs from each condition (EBJ and PL) were annotated with pathway information derived from the whitelist and grouped by KEGG pathway category or literature-defined function. For each pathway, we computed the number of DEGs detected per group and quantified the overlap in gene membership between conditions. To assess whether the degree of gene sharing between groups was greater than expected by chance, we used Fisher's exact test on a 2×2 contingency table of shared vs. unique genes.

2.6. Gene Ontology Enrichment Analysis

Gene Ontology (GO) enrichment analysis was conducted using the enrichGO function from the clusterProfiler package [26] with the org.Hs.eg.db annotation database [17]. DEGs were filtered at an adjusted p-value threshold of < 0.05 and converted from gene symbols to Entrez IDs using bitr (). GO enrichment was run across the Biological Process (BP), Molecular Function (MF), and Cellular Component (CC) ontologies using a contrast-specific background gene list derived from each raw count matrix. Enrichment parameters included a Benjamini–Hochberg adjusted p-value cutoff of 0.05.

To assign directionality to enriched GO terms, contributing gene symbols were decomposed and cross-referenced with DEG direction. Each GO term was annotated as "upregulated", "downregulated", or "mixed" based on the majority direction of its associated genes. The top 10 terms per contrast and ontology were visualized based on $-\log_{10}$(FDR). Cluster-level keywords were automatically extracted from GO term descriptions to summarize biological themes within clusters.

2.7. Gene Set Enrichment Analysis

Gene set enrichment analysis (GSEA) was performed to identify pathways relevant to metabolic flexibility that were altered by EBJ and PL treatments across nutritional states. Genes were ranked by either estimated $\log_2$ fold-change or t-statistics, depending on the contrast, and mapped to Entrez Gene IDs using the bitr () function from the clusterProfiler package with the org.Hs.eg.db annotation database. Enrichment was conducted using the gseKEGG () function, focusing on curated KEGG pathways. Because GSEA is a rank-based method, it considers the distribution of all expressed genes rather than relying on a threshold-defined DEG list. This approach reduces the dependency of pathway enrichment results on absolute DEG counts and enables more robust comparisons across conditions with differing DEG numbers.

To prioritize biologically relevant results, GSEA outputs were filtered using a manually curated whitelist of metabolism- and signaling-related KEGG pathways (n = 51), including canonical pathways (e.g., glycolysis, insulin signaling, AMPK, TCA cycle) as well as additional terms identified through enrichment results and manual review (e.g., pantothenate and CoA biosynthesis, sphingolipid metabolism, oxidative phosphorylation).

Results were further filtered by a significance threshold of FDR-adjusted p-value < 0.1, and pathway directionality was recorded using normalized enrichment scores (NES).

3. Results

3.1. DEG Main Effects and Contrasts

The transcriptomic analysis results are provided in Supplementary Table S2 and visualized in Figure 1. During the fasted-to-fed transition, a total of 1512 genes were identified as differentially expressed (FDR-adjusted $p < 0.05$, $|\log_2 FC| > 0.25$) in the EBJ group, while 350 DEGs were identified in the PL group. Direct comparisons between EBJ and PL in the fed state yielded two DEGs, while no significant DEGs were identified in the fasted state or for the treatment × state interaction term.

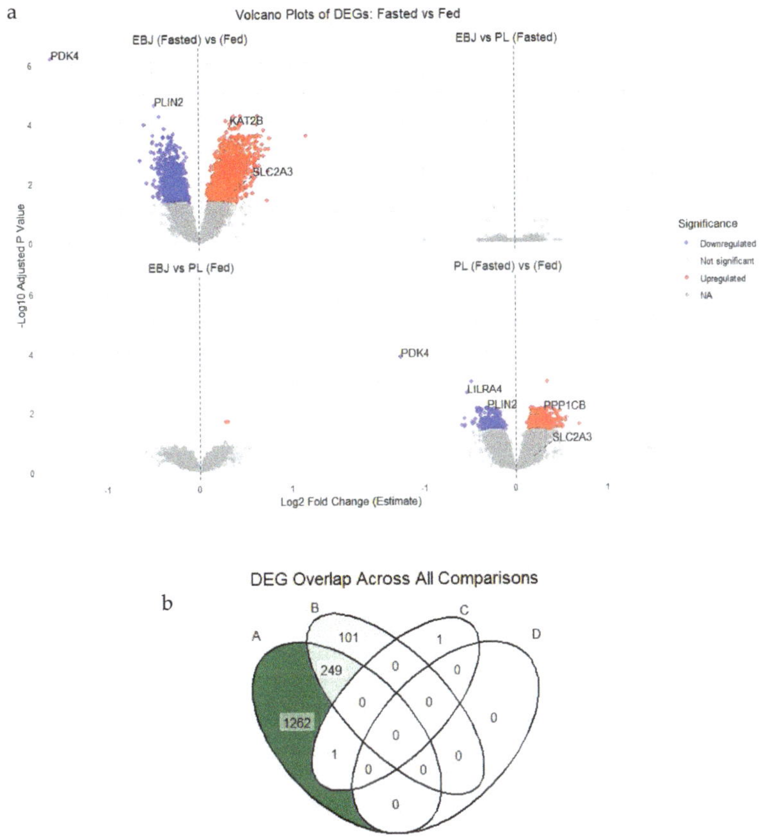

Figure 1. Differentially expressed genes (DEGs) across treatment contrasts. (**a**): Volcano plots of DEGs identified in each of the four contrasts. The x-axis shows the $\log_2$ fold change ($\log_2$FC) in gene expression, and the y-axis shows the $-\log_{10}$ adjusted *p*-value (false discovery rate, FDR). Each point represents a gene: red = significantly upregulated, blue = significantly downregulated, grey = not significant. DEGs were defined as those with FDR-adjusted $p < 0.05$ and $|\log_2 FC| > 0.25$. Gene labels indicate selected DEGs of interest. (**b**): Venn diagram showing overlap of significant DEGs across the four contrasts: (A) EBJ fasted → fed transition, (B) placebo (PL) fasted → fed transition, (C) EBJ vs. PL under fed conditions, and (D) EBJ vs. PL under fasted conditions. Overlapping regions indicate genes shared between contrasts, with counts shaded from white to dark green proportional to the size of the overlap. Data reflect pooled transcriptomic analyses from $n = 10$ participants per group.

In Figure 1a, the distribution of fold changes for EBJ fasted vs. fed comparisons highlights changes ranging from −2.6 to +2.8, with 410 genes exhibiting a $\log_2$FC greater than ±0.32, equating to at least a 1.25-fold change. The overlap of DEGs EBJ and PL feeding responses is shown in Figure 1b, with 249 DEGs shared and 1262 unique to the EBJ group. These findings indicate that while baseline gene expression levels in the fasted state were comparable between EBJ and PL, the EBJ group demonstrated approximately four times more DEGs activated in response to feeding than the PL group.

3.2. Metabolic Flexibility Gene Expression

To examine pathway-level shifts in metabolic gene regulation during the fasted-to-fed transition, differentially expressed genes (DEGs; FDR < 0.05) were mapped to KEGG and curated literature-defined pathways. This analysis yielded 234 metabolic DEGs in the EBJ group and 59 in the PL group, with 44 DEGs shared between groups (Supplementary Table S3). No significant metabolic DEGs were identified in the direct EBJ vs. PL contrast.

To compare the functional distribution of DEGs, Fisher's exact test was applied to identify pathways with significant differences in gene representation between treatment arms (Table 1). Several pathways showed statistically significant enrichment in both groups, but with greater gene-level representation in the EBJ group. This included insulin signaling (FDR = 1.6×10^{-5}), FoxO signaling (FDR = 0.0004), MAPK signaling (FDR = 0.0012), circadian rhythm (FDR = 0.0015), PI3K–Akt signaling (FDR = 0.0090), and autophagy (FDR = 0.0135). Pathways related to cytokine–cytokine receptor interaction (FDR = 0.0153), fatty acid degradation (FDR = 0.0255), and fatty acid biosynthesis (FDR = 0.0270) also showed significantly higher overlap in EBJ-fed samples (Supplementary Table S4 full Fisher's results).

Table 1. Fisher's exact test of pathway enrichment during the fasted-to-fed transition. Counts of significantly differentially expressed genes (DEGs; FDR-adjusted $p < 0.05$, $|\log_2 FC| > 0.25$) for the elderberry juice (EBJ) and placebo (PL) groups, and those shared between groups. Pathways were selected from a whitelist of KEGG metabolic pathways and additional literature-curated gene sets. FDR (false discovery rate) denotes the expected proportion of false positives after multiple-testing correction. Data reflect pooled transcriptomic analyses from n = 10 participants per group.

Pathway	EBJ Count	PL Count	Shared Count	FDR
Insulin Signaling	18	7	6	1.56E-05
FoxO Signaling	8	3	3	<0.001
Literature Curation	4	2	2	0.001
MAPK Signaling	21	8	5	0.001
Circadian Rhythm	4	2	2	0.001
PI3K–Akt Signaling	29	9	5	0.009
Autophagy	17	5	3	0.013
Cytokine–Cytokine Receptor Interaction	19	5	3	0.015

Among the top five significantly regulated genes in both treatment groups (FDR $\leq$ 0.05), three genes were shared: PDK4, PLIN2, and LILRA4, each showing stronger regulation in the EBJ group. PDK4, which encodes pyruvate dehydrogenase kinase 4, was more strongly downregulated in EBJ-fed samples (estimate = −1.61, FDR = 6.3×10^{-7}) compared to PL-fed samples (estimate = −1.25, FDR = 1.6×10^{-4}). PLIN2 (perilipin 2), involved in lipid droplet formation and lipid mobilization, was downregulated by −0.47 (FDR = 2.5×10^{-5}) in EBJ and −0.31 (FDR = 0.0091) in PL. Similarly, LILRA4, which encodes leukocyte immunoglobulin-like receptor A4 and is involved in immune cell signaling, showed greater downregulation in EBJ (estimate = −0.59, FDR = 1.1×10^{-4}) than in PL (estimate = −0.53, FDR = 0.0027).

In addition to these shared genes, EBJ-fed samples uniquely upregulated SLC2A3 (estimate = 0.39, FDR = 0.019), a gene that encodes the glucose transporter protein GLUT3, which is responsible for transporting glucose across cell membranes, and PPARGC1B (estimate = 0.64, FDR = 1.1×10^{-4}), a coactivator of genes involved in mitochondrial biogenesis and energy metabolism. In contrast, the PL group showed unique regulation of ACAA2 (estimate = −0.32, FDR = 0.0091), which encodes acetyl-CoA acyltransferase 2 and is involved in mitochondrial fatty acid β-oxidation, and PPP1CB (estimate = 0.30, FDR = 0.0098), a catalytic subunit of protein phosphatase 1 that contributes to cell cycle regulation, insulin signaling, and circadian processes.

3.3. Gene Ontology Enrichment Analysis

Gene ontology (GO) enrichment analysis was conducted to identify coordinated cellular responses to the fasted-to-fed transition in each treatment group, revealing functional trends in DEGs (Figure 2a,b; Supplementary Table S5).

a

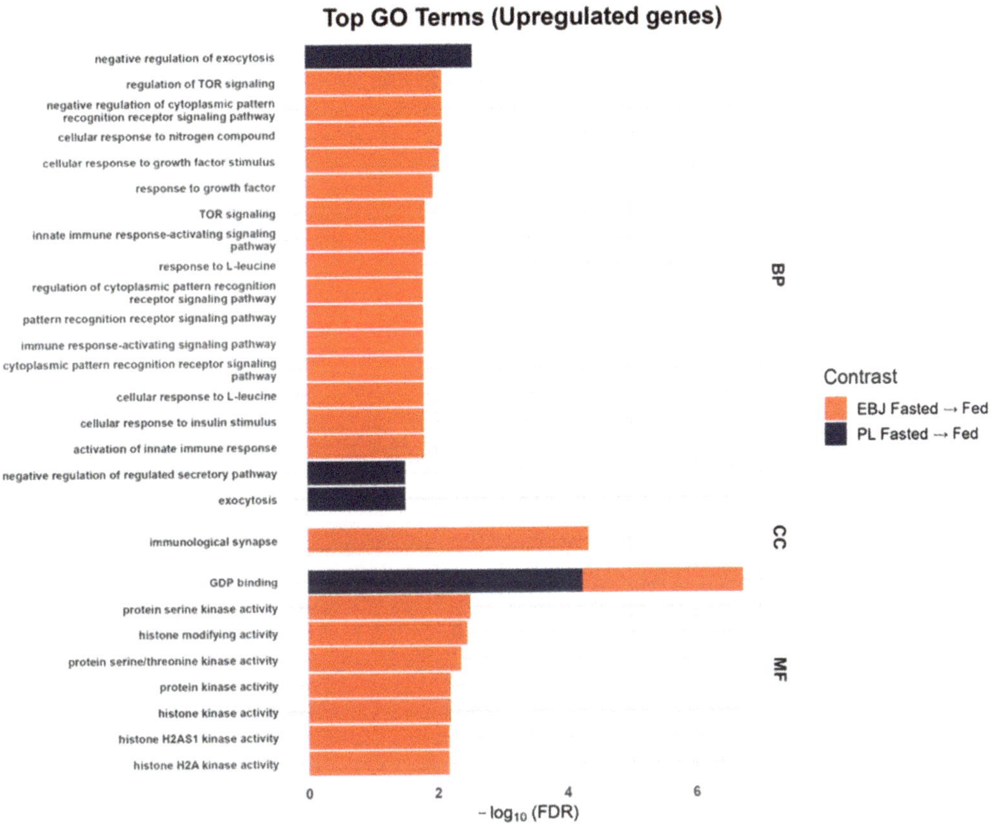

Figure 2. *Cont.*

b

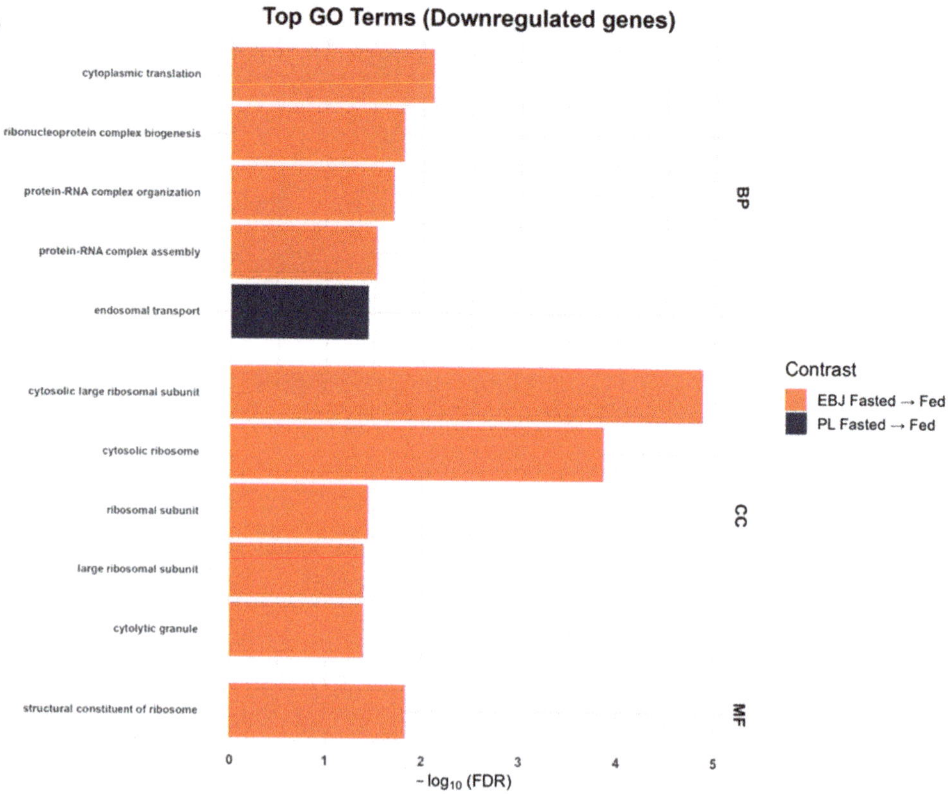

Figure 2. Gene Ontology enrichment for differentially expressed genes (DEGs) in response to feeding. (**a**). Bar plot showing the top Gene Ontology (GO) terms enriched among upregulated DEGs during the fasted-to-fed transition. GO categories are Biological Process (BP), Cellular Component (CC), and Molecular Function (MF). Results are stratified by treatment group (red: elderberry juice, EBJ; black: placebo, PL). Bars represent the $-\log_{10}$ of the false discovery rate (FDR)-adjusted *p*-value for each enriched term. (**b**). GO enrichment for downregulated DEGs in response to feeding, in the same format as Figure (**a**). Data reflect pooled transcriptomic analyses from $n = 10$ participants per group.

In the EBJ group, numerous GO biological process (BP) terms were significantly enriched among upregulated genes (FDR < 0.05), including pathways related to immune signaling, hormone response, and nutrient sensing. Specifically, significant enrichment was observed in cellular response to nitrogen compound (GO:1901699, FDR = 0.0073, n = 133), regulation of TOR signaling (GO:0032006, FDR = 0.0073, n = 48), response to growth factor (GO:0070848, FDR = 0.0102, n = 136), cellular response to insulin stimulus (GO:0032869, FDR = 0.0147, n = 56), and insulin receptor signaling pathway (GO:0008286, FDR = 0.0451, n = 37). Immune-related pathways such as innate immune response-activating signaling pathway (GO:0002758, FDR = 0.0138, n = 78) and pattern recognition receptor signaling pathway (GO:0002221, FDR = 0.0147, n = 73) were also significantly upregulated. In contrast, downregulated processes included ribonucleoprotein complex biogenesis (GO:0022613, FDR = 0.0147, n = 121), protein–RNA complex organization (GO:0071826, FDR = 0.0187, n = 60), and protein–RNA complex assembly (GO:0022618, FDR = 0.0280, n = 57).

For the Cellular Component (CC) category, downregulated genes in the EBJ group were significantly enriched in multiple ribosome-related compartments, including the cytosolic large ribosomal subunit (GO:0022625, FDR = 1.25×10^{-5}, n = 29), cytosolic ribosome (GO:0022626, FDR = 1.29 × 10^{-4}, n = 44), ribosomal subunit (GO:0044391, FDR = 3.37 × 10^{-2}, n = 55), large ribosomal subunit (GO:0015934, FDR = 3.72 × 10^{-2}, n = 37), and cytolytic granule (GO:0044194, FDR = 3.72 × 10^{-2}, n = 9). The immunological synapse (GO:0001772, FDR = 4.36 × 10^{-5}, n = 25) was significantly enriched among upregulated genes.

Within the Molecular Function (MF) category, upregulated genes in the EBJ group were significantly enriched for several kinase-related activities, including protein serine/threonine kinase activity (GO:0004674, FDR = 4.19 × 10^{-3}, n = 104), protein kinase activity (GO:0004672, FDR = 6.08 × 10^{-3}, n = 127), histone kinase activity (GO:0035173, FDR = 6.09 × 10^{-3}, n = 68), and histone H2A kinase activity (GO:0140995, FDR = 6.45 × 10^{-3}, n = 65). Additional significant enrichment was observed for GDP binding (GO:0019003, FDR = 2.98 × 10^{-3}, n = 27) and histone-modifying activity (GO:0140993, FDR = 3.30 × 10^{-3}, n = 109). In contrast, the structural constituent of the ribosome (GO:0003735, FDR = 1.37 × 10^{-2}, n = 50) was enriched among downregulated genes.

In the placebo group, GO enrichment analysis indicated significant changes in the BP categories in response to feeding. Upregulated BP included negative regulation of exocytosis (GO:0045920, FDR = 0.0025, n = 10) and negative regulation of the regulated secretory pathway (GO:1903306, FDR = 0.0299, n = 7), both of which included RAP and RAB GTPase genes. Positive regulation of neuron projection development (GO:0010976, FDR = 0.0299, n = 17) was also enriched, though regulation within this term was mixed. Broader secretory pathway terms, such as exocytosis (GO:0006887, FDR = 0.0299, n = 29) and endosomal transport (GO:0016197, FDR = 0.0359, n = 28), were enriched, with the latter primarily associated with downregulated genes.

Within the MF category for the placebo group, GDP binding (GO:0019003, FDR = 5.85 × 10^{-5}, n = 15) was significantly enriched among upregulated genes, encompassing multiple small GTPases (RAB8B, RAP1A, RAP1B, RHEB), suggesting alterations in vesicular trafficking activity during the fed state.

PL did not show any significant changes in the CC category.

3.4. Gene Set Enrichment Analysis

To explore coordinated transcriptional responses to feeding, we performed KEGG GSEA on ranked gene expression data from fasted and fed samples in both the EBJ and PL arms (Supplementary Table S6). Enrichment was performed using the gseKEGG () function, and results were filtered using a manually curated whitelist of 51 KEGG pathways relevant to metabolic flexibility. Pathways of interest included canonical metabolic and signaling routes (e.g., insulin signaling, oxidative phosphorylation, AMPK, TCA cycle) and were retained if the FDR-adjusted p-value was below 0.1 (Supplementary Table S7).

In the EBJ group, 27 pathways met the significance threshold (FDR < 0.1), of which 24 had FDR < 0.05. Figure 3 illustrates a dotplot of the top 20 pathways. Upregulated pathways included FoxO signaling (NES = 2.15, FDR = 8.67 × 10^{-7}), insulin signaling (NES = 2.00, FDR = 3.79 × 10^{-5}), PI3K–Akt signaling (NES = 1.65, FDR = 0.0003), mTOR signaling (NES = 1.76, FDR = 0.0012), AMPK signaling (NES = 1.68, FDR = 0.0037), cAMP signaling (NES = 1.72, FDR = 0.0013), and cGMP-PKG signaling (NES = 1.82, FDR = 0.0003). Additional significantly upregulated pathways included autophagy (NES = 1.99, FDR = 4.20 × 10^{-6}), Toll-like receptor signaling (NES = 2.05, FDR = 4.82 × 10^{-5}), HIF-1 signaling (NES = 1.63, FDR = 0.0064), and adipocytokine signaling (NES = 1.64, FDR = 0.020).

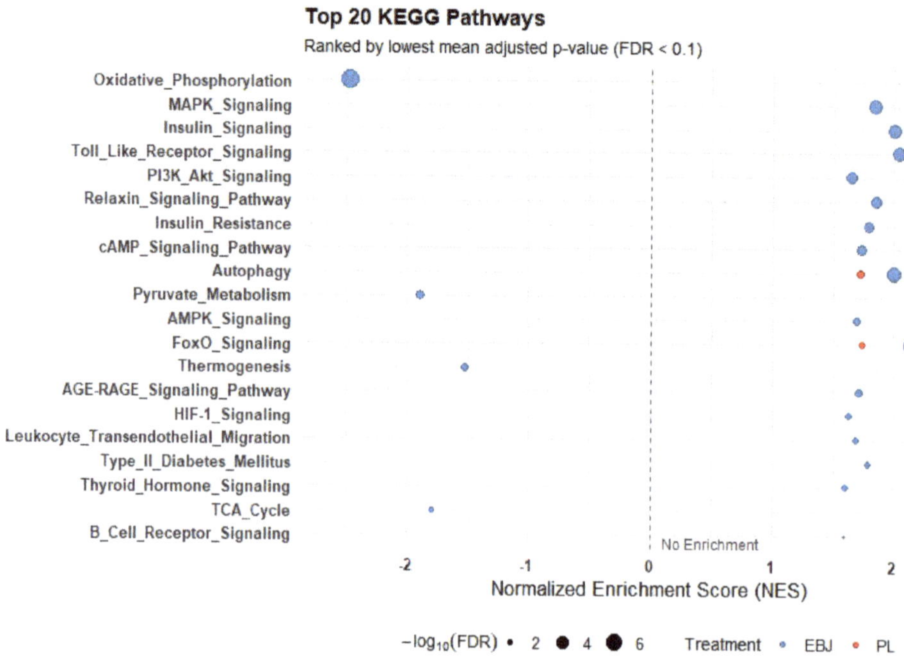

Figure 3. Top KEGG pathways identified by gene set enrichment analysis. Gene set enrichment analysis (GSEA) of the top 20 Kyoto Encyclopedia of Genes and Genomes (KEGG) pathways in peripheral blood mononuclear cells (PBMCs) following elderberry juice (EBJ) or placebo (PL) treatment. Pathways are ranked by the lowest mean adjusted *p*-value across both groups [false discovery rate (FDR) < 0.1]. GSEA evaluates the distribution of all expressed genes ranked by fold-change or test statistic. Each dot represents a pathway–treatment combination, with the *x*-axis showing the normalized enrichment score (NES), a standardized metric reflecting the degree to which a pathway's genes are overrepresented at the top or bottom of the ranked list. Dot size corresponds to statistical significance [$-\log_{10}$(FDR)], and color indicates treatment group (blue = EBJ, red = PL). Positive NES values indicate pathway enrichment in the fasted versus fed state, while negative NES values indicate relative downregulation. The vertical dashed line at NES = 0 denotes no enrichment. Data reflect pooled transcriptomic analyses from $n = 10$ participants per group.

Downregulated pathways in the EBJ group included oxidative phosphorylation (NES = −2.47, FDR = 1.16×10^{-8}), TCA cycle (NES = −1.79, FDR = 0.011), pyruvate metabolism (NES = −1.89, FDR = 0.0031), fatty acid degradation (NES = −1.55, FDR = 0.041), and glycolysis/gluconeogenesis (NES = −1.47, FDR = 0.058).

In the PL group, seven pathways passed the FDR < 0.1 threshold. These included upregulation of FoxO signaling (NES = 1.74, FDR = 0.0075), autophagy (NES = 1.72, FDR = 0.0056), mTOR signaling (NES = 1.45, FDR = 0.068), and cGMP-PKG signaling (NES = 1.56, FDR = 0.039). Downregulated pathways included glycolysis/gluconeogenesis (NES = −1.52, FDR = 0.097) and fructose and mannose metabolism (NES = −1.64, FDR = 0.100).

4. Discussion

In this study, we examined transcriptomic markers of this substrate switching response in PBMCs following an EBJ intervention, using samples from a previously published short-term clinical study [10]. PBMCs, although primarily immune cells, express a high proportion of the human genome and interact dynamically with metabolic tissues. Through receptors for hormones such as insulin and leptin, PBMCs capture systemic signals that influence metabolic pathways. This positions them as practical "sentinels" for reflecting transcriptional adaptations in key tissues, including adipose, liver, and muscle, which are challenging to biopsy in clinical trials [27]. Prior work shows that PBMCs can mirror fasting-induced changes in lipid metabolism genes observed in adipose tissue and detect diet-induced metabolic shifts, supporting their utility as accessible surrogates for systemic responses in nutrigenomic studies [22,27,28]. At the same time, it is important to recognize their limitations. PBMCs are immune-derived cells, and while they mirror systemic signals, they cannot fully substitute for transcriptional changes occurring in primary metabolic tissues. Thus, while PBMCs provide valuable and biologically coherent insight into systemic nutritional adaptations, their role should be viewed as complementary rather than equivalent to direct tissue profiling. Future work incorporating adipose or muscle biopsies would be required to confirm tissue-level adaptations.

4.1. Systemic Absorption and Bioavailability of Anthocyanins from EBJ

In this study, participants consumed American black elderberry juice (*Sambucus nigra* spp. *canadensis*), which contains principally acylated anthocyanins, constituting approximately 70% of the total anthocyanin content when fully ripened, as confirmed in our previous study [9,10]. The prominent acylated anthocyanin is cyanidin-3-(E)-*p*-coumaroyl-sambubioside-5-glucoside, compared to the non-acylated cyanidin 3-O-sambubioside, the predominant form in the European elderberry (*Sambucus nigra*). The latter bears a free hydroxyl group at C-5 and lacks acyl functionalities in the structure, as noted by several separate studies investigating the profiles of the European black elderberry [29–32]. This distinction in anthocyanin composition underscores the critical difference between the two species, as acylation increases stability (to heat, light, and pH) and alters absorption routes relative to non-acylated forms [30].

Acylated anthocyanins are absorbed in the gastrointestinal tract through specific transporters. Computational and in vitro studies demonstrate a preferential interaction with glucose transporter GLUT3 compared to the GLUT1 preference of nonacylated anthocyanins [33,34]. This preferential GLUT3 binding occurs due to structural features of acylated anthocyanins that facilitate binding through both hydrophobic (CH–π and π–π stacking) and hydrophilic (hydrogen bonding) interactions essential for transmembrane transport [34].

Experimentation of GLUT involvement in acylated anthocyanin transport was described by Oliveira et al. [34], who used gold nanoparticles to selectively knockdown GLUT1 and GLUT3 in human gastric epithelial cells. They demonstrated that these transporters account for ~60% of anthocyanin gastric transport, including acylated forms from purple sweet potato (Pn3HBsoph5glc and Pn3HBCsoph5glc), though with lower efficiency than non-acylated counterparts due to steric hindrance. The glucose moiety remained essential for binding regardless of acylation, indicating that acylated anthocyanins like those in American black elderberry can interact with glucose transporters.

Consistent with this purported mechanism, our PBMC transcriptome analysis revealed significant upregulation of *SLC2A3* (GLUT3) at 120 min after EBJ consumption, which may indicate transporter activation extending to systemic circulation beyond gastric interactions. As a high-affinity glucose transporter expressed in leukocytes, this change is consistent with potential modulation of GLUT3 expression in circulating immune cells by EBJ anthocyanins [35]. Overall, the specific anthocyanin profile of American black elderberry and its enrichment in acylated forms is plausibly linked to observed metabolic effects, though direct confirmation in human tissues is needed.

4.2. Elderberry Juice and Blood Glucose Homeostasis

In our study, EBJ-fed samples exhibited significant upregulation of key components in insulin signaling and glucose metabolism. This included SLC2A3 (GLUT3) upregulation, which facilitates cellular glucose uptake, RAB10, a Rab GTPase involved in vesicle trafficking for insulin-mediated glucose transport, and PDPK1, a kinase that activates AKT in the PI3K–AKT signaling pathway. In vitro evidence suggests that acylated anthocyanins may induce stronger activation of the PI3K/AKT pathway than their nonacylated counterparts [33].

In the EBJ group, downregulation of PDK2 and PDK4, negative regulators of the pyruvate dehydrogenase complex (PDC), may have facilitated greater glucose utilization. This downregulation facilitates greater entry of pyruvate into the TCA cycle for energy production, allowing for more efficient glucose metabolism following a high-glucose meal. Additionally, we observed upregulation of glycolytic genes, including HK2, PFKFB2, and PFKFB3, suggesting that the glycolytic pathway was also enhanced. These gene expression changes are supported by the 24% reduction in postprandial glucose incremental area under the curve (iAUC) observed in our clinical trial, providing a partial mechanistic basis for the glucose-lowering effects of EBJ [10]. Anthocyanins also reportedly slow intestinal absorption of glucose at the brush border of enterocytes [24]. Therefore, mechanistic events related to intestinal inhibition of glucose absorption by elderberry anthocyanins are also possibly involved but are beyond the scope of the current study.

In contrast, samples from the placebo group showed similar downregulation of PDK4, but this occurred without accompanying reductions in PDK2 or increases in glycolytic genes. Such a pattern may suggest less effective glucose metabolism due to the lack of signaling enhanced by the anthocyanins in the EBJ. Pathway-level analysis indicated that both groups affected glycolysis and gluconeogenesis pathways. However, EBJ uniquely activated compensatory signaling pathways, including insulin signaling, which facilitates glucose uptake, and AMPK signaling, involved in energy switching and fatty acid oxidation. This too is corroborated by the observations on improved insulin sensitivity and reduced respiratory quotient in our previous clinical study.

These findings are consistent with the idea that EBJ may support coordination of glucose-handling pathways and contribute to metabolic flexibility in individuals with overweight or obesity. The differential transcriptomic response suggests that acylated anthocyanins from EJB could influence glucose metabolism, pointing to a potential role in managing metabolic health.

4.3. Lipid Metabolism, FAO Suppression, and Mitochondrial Function

In the fed state, insulin drives anabolic lipid metabolism by promoting de novo lipogenesis, a process that balances nutrient storage and metabolic flexibility [36]. Our study revealed distinct metabolic responses in the EBJ group, characterized by a comprehensive modulation of lipid metabolism and mitochondrial function.

The EBJ group demonstrated significant upregulation of key genes involved in lipid metabolism. ACSL1 and ACSL4 catalyze the activation of long-chain fatty acids for triglyceride synthesis, while ELOVL5 and HACD2/HACD4 facilitate fatty acid chain elongation and lipid diversity. FAR1 supports fatty acid reductase activity, and PPARGC1B is the master regulator of mitochondrial biogenesis and metabolic adaptation. These changes were further supported by coactivators RXRA and NCOA2, which enhance nuclear receptor signaling in lipid metabolism. KEGG pathway analysis confirmed these findings, showing upregulation of glycerophospholipid metabolism and downregulation of fatty acid degradation.

In contrast, the placebo group exhibited only partial gene upregulation, primarily in ACSL4 and FAR1, suggesting a less comprehensive metabolic response.

4.4. Fatty Acid Oxidation and Mitochondrial Modulation

Both groups showed downregulation of FAO genes, including CPT1A and SLC25A20, consistent with insulin's metabolic effects in the fed state. Notably, the EBJ group exhibited significant downregulation of oxidative phosphorylation, involving critical mitochondrial genes with specific metabolic roles. NDUFV1, a key component of Complex I in the electron transport chain, plays a crucial role in transferring electrons from NADH to ubiquinone, directly impacting energy production. COX3, the final enzyme in the electron transport chain, catalyzes the reduction of molecular oxygen to water, representing the culmination of cellular respiration. The coordinated downregulation of these genes suggests a strategic metabolic adaptation that may prevent nutrient overload, reduce reactive oxygen species (ROS) accumulation, and minimize cellular stress during metabolic adaptation [37]. The above two sections describe a transcriptomic enhancement of lipid synthesis and storage, yet our clinical study observations demonstrated higher fat oxidation over the course of a 3 h postprandial state when study volunteers were fed a high-sugar meal with EBJ compared to a placebo [10]. These transcriptomic and clinical observations may appear contradictory but could potentially be reconciled through the following hypothesis: the dampened insulin response, enhanced glucose handling, and potentially slowed intestinal absorption of the challenge meal's glucose bolus may help explain why the EBJ treatment led to a comparatively increased whole-body fat oxidation state compared to placebo. At the same time, the transcriptomic analyses suggest the possibility of enhanced switching of metabolic fuels—and thus improved insulin sensitivity—as described below.

4.5. Insulin and Nutrient-Sensing Signaling

In both EBJ and placebo groups, transcriptional patterns indicated distinct responses to insulin signaling. In EBJ-fed samples, upregulated genes such as IGF1R, GRB10, and GAB1 indicated enhanced insulin receptor function, supported by GO enrichment for insulin receptor signaling (GO:0008286) and response to insulin (GO:0032868). Activation of the PI3K–AKT pathway was evident through components like PDPK1 and RAB10, along with pathway enrichment linking downstream to mTOR and FoxO signaling. This signaling profile reflects upstream insulin components inhibiting FoxO1 via AKT phosphorylation, thereby promoting anabolic responses [38]. Additionally, an anthocyanin-rich diet enhances insulin sensitivity, as discussed by Randeni et al. [39], who highlighted how anthocyanins modulate the PI3K/AKT pathway, facilitating improved glucose uptake and metabolic responses.

In contrast, placebo-fed samples displayed mixed regulation in insulin-related pathways, including FOXO3, mTOR and FoxO enrichment upregulation, but no significant PI3K–AKT activation. This lack of coordinated anabolic gene expression indicates incomplete adaptation in the placebo group, emphasizing a more robust insulin-driven substrate switching observed in EBJ-fed samples.

4.6. Study Limitations

The RNA-seq cohort was modest (n = 10 participants; 40 libraries), which limits external generalizability and precludes adequately powered subgroup or interaction analyses. Nevertheless, the design and analytic framework support internal validity. The 2×2 crossover provided four repeated measures per participant, reducing between-person variability and increasing efficiency for treatment contrasts. We modeled repeated measures with lmerSeq, a linear mixed-effects approach specifically developed for small-n RNA-seq designs, which has been shown in simulations and real whole-blood datasets to maintain nominal false discovery rate control and higher power than alternative methods [20]. Broadly, benchmarking studies show that replication increases statistical power more effectively than sequencing depth, with ~6–12 replicates often sufficient depending on design [40]. Similar nutrition-focused crossover transcriptomic studies have successfully reported biologically coherent findings with sample sizes in this same range or smaller (n = 6–14) [41–43]. However, our interpretations draw on supportive in vitro, computational, and animal-based research for a mechanistic context, notably with anthocyanin acetylation and transporter interaction. These mechanistic interpretations require direct human evidence. Taken together, our findings should be regarded as exploratory and hypothesis-generating, but are supported by design efficiency, appropriate methods, and field precedent.

5. Conclusions

This study provides a comprehensive transcriptomic analysis of American black elderberry juice's effects on metabolic flexibility in human PBMCs in response to a high sugar test meal. Our findings reveal that elderberry juice (EBJ) consumption may enhance the transcriptional response to feeding, with approximately four times more differentially expressed genes (1512 vs. 350) compared to placebo during the fasted-to-fed transition. This amplified transcriptional plasticity potentially represents a molecular signature of improved metabolic flexibility. The marked enrichment of nutrient-sensing and insulin signaling pathways following EBJ consumption aligns with our previous clinical findings showing improved glucose tolerance and higher fat oxidation compared to placebo [10]. Our GSEA results demonstrate that EBJ upregulated key nutrient-sensing pathways (FoxO, insulin, mTOR, AMPK, cAMP/cGMP-PKG) and autophagy, while simultaneously affecting energy metabolism pathways (oxidative phosphorylation, TCA cycle, glycolysis). This pattern suggests that EBJ enhances cellular energy efficiency by promoting dynamic fuel switching and optimizing metabolic resource allocation instead of increasing overall metabolic rate, which was not observed in our clinical findings. The transcriptional changes in key metabolic genes provide mechanistic insights into EBJ's physiological effects. Particularly notable was the stronger downregulation of PDK4 (pyruvate dehydrogenase kinase 4) in EBJ-fed samples compared to placebo, indicating enhanced suppression of PDK4's inhibitory effect on carbohydrate oxidation. Paired with a reduction in genes responsible for electron transport chain enzymes, this could suggest an enhancement in replenishing TCA cycle intermediates, or protection of the mitochondria against ROS, but molecular investigations would need to confirm this. These insights stand in juxtaposition with the increased fat oxidation observed in our previous study [10], where EBJ consumption significantly lowered the respiratory quotient and, therefore, increased fat utilization during both postprandial and exercise conditions; however, a dampened insulin response in the EBJ treatment hypothetically explains this disparity between transcriptomics and clinical observations. The upregulation of PPARGC1B and AMPK, key regulators of mitochondrial biogenesis and fatty acid oxidation, shows that EBJ enhances overall oxidative capacity, further supporting metabolic flexibility. Our findings are consistent with recent research on elderberry anthocyanins' bioavailability and metabolic effects. The rapid absorption of anthocyanins in the stomach via transporters like GLUTs and bilitranslocase [44] potentially explains how elderberry compounds can exert acute effects on gene expression in peripheral tissues. Notably, our finding that SLC2A3 (GLUT3) was upregulated in PBMCs after EBJ intervention aligns with our previous discussion [24], where we identified GLUT3 as a major transporter involved in anthocyanin absorption in gastric cells, and the present study extends its potential modulation to white blood cells. These converging results suggest that anthocyanin-rich foods may acutely shape glucose transporter expression, potentially supporting both anthocyanin bioavailability and glucose metabolism at multiple biological sites. These results support exploring EBJ as a practical dietary adjunct for enhancing metabolic flexibility—including improved glucose handling, insulin sensitivity, and fat oxidation—in overweight individuals, potentially reducing reliance on pharmacological options for managing metabolic health. Nevertheless, given the modest RNA-seq cohort (n = 10), these transcriptomic findings should be considered exploratory and hypothesis-generating, with confirmation warranted in larger, adequately powered studies.

Supplementary Materials: The following supporting information can be downloaded at: https://www.mdpi.com/article/10.3390/nu17193142/s1, Table S1: Custom metabolic flexibility gene whitelist constructed from 38 KEGG pathways related to energy metabolism, nutrient sensing, redox regulation, and mitochondrial function; Table S2: Full transcriptomic analysis results for all genes; Table S3: Metabolic flexibility–related differentially expressed genes (DEGs) identified during the fasted-to-fed transition in EBJ and PL groups; Table S4: Fisher's exact test results for differential pathway representation between treatment arms; Table S5: Gene Ontology enrichment results for DEGs in each treatment group; Table S6: KEGG gene set enrichment analysis (GSEA) results for all pathways in EBJ and PL groups; Table S7: Filtered KEGG GSEA results for curated metabolic flexibility–related pathways (FDR < 0.1).

Author Contributions: Conceptualization, P.M.S.; methodology, C.T. and P.M.S.; validation, C.T. and P.M.S.; formal analysis, C.T.; investigation, C.T. and P.M.S.; data curation, C.T. and P.M.S.; writing—original draft preparation, C.T. and P.M.S.; writing—review and editing, C.T., A.J.E., and P.M.S.; visualization, C.T.; supervision, P.M.S.; project administration, A.J.E. and P.M.S.; funding acquisition, A.J.E. and P.M.S. All authors have read and agreed to the published version of the manuscript.

Funding: The human clinical trial research was funded by the United States Department of Agriculture (National Institute of Food and Agriculture, grant number 2020-67018-30851), which also funded the APC. The funding agencies had no role in the design, analysis, interpretation, or reporting of our findings.

Institutional Review Board Statement: The study was conducted in accordance with the Declaration of Helsinki, and the study protocol was approved by the Washington State University (WSU) Institutional Review Board (Pullman, WA, USA) under protocol number 18597 (approved on 30 December 2020).

Informed Consent Statement: Written informed consent was obtained from all subjects involved in the study.

Data Availability Statement: Research data from measures of human transcriptomics are available in Supplementary Tables S1–S7 described above.

Acknowledgments: We thank the human study volunteers who made this investigation possible and for the expert technical assistance only made possible by Nicholas Dunn.

Conflicts of Interest: The authors declare no conflicts of interest.

Abbreviations

The following abbreviations are used in this manuscript:

AMPK	AMP-activated protein kinase
BP	Biological Process (Gene Ontology category)
CC	Cellular Component (Gene Ontology category)
C3GE	Cyanidin-3-glucoside equivalents
DEG	Differentially expressed gene
EBJ	Elderberry juice
FAO	Fatty acid oxidation

FC	Fold change
FDR	False discovery rate
FoxO	Forkhead box O
GSEA	Gene set enrichment analysis
GO	Gene Ontology
HK2	Hexokinase 2
KEGG	Kyoto Encyclopedia of Genes and Genomes
MAPK	Mitogen-activated protein kinase
MF	Molecular Function (Gene Ontology category)
mTOR	Mechanistic target of rapamycin
MTT	Meal tolerance test
NES	Normalized enrichment score
PBMC	Peripheral blood mononuclear cell
PDK2	Pyruvate dehydrogenase kinase 2
PDK4	Pyruvate dehydrogenase kinase 4
PI3K–AKT	Phosphoinositide 3-kinase–protein kinase B
PL	Placebo
PPARGC1B	Peroxisome proliferator-activated receptor gamma coactivator 1-beta
RQ	Respiratory quotient
TCA	Tricarboxylic acid
TOR	Target of rapamycin
VST	Variance-stabilizing transformation

References

1. Galgani, J.E.; Bergouignan, A.; Rieusset, J.; Moro, C.; Nazare, J.A. Editorial: Metabolic Flexibility. *Front. Nutr.* **2022**, *9*, 946300. [CrossRef] [PubMed]
2. Palmer, B.F.; Clegg, D.J. Metabolic Flexibility and Its Impact on Health Outcomes. *Mayo Clin. Proc.* **2022**, *97*, 761–776. [CrossRef] [PubMed]
3. Smith, R.L.; Soeters, M.R.; Wüst, R.C.I.; Houtkooper, R.H. Metabolic Flexibility as an Adaptation to Energy Resources and Requirements in Health and Disease. *Endocr. Rev.* **2018**, *39*, 489–517. [CrossRef] [PubMed]
4. Goodpaster, B.H.; Sparks, L.M. Metabolic flexibility in health and disease. *Cell Metab.* **2017**, *25*, 1027–1036. [CrossRef]
5. Tareen, S.H.; Kutmon, M.; Arts, I.C.; De Kok, T.M.; Evelo, C.T.; Adriaens, M.E. Logical modelling reveals the PDC-PDK interaction as the regulatory switch driving metabolic flexibility at the cellular level. *Genes Nutr.* **2019**, *14*, 27. [CrossRef]
6. Nistor, M.; Pop, R.; Daescu, A.; Pintea, A.; Socaciu, C.; Rugina, D. Anthocyanins as Key Phytochemicals Acting for the Prevention of Metabolic Diseases: An Overview. *Molecules* **2022**, *27*, 4254. [CrossRef]
7. Riordan, J.; Solverson, P. Berry Anthocyanins in Rodent and Human Obesity and Diabetes: A Review of the Evidence. *BioMed* **2022**, *2*, 210–237. [CrossRef]
8. Sharma, S.; Pandita, G.; Bhosale, Y.K. Anthocyanin: Potential tool for diabetes management and different delivery aspects. *Trends Food Sci. Technol.* **2023**, *140*, 104170. [CrossRef]
9. Osman, A.G.; Avula, B.; Katragunta, K.; Ali, Z.; Chittiboyina, A.G.; Khan, I.A. Elderberry Extracts: Characterization of the Polyphenolic Chemical Composition, Quality Consistency, Safety, Adulteration, and Attenuation of Oxidative Stress- and Inflammation-Induced Health Disorders. *Molecules* **2023**, *28*, 3148. [CrossRef]
10. Teets, C.; Ghanem, N.; Ma, G.; Minj, J.; Perkins-Veazie, P.; Johnson, S.A.; Etter, A.J.; Carbonero, F.G.; Solverson, P.M. A One-Week Elderberry Juice Intervention Augments the Fecal Microbiota and Suggests Improvement in Glucose Tolerance and Fat Oxidation in a Randomized Controlled Trial. *Nutrients* **2024**, *16*, 3555. [CrossRef]
11. Abueg, L.A.L.; Afgan, E.; Allart, O.; Awan, A.H.; Bacon, W.A.; Baker, D.; Bassetti, M.; Batut, B.; Bernt, M.; Blankenberg, D.; et al. The Galaxy platform for accessible, reproducible, and collaborative data analyses: 2024 update. *Nucleic Acids Res.* **2024**, *52*, W83–W94. [CrossRef] [PubMed]
12. Bolger, A.M.; Lohse, M.; Usadel, B. Trimmomatic: A flexible trimmer for Illumina sequence data. *Bioinformatics* **2014**, *30*, 2114–2120. [CrossRef] [PubMed]
13. Kopylova, E.; Noé, L.; Touzet, H. SortMeRNA: Fast and accurate filtering of ribosomal RNAs in metatranscriptomic data. *Bioinformatics* **2012**, *28*, 3211–3217. [CrossRef] [PubMed]
14. Kim, D.; Paggi, J.M.; Park, C.; Bennett, C.; Salzberg, S.L. Graph-based genome alignment and genotyping with HISAT2 and HISAT-genotype. *Nat. Biotechnol.* **2019**, *37*, 907–915. [CrossRef] [PubMed]

15. Liao, Y.; Smyth, G.K.; Shi, W. featureCounts: An efficient general purpose program for assigning sequence reads to genomic features. *Bioinformatics* **2014**, *30*, 923–930. [CrossRef]
16. Love, M.I.; Huber, W.; Anders, S. Moderated estimation of fold change and dispersion for RNA-seq data with DESeq2. *Genome Biol.* **2014**, *15*, 550. [CrossRef]
17. Carlson, M. org.Hs.eg.db: Genome Wide Annotation for Human. Available online: https://bioconductor.org/packages/org.Hs.eg.db/ (accessed on 7 August 2025).
18. Lim, C.-Y.; In, J. Considerations for crossover design in clinical study. *Korean J. Anesthesiol.* **2021**, *74*, 293–299. [CrossRef]
19. Duda, J.C.; Drenda, C.; Kästel, H.; Rahnenführer, J.; Kappenberg, F. Benefit of using interaction effects for the analysis of high-dimensional time-response or dose-response data for two-group comparisons. *Sci. Rep.* **2023**, *13*, 20804. [CrossRef]
20. Vestal, B.E.; Wynn, E.; Moore, C.M. lmerSeq: An R package for analyzing transformed RNA-Seq data with linear mixed effects models. *BMC Bioinform.* **2022**, *23*, 489. [CrossRef]
21. Laurent, G.S.; Shtokalo, D.; Tackett, M.R.; Yang, Z.; Vyatkin, Y.; Milos, P.M.; Seilheimer, B.; McCaffrey, T.A.; Kapranov, P. On the importance of small changes in RNA expression. *Methods* **2013**, *63*, 18–24. [CrossRef]
22. Costa, A.; van der Stelt, I.; Reynés, B.; Konieczna, J.; Fiol, M.; Keijer, J.; Palou, A.; Romaguera, D.; van Schothorst, E.M.; Oliver, P. Whole-Genome Transcriptomics of PBMC to Identify Biomarkers of Early Metabolic Risk in Apparently Healthy People with Overweight-Obesity and in Normal-Weight Subjects. *Mol. Nutr. Food Res.* **2023**, *67*, 2200503. [CrossRef] [PubMed]
23. Tareen, S.H.K.; Adriaens, M.E.; Arts, I.C.W.; De Kok, T.M.; Vink, R.G.; Roumans, N.J.T.; Van Baak, M.A.; Mariman, E.C.M.; Evelo, C.T.; Kutmon, M. Profiling Cellular Processes in Adipose Tissue During Weight Loss Using Time Series Gene Expression. *Genes* **2018**, *9*, 525. [CrossRef] [PubMed]
24. Solverson, P. Anthocyanin Bioactivity in Obesity and Diabetes: The Essential Role of Glucose Transporters in the Gut and Periphery. *Cells* **2020**, *9*, 2515. [CrossRef] [PubMed]
25. Tareen, S.H.K.; Kutmon, M.; Adriaens, M.E.; Mariman, E.C.M.; De Kok, T.M.; Arts, I.C.W.; Evelo, C.T. Exploring the cellular network of metabolic flexibility in the adipose tissue. *Genes. Nutr.* **2018**, *13*, 17. [CrossRef]
26. Yu, G.; Wang, L.-G.; Han, Y.; He, Q.-Y. clusterProfiler: An R Package for Comparing Biological Themes Among Gene Clusters. *OMICS J. Integr. Biol.* **2012**, *16*, 284–287. [CrossRef]
27. Reynés, B.; Priego, T.; Cifre, M.; Oliver, P.; Palou, A. Peripheral blood cells, a transcriptomic tool in nutrigenomic and obesity studies: Current state of the art. *Compr. Rev. Food Sci. Food Saf.* **2018**, *17*, 1006–1020. [CrossRef]
28. O'Grada, C.M.; Morine, M.J.; Morris, C.; Ryan, M.; Dillon, E.T.; Walsh, M.; Gibney, E.R.; Brennan, L.; Gibney, M.J.; Roche, H.M. PBMCs reflect the immune component of the WAT transcriptome—implications as biomarkers of metabolic health in the postprandial state. *Mol. Nutr. Food Res.* **2014**, *58*, 808–820. [CrossRef]
29. Inami, O.; Tamura, I.; Kikuzaki, H.; Nakatani, N. Stability of anthocyanins of Sambucus canadensis and Sambucus nigra. *J. Agric. Food Chem.* **1996**, *44*, 3090–3096. [CrossRef]
30. Jokioja, J.; Yang, B.; Linderborg, K.M. Acylated anthocyanins: A review on their bioavailability and effects on postprandial carbohydrate metabolism and inflammation. *Compr. Rev. Food Sci. Food Saf.* **2021**, *20*, 5570–5615. [CrossRef]
31. Pascariu, O.-E.; Israel-Roming, F. Bioactive Compounds from Elderberry: Extraction, Health Benefits, and Food Applications. *Processes* **2022**, *10*, 2288. [CrossRef]
32. Lee, J.; Finn, C.E. Anthocyanins and other polyphenolics in American elderberry (*Sambucus canadensis*) and European elderberry (*S. nigra*) cultivars. *J. Sci. Food Agric.* **2007**, *87*, 2665–2675. [CrossRef] [PubMed]
33. Chen, K.; Kortesniemi, M.K.; Linderborg, K.M.; Yang, B. Anthocyanins as Promising Molecules Affecting Energy Homeostasis, Inflammation, and Gut Microbiota in Type 2 Diabetes with Special Reference to Impact of Acylation. *J. Agric. Food Chem.* **2023**, *71*, 1002–1017. [CrossRef] [PubMed]
34. Oliveira, H.; Roma-Rodrigues, C.; Santos, A.; Veigas, B.; Brás, N.; Faria, A.; Calhau, C.; de Freitas, V.; Baptista, P.V.; Mateus, N. GLUT1 and GLUT3 involvement in anthocyanin gastric transport-Nanobased targeted approach. *Sci. Rep.* **2019**, *9*, 789. [CrossRef] [PubMed]
35. Mueckler, M.; Thorens, B. The SLC2 (GLUT) family of membrane transporters. *Mol. Asp. Med.* **2013**, *34*, 121–138. [CrossRef] [PubMed]
36. Hsiao, W.Y.; Guertin, D.A. De Novo Lipogenesis as a Source of Second Messengers in Adipocytes. *Curr. Diab. Rep.* **2019**, *19*, 138. [CrossRef]
37. Jiang, S.; Liu, H.; Li, C. Dietary Regulation of Oxidative Stress in Chronic Metabolic Diseases. *Foods* **2021**, *10*, 1854. [CrossRef]
38. Yang, W.; Jiang, W.; Guo, S. Regulation of macronutrients in insulin resistance and glucose homeostasis during type 2 diabetes mellitus. *Nutrients* **2023**, *15*, 4671. [CrossRef]
39. Randeni, N.; Luo, J.; Xu, B. Critical Review on Anti-Obesity Effects of Anthocyanins Through PI3K/Akt Signaling Pathways. *Nutrients* **2025**, *17*, 1126. [CrossRef]

40. Schurch, N.J.; Schofield, P.; Gierliński, M.; Cole, C.; Sherstnev, A.; Singh, V.; Wrobel, N.; Gharbi, K.; Simpson, G.G.; Owen-Hughes, T. How many biological replicates are needed in an RNA-seq experiment and which differential expression tool should you use? *RNA* **2016**, *22*, 839–851. [CrossRef]
41. Smolders, L.; Mensink, R.P.; Boekschoten, M.V.; De Ridder, R.J.J.; Plat, J. The acute effects on duodenal gene expression in healthy men following consumption of a low-fat meal enriched with theobromine or fat. *Sci. Rep.* **2018**, *8*, 1700. [CrossRef]
42. Sagaya, F.M.; Hurrell, R.F.; Vergères, G. Postprandial blood cell transcriptomics in response to the ingestion of dairy products by healthy individuals. *J. Nutr. Biochem.* **2012**, *23*, 1701–1715. [CrossRef]
43. Davis, R.; Murgia, C.; Dordevic, A.L.; Bonham, M.P.; Huggins, C.E. Diurnal variation in gene expression of human peripheral blood mononuclear cells after eating a standard meal compared with a high protein meal: A cross-over study. *Clin. Nutr.* **2021**, *40*, 4349–4359. [CrossRef]
44. Gui, H.; Sun, L.; Liu, R.; Si, X.; Li, D.; Wang, Y.; Shu, C.; Sun, X.; Jiang, Q.; Qiao, Y.; et al. Current knowledge of anthocyanin metabolism in the digestive tract: Absorption, distribution, degradation, and interconversion. *Crit. Rev. Food Sci. Nutr.* **2023**, *63*, 5953–5966. [CrossRef]

nutrients

Article

Combined Effects of Exercise and Broccoli Supplementation on Metabolic and Lipoprotein Biomarkers in Adults with Type 2 Diabetes: A Randomized Controlled Trial

Maryam Delfan [1,*], Masoumeh Gharedaghi [1], Farzaneh Zeynali [1], Rawad El Hage [2], Anthony C. Hackney [3], Halil İbrahim Ceylan [4], Ayoub Saeidi [5], Ismail Laher [6], Nicola Luigi Bragazzi [7,*,†] and Hassane Zouhal [8,9,*,†]

1 Department of Exercise Physiology, Faculty of Sport Sciences, Alzahra University, Tehran 15847-15414, Iran; gharedaghimasum@gmail.com (M.G.); f.zeynali@alzahra.ac.ir (F.Z.)
2 Department of Physical Education, Division of Education, Faculty of Arts and Sciences, University of Balamand, Tripoli P.O. Box 100, Lebanon
3 Department of Exercise & Sport Science, University of North Carolina, Chapel Hill, NC 27599, USA
4 Department of Physical Education of Sports Teaching, Faculty of Sports Sciences, Atatürk University, 25240 Erzurum, Türkiye; halil.ceylan@atauni.edu.tr
5 Department of Physical Education and Sport Sciences, Faculty of Humanities and Social Sciences, University of Kurdistan, Sanandaj 66177-15175, Iran
6 Department of Anesthesiology, Pharmacology, and Therapeutics, Faculty of Medicine, University of British Columbia, Vancouver, BC V6T 1Z3, Canada
7 Laboratory for Industrial and Applied Mathematics (LIAM), Department of Mathematics and Statistics, York University, Toronto, ON M3J 1P3, Canada
8 International Institute of Sport Sciences (2I2S), 35850 Irodouer, France
9 Laboratoire Optimisation de la Performance Sportive (LR09SEP01) Centre National de la Médecine et des Sciences des Sports, Tunis 1004, Tunisia
* Correspondence: m.delfan@alzahra.ac.ir (M.D.); robertobragazzi@gmail.com (N.L.B.); hassane.zouhal@gmail.com (H.Z.)
† These authors contributed equally to this work.

Abstract: Aim: To investigate the synergistic effects of exercise training and *Brassica oleracea* var. italica (broccoli sprout) supplementation on Apolipoprotein A-I, B-100, and J levels in men with Type 2 diabetes mellitus (T2DM). **Methods:** Forty-four males with T2DM were randomly assigned to four groups: Control (CG), Supplement (SG), Training (TG), and Training + Supplement (TSG) groups. Participants in the supplement groups (SG and TSG) received 10 g of broccoli supplement after meals for 12 weeks, while those in the training groups (TG and TSG) participated in a structured exercise program (resistance and aerobic), performed three times per week for 12 weeks, at intensities of 60–70% one-repetition maximum (1RM) for resistance training and 60–70% peak oxygen uptake (VO_{2peak}) for aerobic training. **Results:** Circulating levels of apolipoproteins improved after 12 weeks in the TSG, TG, and SG groups. However, the TSG group exhibited the most pronounced improvements across metabolic and lipoprotein markers, reflecting an additive effect of both interventions. Specifically, the TSG group demonstrated absolute reductions in ApoB-100 (−48.30 ± 7.20 mg/dL) and ApoJ (−44.05 ± 5.76 mg/dL), along with an increase in ApoA-I (+44.92 ± 6.05 mg/dL). Main effect analysis revealed that exercise training elicited the most substantial improvements across metabolic and lipoprotein markers, with large effect sizes for glucose (η^2p = 0.787), insulin (η^2p = 0.640), HOMA-IR (η^2p = 0.856), ApoA-I (η^2p = 0.685), ApoB-100 (η^2p = 0.774), ApoJ (η^2p = 0.848), and HDL-C (η^2p = 0.535). Supplementation showed moderate effects, particularly on HOMA-IR (η^2p = 0.370), ApoA-I (η^2p = 0.383), and ApoB-100 (η^2p = 0.334), supporting an additive but exercise-dominant benefit. The combined intervention group (TSG) showed the most pronounced improvements across all measured outcomes, with large effect sizes for ApoA-I (η^2p = 0.883), glucose (η^2p = 0.946), insulin (η^2p = 0.881), HOMA-IR (η^2p = 0.904), and ApoJ

(η^2p = 0.852). **Conclusions:** The effects of combining training and broccoli sprout supplementation on apolipoprotein levels are likely to result from the activation of two separate pathways, one from training and the other from supplementation. This dual-modality intervention could serve as an effective complementary strategy in managing metabolic and cardiovascular risk factors for individuals with T2DM. However, the magnitude of change induced by the combination of exercise training and broccoli supplementation was largely driven by the training component, with supplementation providing complementary but less consistent benefits.

Keywords: concurrent training; broccoli supplementation; apolipoproteins; diabetes mellitus

1. Introduction

Type 2 diabetes mellitus (T2DM) is a commonly diagnosed metabolic disease associated with high mortality worldwide [1,2]. Insulin resistance (IR), a hallmark of T2DM, is responsible for hyperglycemia, hyperinsulinemia, oxidative stress, and dyslipidemia [1]. These metabolic disturbances have detrimental effects on the lipid profile in patients with T2DM. Lipoprotein abnormalities, such as high levels of low-density lipoprotein cholesterol (LDL-C) and triglycerides and low levels of high-density lipoprotein cholesterol (HDL-C) contribute to the progression of cardiovascular disease (CVD) [2,3]. Emerging evidence suggests that measuring circulating apolipoproteins may offer greater predictive value than traditional lipid parameters in assessing the risk of T2DM, thereby providing novel insights not only into disease pathophysiology but also into potential pharmacological targets for the development of more precise, mechanism-based therapies and interventions [2].

Apolipoproteins are a class of proteins that play crucial roles in the structure, function, metabolism, and regulation of lipoproteins [4]. Among the various apolipoproteins, Apolipoprotein A (ApoA-I), Apolipoprotein B100 (ApoB-100), and Apolipoprotein J (ApoJ) have been extensively studied due to their association with cardiovascular health [5]. ApoA-I is the most abundant protein component of HDL and plays a role in glucose uptake by the skeletal muscle and heart [6]. Reduced plasma levels of ApoA-I in T2DM may be due to decreased responsiveness of the ApoA-I gene to insulin or the reduction in plasma HDL levels [7]. ApoB-100 is a significant structural component of atherogenic lipoproteins, such as LDL, very-low-density lipoproteins (VLDL), and intermediate-density lipoproteins (IDL) [8]. Increased levels of ApoB-100 are associated with the development of atherosclerosis plaques [9]. Another important apolipoprotein is ApoJ, also known as clusterin [10]. It interacts with specific receptors, including the HDL-C receptor, LDL-related protein 2 (LRP2), ApoE receptor 2 (ApoER2), and the VLDL receptor (VLDLR). ApoJ is involved in the pathophysiology of several metabolic conditions, including obesity, T2DM, and CVD [5,10]. Increased circulating levels of ApoJ have been reported in individuals with T2DM, obesity, and systemic inflammation—conditions commonly characterized by insulin resistance [11].

Non-pharmacological strategies for managing T2DM emphasize lifestyle interventions, such as a healthy diet and regular physical activity [12,13]. Herbal supplements also have a role in the management of T2DM [14]. Broccoli and broccoli sprouts contain bioactive compounds, including antioxidant vitamins, minerals such as selenium, phenolic compounds, and glucosinolates like indole-3-carbinol [15]. A four-week intake of broccoli (10 g/d) reduces serum insulin levels and improves the homeostatic model assessment for insulin resistance (HOMA-IR) in individuals with T2DM [16]. Sulforaphane (SFN), another key compound in broccoli, reduces lipid peroxidation, enhances total antioxidant capacity, and decreases oxidative stress in individuals with T2DM by activating antioxidant pathways [17]. Furthermore, SFN improves muscle strength, function, and exercise capacity while protecting muscles from oxidative damage and inflammation [18]. Additionally, broccoli supplementation has been shown to reduce exercise-induced muscle soreness and lower oxidative stress indicators in individuals with T2DM [19].

Aerobic exercise improves peak oxygen uptake (VO_{2peak}), IR, glycated hemoglobin (HbA1c), and triglyceride levels [20]. Resistance exercise decreases fat mass and blood pressure, increases muscle strength, promotes muscle rehabilitation, and enhances glucose transporter type 4 (GLUT-4) expression in individuals with T2DM and obesity [21,22]. Combining aerobic and resistance exercises may have a synergistic effect on T2DM and obesity [22,23]. It can increase HDL-C levels and decrease plasma ApoJ levels by reducing body weight, total fat mass, and improving skeletal muscle mass in individuals with T2DM [24].

In short, exercise can improve various health parameters in patients with T2DM [25]. Additionally, studies indicate that taking dietary supplements can have a positive impact on overall physical health [17,26]. However, only a few studies have examined the effect of combining exercise and nutritional supplements on patients with T2DM [27]. Some studies suggest that combining dietary supplements with regular exercise could help maximize their synergistic effects [27]. Nonetheless, there is insufficient research to demonstrate how the combination of exercise and dietary supplements affects T2DM. While previous studies have independently examined the effects of broccoli supplementation and combined training on apolipoproteins [17,24], the synergistic effects of these two interventions remain unclear. For example, in postmenopausal women with T2DM, twelve weeks of combined aerobic and resistance training significantly reduced circulating levels of ApoJ and improved indices of IR [27]. Separately, a previous review study reported that broccoli sprout supplementation (rich in SFN) decreased oxidative stress, lipid peroxidation, serum triglycerides, IR, and inflammatory markers in patients with T2DM [17]. Therefore, the main objective of this study was to investigate the combined effects of broccoli sprout supplementation and exercise training on circulating levels of ApoA-I, ApoB-100, and ApoJ in men with T2DM. A secondary objective was to assess the impact of the intervention on glycemic markers, such as fasting blood glucose (FBG) and HOMA-IR, to explore potential metabolic interactions beyond lipid-related outcomes. Due to limited access to eligible female participants and to minimize sex-related biological variability in metabolic and hormonal responses, the present study was conducted solely on males.

2. Methods

2.1. Participants

A total of 80 individuals volunteered to participate in the study following extensive recruitment efforts conducted across public spaces, research laboratories, sports clubs, and social media platforms. Of these, 20 individuals were excluded for not meeting the established inclusion criteria (Figure 1). All participants underwent medical screening by a certified cardiologist to confirm their health status and suitability for participation.

This study was a 12-week randomized controlled trial involving four intervention groups. Participants were assigned to one of the four groups using simple randomization. The randomization sequence was generated using SPSS version 26. To ensure allocation concealment, group assignments were performed by an independent researcher who was not involved in delivering the intervention or assessing outcomes.

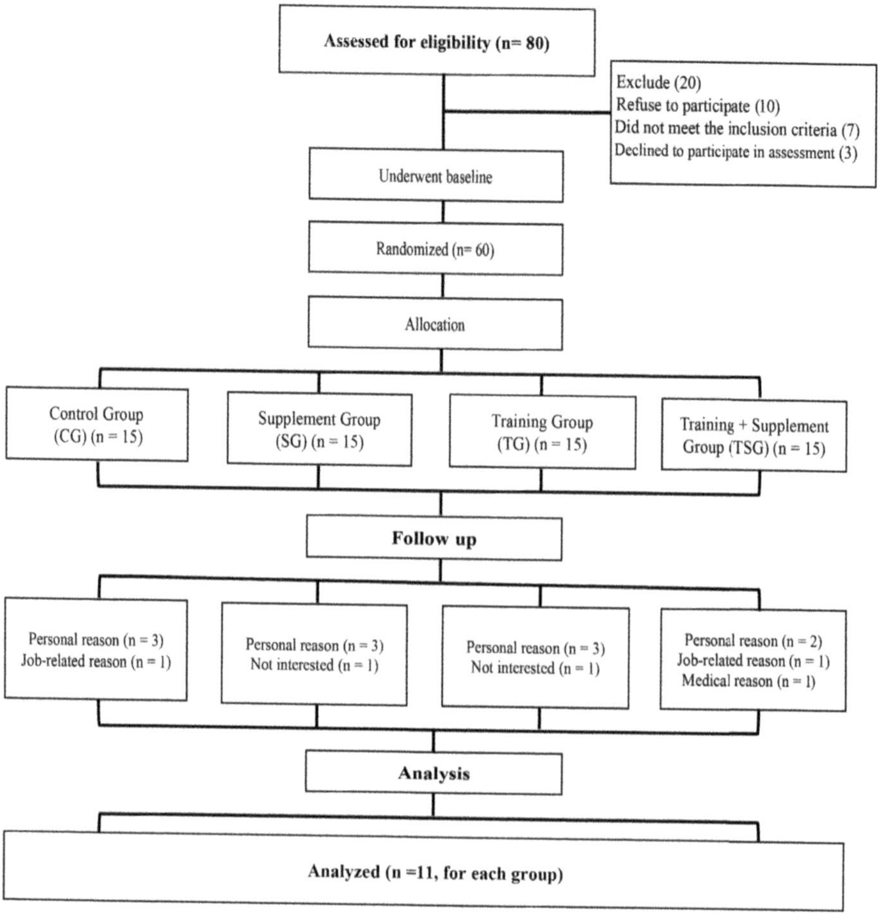

Figure 1. Pictorial flowchart of the experimental design of the present study.

The study protocol was reviewed and approved by the Ethics Committee of the Sport Sciences Research Institute, Tehran, Iran (Ethics code: IR.SSRC.REC.1401.142), and all procedures were conducted in accordance with the most recent version of the Declaration of Helsinki [28].

Inclusion criteria: Participants had to be males between the ages of 40 and 60, diagnosed with T2DM according to the American Diabetes Association guidelines, have had T2DM for more than two years, have FBG levels of 126 mg/dL or higher, and be receiving oral hypoglycemic medications.

Exclusion criteria: Participants with cardiac pathologies, hypertension (defined as blood pressure exceeding 160/90 mmHg), musculoskeletal diseases, proliferative diabetic retinopathy, advanced nephropathy, FBG levels exceeding 270 mg/dL, those receiving insulin injections, and individuals taking lipid- and blood-pressure-lowering medications were excluded from the study. This exclusion criterion was implemented to minimize the confounding effects of pharmacological interventions and to ensure that any observed changes could be attributed to the study intervention. All participants were under regular medical supervision, and those requiring statin or antihypertensive therapy according to clinical guidelines were excluded from participation due to ethical considerations.

2.2. Experimental Design

2.2.1. Baseline Evaluations

All participants attended a familiarization session one week before the initiation of the training protocols. During this session, the study procedures were clearly explained, and participants completed the Physical Activity Readiness Questionnaire (PAR-Q). In addition, each participant's height and weight were measured to calculate their body mass index (BMI).

2.2.2. Study Design

Following the baseline evaluations, the 60 eligible participants were randomly allocated to four study groups of 15 individuals each: the Control Group (CG), the Supplement Group (SG), the Training Group (TG), and the Training + Supplement Group (TSG).

Participants in the intervention groups were closely monitored for adherence. Following the American College of Sports Medicine's guideline of at least 80% adherence as adequate participation in exercise programs [29], individuals who missed more than seven of the 36 training sessions were excluded from the analysis. Supplement adherence was defined as consuming at least 80% of the assigned doses. Therefore, the adherence rate among the remaining participants in the TG, SG, and TSG groups was considered to be 100%.

Furthermore, during the course of the protocol, several participants were excluded from the study due to either personal reasons—such as voluntary withdrawal, scheduling conflicts, or difficulty complying with study instructions—or medical reasons, including previously undisclosed conditions or newly arising health issues. These exclusions were made to protect participant safety and to ensure the validity and consistency of the data collected.

During the third session, each group received comprehensive instructions on how to perform their respective training protocols. Following baseline measurements, both training groups (TG and TSG) commenced a structured 12-week exercise program. During the study, participants were asked to carefully record their food intake over three consecutive days, including two weekdays and one weekend day. These records calculated total daily caloric intake (in kilocalories) and the amounts of carbohydrates, fats, and proteins (in grams). Dietary data were analyzed using Diet Analysis Plus software, version 10 (Cengage, Boston, MA, USA) (Table 1). Those assigned to the control and supplement groups were advised to continue their daily routines throughout the study. All measurements were taken roughly at the same time each day (with a deviation of about 1 h) and under consistent environmental conditions (approximately 20 °C and ~55% humidity).

Table 1. Mean ± SD values of nutritional intake in the four study groups.

Groups	Energy (kcal/d)	CHO (g/d)	Fat (g/d)	Protein (g/d)
CG	2383.1 ± 106.6	305.1 ± 36.1	77.0 ± 15.7	117.3 ± 17
SG	2385.6 ± 157.0	304.6 ± 34.8	76.9 ± 14.2	118.7 ± 19.2
TG	2340.3 ± 213.4	291.6 ± 29.5	76.9 ± 14.5	117.0 ± 18.9
TSG	2358.0 ± 193.2	295.5 ± 32.4	79.1 ± 14.6	116.3 ± 17.8

CG: Control Group, SG: Supplement Group, TG: Training Group, TSG: Training + Supplement Group, CHO: Carbohydrate.

2.2.3. Peak Oxygen Uptake, Blood Pressure, Heart Rates, and One-Repetition Maximum Assessments

A modified Bruce protocol using a motorized treadmill (Pulsar 3p, H/p/Cosmos, Nussdorf-Traunstein, Germany) with a gas analyzer system (Metalyzer 3B Analyzer, Cortex Biophysik, Leipzig, Germany) was used to estimate VO_{2peak} [30]. Systolic and diastolic blood pressure measurements were obtained using an automated device (Omron M6 Comfort HEM-7221-E, Omron Healthcare, Kyoto, Japan). Simultaneously, heart rate (HR, beats per minute) was continuously measured using a heart rate monitoring device (Polar Electro, Espoo, Finland). The intensity of aerobic exercise was determined based on the individual's VO_{2peak}. A 1-repetition maximum (1-RM) method was used to assess muscle strength for all strength exercises; the 1-RM measurement occurred during the final familiarization session. Patients engaged in a 5-min warm-up before the exercises to prevent injuries, and they were instructed to lift the maximum amount of weight they could manage for 6–8 repetitions for each exercise. Subsequently, the 1-RM value was calculated using the Brzycki formula [31].

2.2.4. Training Protocols

The exercise training sessions for patients with T2DM (TG and TSG groups) were closely supervised by exercise physiologists and endocrinologists, ensuring professional oversight. These sessions consisted of both aerobic and resistance exercises, meticulously planned in terms of volume and intensity for patients with T2DM [32]. Each session began with a 5- to 10-min warm-up period, which included walking and running on a treadmill at 50–60% of the participants' maximum heart rate (HR_{max}), followed by 45 min of resistance training that involved nine specific movements targeting both the upper and lower body. These movements included the leg press, knee flexion, knee extension, chest press, lat pull-down, abdominal crunches, biceps curls, triceps press down, and shoulder press. The resistance exercises were performed at 60–70% of the patients' 1-RM. In addition to resistance training, aerobic exercises were incorporated, lasting 30 min and maintained at 60–70% of the patients' VO_{2peak}. These aerobic sessions were conducted on a motorized treadmill (Pulsar 3p, H/p/Cosmos, Nussdorf-Traunstein, Germany). The duration of aerobic exercise gradually increased from 10 min in the first week to 30 min by the eighth week and remained at this level throughout the study (Table 2). The 1-RM and VO_{2peak} tests were repeated every four weeks to adhere to the principle of overloading.

Table 2. Combined training protocols (aerobic + resistance exercise) for TG and TSG groups over 12 weeks.

	Aerobic Training			Resistance Training			
Weeks	**Durations (Min/Sessions)**	**Intensity (VO_{2peak})**	**Sessions (per Week)**	**Sets**	**Repetition**	**1-RM**	**Sessions (per Week)**
1–2	10	60%	3	3	12–15	60–68%	3
2–4	15	65%	3	3	12–15	60–65%	3
4–6	20	70%	3	3	8–10	70%	3
6–8	25	70%	3	3	8–10	70%	3
8–12	30	70%	3	3	8–10	70%	3

Notes: 1-RM, one-repetition maximum.

2.2.5. Supplementation of Broccoli Sprout and Placebo

Neither the participants nor the researchers were aware of the supplement assignments. This study used a broccoli sprout powder supplement (Cyvex Nutrition Company, Irvine, CA, USA). The dosage of SFN administered was 225 μmol per 10 g/d of the broccoli sprout powder supplement. The SG and TSG group participants were instructed to consume one packet of the broccoli sprout supplement (10 g) daily for 12 weeks [33,34]. Comparable amounts of placebo were also provided for both the CG and TG. The placebo was formulated using a mixture of 5 g of cornstarch powder and spinach powder (in a 10:1 ratio) and prepared to resemble the appearance of the broccoli sprout supplement. Supplement adherence was defined as participants consuming at least 80% of their assigned doses (i.e., 67 packets).

2.2.6. Biochemical Analysis

All testing was conducted under standard conditions between 8 a.m. and 10 a.m. Blood samples were taken (after 12 h of fasting) from the right arm 48 h before the first exercise session and 48 h after the last session. Blood samples were collected in EDTA tubes for plasma isolation, centrifuged at 3500 rpm for 15 min, and stored at −80 °C. Glucose assay kits measured glucose levels with a sensitivity of 1 mg/dL. Insulin levels were assessed using a radioimmunoassay kit (Diagnostic Systems Laboratories, Webster, TX, USA). The HOMA-IR was used to estimate the insulin resistance index, using the following formula: fasting plasma glucose (mmol/L) × fasting plasma insulin (μU/mL)/22.5 [35]. Plasma triglycerides, LDL-C, HDL-C, and total cholesterol (TC) levels were measured using a standard biochemical analyzer (DAX 96; Bayern Diagnostics, Milan, Italy). The plasma concentrations of ApoA-I, ApoB-100, and ApoJ were assessed with ELISA kits (Zellbio, Lonsee, Germany). The coefficients of variation were 1.2% for glucose, 1.8% for insulin, 2.9% for HOMA-IR, and less than 5% for HDL-C, LDL-C, TC, and triglycerides.

2.2.7. Statistical Analysis

A power analysis was conducted using the software G*Power Version 3.1.9.6 (Kiel, Germany) to calculate the sample size. The input parameters were an alpha level of 0.05 and 95% statistical power. The study by Delfan et al. [36] was used as a reference, as it employed a similar study design. From this study, we extracted the effect size measure, Cohen's f = 0.88, for the outcome insulin and included it in our a priori power analysis. The results of the power analysis indicated that a total of 12 participants per group would be needed to achieve significant group-by-time interactions. To account for potential dropouts, 15 participants were initially recruited in each group. Statistical analysis was performed using GraphPad Prism software version 8.4.0 (GraphPad Software, Boston, MA, USA). The data were initially assessed for their distribution using the Kolmogorov–Smirnov test, and the results were analyzed with three-way ANOVA with repeated measures (2 × 2 × 2; supplementation [broccoli vs. placebo] × training [yes vs. no] × time [baseline vs. end]). The partial eta squared for main effects was calculated from the ANOVA ($\eta^2 p$) and was interpreted as follows: 0.01 = small effect, 0.06 = medium effect, and 0.14 = large effect [37]. When a significant interaction was found, the Bonferroni post hoc test was performed to determine differences between groups [SG, TG, TSG, and CG]. Data are shown as mean ± SD; $p < 0.050$ was considered statistically significant.

3. Results

3.1. Anthropometry

A total of 16 participants (n = 4 per group) withdrew from the study due to medical issues, work-related constraints, or a lack of sustained interest, resulting in 44 participants remaining in the study (n = 11 per group) for the final analysis. The groups were comparable in terms of age, ethnicity, duration of diabetes, and medication use. There were no differences ($p > 0.050$) in body mass and BMI between the study groups at the beginning of the study (Table 3). Weight reductions were evident in both training groups compared to the pre-test measurements ($p < 0.0007$). Additionally, BMI alterations were observed from baseline to 12 weeks in both the TG and TSG groups; however, significance was evident only in the TSG group ($p = 0.021$).

Table 3. Body mass and BMI of the study groups.

	CG			SG			TG			TSG		
	Pre-Test	**Post-Test**	p	**Pre-Test**	**Post-Test**	p	**Pre-Test**	**Post-Test**	p	**Pre-Test**	**Post-Test**	p
Body mass (kg)	86.35 ± 3.34	86.74 ± 2.99	0.789	85.09 ± 4.93	85.89 ± 3.47	0.628	86.96 ± 4.39	79.69 ± 3.31	0.0007 *	86.67 ± 4.46	79.10 ± 4.86	0.0007 *
BMI (kg/m^2)	28.34 ± 0.96	28.46 ± 0.96	0.777	27.39 ± 1.26	27.44 ± 1.58	0.947	28.51 ± 1.73	27.34 ± 1.41	0.065	28.07 ± 1.12	26.18 ± 1.83	0.021 *

Notes: BMI: Body Mass Index, CG: Control Group, SG: Supplement Group, TG: Training Group, TSG: Training + Supplement Group, * $p < 0.05$.

3.2. *Glucose, Insulin, and HOMA-IR*

There was a main effect of training ($p < 0.001$, η^2p: 0.787) and time ($p < 0.001$, η^2p: 0.946) on blood glucose concentration, while the main effect of supplementation did not reach statistical significance for this variable ($p = 0.075$, η^2p: 0.283). The post hoc analysis revealed that despite comparable values before the interventions across all four groups, only the SG, TG, and TSG reduced blood glucose concentrations after the intervention (all $p < 0.050$, Figure 2A). At the end of the interventions, blood glucose concentration in the CG were higher than in the TG and TSG ($d = 0.96$, $p < 0.01$ and $d = 1.19$, $p < 0.01$, respectively) and those in the SG were also higher than in the TG and TSG ($d = 0.93$, $p < 0.01$ and $d = 1.16$, $p < 0.01$, respectively). However, there were no differences in blood glucose concentration between the TG and TSG at the end of the interventions ($d = 0.87$, $p = 0.065$).

There was a main effect of training ($p = 0.002$, η^2p: 0.640) and time ($p < 0.001$, η^2p: 0.881) on insulin concentration, while the main effect of supplementation did not reach statistical significance for this variable ($p = 0.051$, η^2p: 0.330). The post hoc analysis revealed that despite comparable values before the interventions across all four groups, only the SG, TG, and TSG reduced insulin concentrations after the intervention (all $p < 0.050$, Figure 2B). At the end of the interventions, insulin concentration in the CG was higher than in the SG, TG, and TSG ($d = 2.92$, $p < 0.01$, $d = 3.95$, $p < 0.01$, and $d = 3.71$, $p < 0.01$, respectively) and in the SG it was higher than in the TSG ($d = 2.75$, $p < 0.01$), without differences between the TG and TSG ($d = 0.96$, $p = 0.252$).

There was a main effect of supplementation ($p = 0.036$, η^2p: 0.370), training ($p < 0.001$, η^2p: 0.856), and time ($p < 0.001$, η^2p: 0.904) onHOMA-IR. The post hoc analysis revealed that despite comparable HOMA-IR values before the interventions across all four groups, only the SG, TG, and TSG reduced HOMA-IR after the intervention (all $p < 0.050$, Figure 2C). At the end of the interventions, HOMA-IR in the CG was higher than in the SG, TG, and TSG ($d = 1.36$, $p < 0.05$, $d = 1.41$, $p < 0.01$ and $d = 1.36$, $p < 0.01$, respectively) and in the SG it was higher than in the TG ($d = 0.65$, $p < 0.05$) and in the TSG ($d = 1.03$, $p < 0.01$), without differences between the TG and TSG ($d = 0.71$, $p = 0.084$).

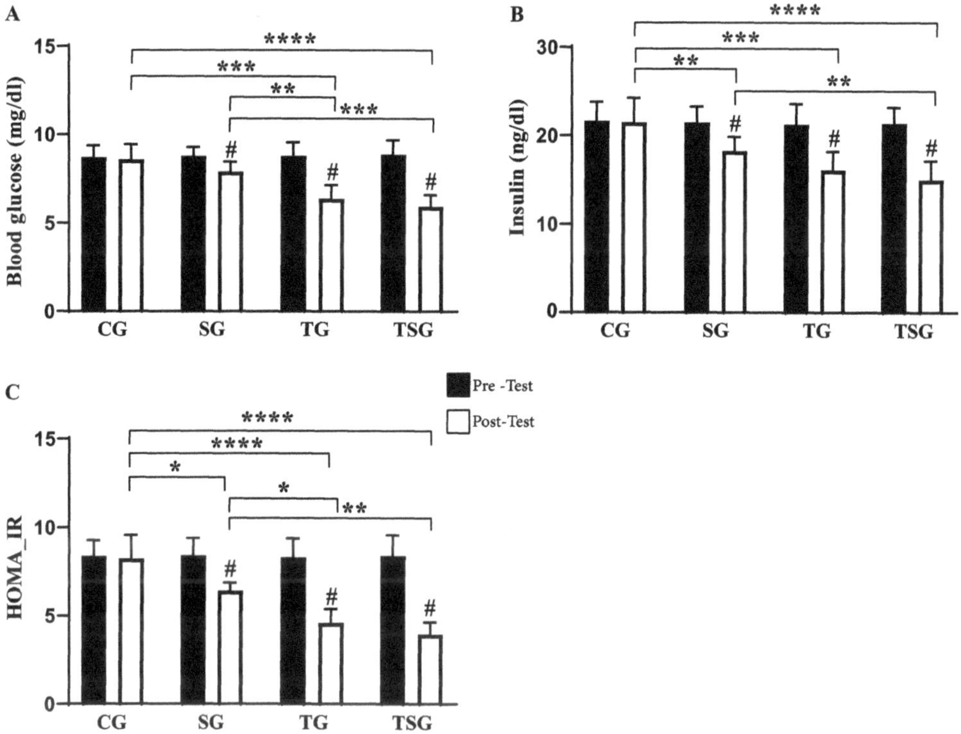

Figure 2. Pre-test and post-test intervention values of (**A**) fasting glucose, (**B**) insulin, and (**C**) HOMA-IR in CG: Control Group, SG: Supplement Group, TG: Training Group, TSG: Training + Supplement Group. # indicates a significant difference from baseline. * Significant differences: * $p < 0.05$, ** $p < 0.01$, *** $p < 0.001$, **** $p < 0.0001$.

3.3. Lipid Profile

There was a main effect of time ($p < 0.001$, η^2p: 0.929) on TG concentration with no effect of training ($p = 0.661$, η^2p: 0.020) or supplementation for this variable ($p = 0.694$, η^2p: 0.016). The post hoc analysis revealed that TG values before the interventions were similar across all four groups, but only the SG, TG, and TSG reduced TG after the intervention (all $p < 0.050$, Figure 3A). However, post-intervention values of TG were similar across all four groups.

There was a main effect of supplementation ($p = 0.039$, η^2p: 0.360) and time ($p < 0.001$, η^2p: 0.826) on TC concentration, while the main effect training did not reach statistical significance for this variable ($p = 0.179$, η^2p: 0.173). The post hoc analysis revealed that TG values before the interventions were similar across all four groups but only the SG, TG, and TSG reduced TC after the intervention (all $p < 0.050$, Figure 3B). At the end of the interventions, TG in the CG was higher than in the SG ($d = 1.95$, $p < 0.01$), TG ($d = 2.01$, $p < 0.01$), and TSG ($d = 2.31$, $p < 0.01$).

There was a main effect of time ($p < 0.001$, η^2p: 0.945) on LDL-C concentration with no effect of training ($p = 0.183$, η^2p: 0.170) or supplementation for this variable ($p = 0.256$, η^2p: 0.127). The post hoc analysis revealed that LDL-C values before the interventions were similar across all four groups but only the SG, TG, and TSG reduced LDL-C after the intervention (all $p < 0.050$, Figure 3C). At the end of the interventions, LDL-C in the CG was higher than in the TG ($d = 1.56$, $p < 0.05$) and TSG ($d = 2.12$, $p < 0.01$).

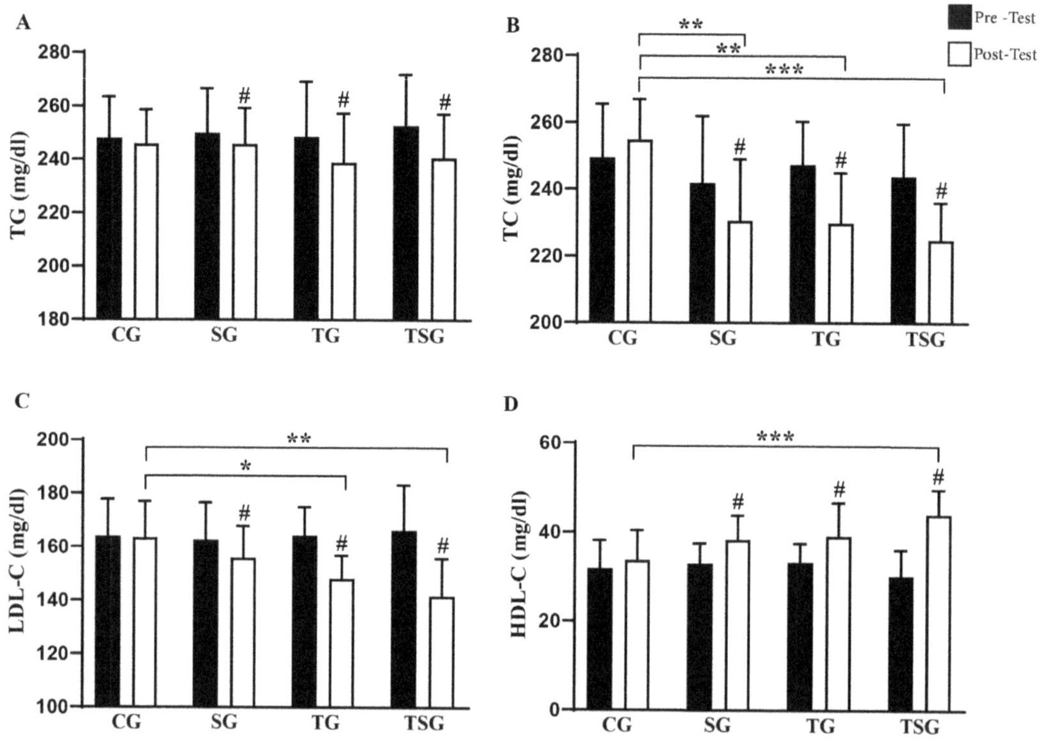

Figure 3. Pre-test and post-test values for lipid profile. (**A**) TG: Triglycerides. (**B**) TC: Total Cholesterol (**C**) LDL-C: Low-Density Lipoprotein Cholesterol and (**D**) HDL-C: high-density lipoprotein cholesterol in CG: Control Group, SG: Supplement Group, TG: Training Group, TSG: Training + Supplement Group. # indicates a significant difference from baseline. Significant differences: * $p < 0.05$, ** $p < 0.01$, *** $p < 0.001$.

There was a main effect of training ($p = 0.007$, η^2p: 0.535) and time ($p < 0.001$, η^2p: 0.939) on HDL-C concentration, while the main effect of supplementation did not reach statistical significance for this variable ($p = 0.338$, η^2p: 0.092). The post hoc analysis revealed that HCL-C values before the interventions were similar across all four groups but only the SG, TG, and TSG increased HDL-C after the intervention (all $p < 0.050$, Figure 3D). At the end of the interventions, HDL-C in the CG was only lower than in the TSG ($d = 8.76$, $p < 0.01$).

3.4. ApoA-I, ApoB-100, and ApoJ

There was a main effect of supplementation ($p < 0.032$, η^2p: 0.383), training ($p < 0.001$, η^2p: 0.685), and time ($p < 0.001$, η^2p: 0.883) on ApoA-I concentration. The post hoc analysis revealed that despite comparable values before the interventions across all four groups, only the SG, TG, and TSG increased ApoA-I concentrations after the intervention (all $p < 0.050$, Figure 4A). At the end of the interventions, ApoA-I in the CG were than lower in the SG ($d = 1.67$, $p < 0.01$), TG ($d = 2.45$, $p < 0.01$), and TSG ($d = 1.48$, $p < 0.01$), without differences among these three groups.

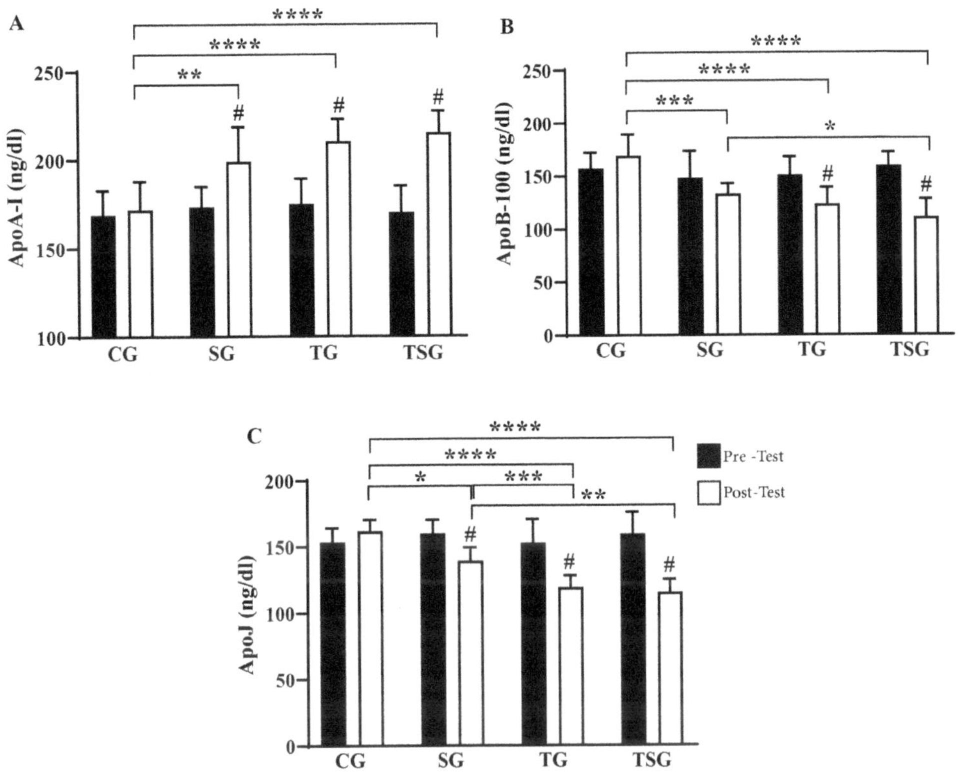

Figure 4. Pre-test and post-test values (mean ± SD) for (**A**) ApoA-I, (**B**) ApoB-100, and (**C**) ApoJ in CG: Control Group, SG: Supplement Group, TG: Training Group, TSG: Training + Supplement Group. # indicates a significant difference from baseline. * Significant differences: * $p < 0.05$, ** $p < 0.01$, *** $p < 0.001$, **** $p < 0.0001$.

There was a main effect of supplementation ($p < 0.049$, η^2p: 0.334), training ($p < 0.001$, η^2p: 0.774), and time ($p < 0.001$, η^2p: 0.684) on ApoB-100 concentration. The post hoc analysis revealed that despite comparable values before the interventions across all four groups, only the TG and TSG reduced ApoB-100 concentrations after the intervention (all $p < 0.050$, Figure 4B). At the end of the interventions, ApoB-100 in the CG were higher than in the SG ($d = 1.80$, $p < 0.01$), TG ($d = 1.68$, $p < 0.01$), and TSG ($d = 2.57$, $p < 0.01$). Additionally, ApoB-100 concentrations in the SG were higher than in the TSG ($d = 1.75$, $p = 0.02$).

There was a main effect of training ($p < 0.001$, η^2p: 0.848) and time ($p < 0.001$, η^2p: 0.852) on ApoJ concentration, while the effect of supplementation did not reach statistical significance ($p = 0.103$, η^2p: 0.244) The post hoc analysis revealed that despite comparable values before the interventions across all four groups, only the SG, TG, and TSG reduced ApoJ concentrations after the intervention (all $p < 0.050$, Figure 4C). At the end of the interventions, ApoJ concentrations in the CG were higher than in the SG ($d = 0.85$, $p < 0.05$), TG ($d = 1.34$, $p < 0.01$) and TSG ($d = 2.51$, $p < 0.01$). Additionally, ApoJ concentrations in the SG were higher than in the TG ($d = 1.68$, $p = 0.03$) and TSG ($d = 1.75$, $p < 0.01$).

4. Discussion

Our study demonstrated that a 12-week intervention combining exercise training and broccoli sprout supplementation elicited significant improvements in key metabolic and lipoprotein biomarkers in men with T2DM. Notably, the three-way ANOVA revealed robust main effects of training across nearly all variables, including glucose, insulin, HOMA-IR, ApoA-I, ApoB-100, ApoJ, and HDL-C, with large effect sizes (η^2p ranging from 0.535 to 0.856). Broccoli sprout supplementation also contributed to improvements, particularly in HOMA-IR, TC, ApoA-I, and ApoB-100, though its effects were generally more modest. The combined intervention group (TSG) consistently showed the greatest magnitude of change, suggesting additive benefits in some variables. However, the marginal differences between the TSG and TG groups imply that the majority of the observed benefits may be attributed to the training component. These findings underscore the dominant role of structured exercise training in modulating metabolic health in T2DM, while also highlighting the complementary value of broccoli sprout supplementation.

Circulating levels of ApoA-I increased in the SG, TG, and TSG compared to the CG, with the most significant increases observed in the TG and TSG. This aligns with previous findings that combined exercise training increased ApoA-I levels [38]. Although we did not directly measure the underlying molecular mediators, we hypothesize that this change in ApoA-I levels could result from combined training elevating ATP-binding cassette transport (ABC) proteins, including the A group (ABCA) and ABC group (ABCG), which can increase *ApoA* gene expression [39]. Another study reported that a 17-week diet supplemented with 10% (w/w) broccoli florets or broccoli stalks in male mice (7–8 weeks old) increased the levels of peroxisome proliferator-activated receptor α (PPARα) and adenosine monophosphate-activated protein kinase (AMPK) [40]. While we did not assess PPARα or AMPK activation in our study, their involvement is proposed as a possible mechanism for the observed changes and warrants investigation in future research. PPARα activation has been reported to increase liver *ApoA-I* mRNA levels [41]. The regulatory function of PPARα on gene expression of HDL apolipoproteins may have important clinical implications [41]. Higher ApoA-I levels are inversely associated with cardiovascular risk, indicating a protective effect, particularly in individuals with T2DM. From a clinical perspective, the increase in ApoA-I levels observed in our study approaches the upper reference range for men (above 120 mg/dL), a threshold associated with enhanced reverse cholesterol transport and reduced cardiovascular risk. This suggests that the elevation in ApoA-I may be clinically beneficial, especially for participants with low baseline levels [42].

Circulating levels of ApoB-100 decreased in the SG, TG, and TSG compared to the CG, with decreases in the TSG being statistically significant compared to the SG. A study investigating the secretion of ApoB-100 from HepG2 cells treated with indole-3-carbinol reported that it could inhibit the secretion of ApoB-100. This improvement may be explained by the finding that it suppresses the protein expression of sterol regulatory element-binding protein (SREBP)-1. A reduction in lipid synthesis caused by indole-3-carbinol could potentially decrease the amount of lipid substrates required for ApoB-100 assembly [15]. Research has shown that 24 weeks of combined training (aerobic and resistance training) decreased plasma ApoB-100 concentrations in middle-aged obese women, indicating the positive effects of these training methods in preventing CVD [38]. This finding may be related to increased insulin sensitivity, as findings suggest that combined training (aerobic and resistance training) increased IRS-1 expression by 90% [22]. The increase in IRS-1 expression leads to improved insulin signaling through the MAPK (mitogen-activated protein kinase) activation pathway, and a reduction in MTTP (microsomal triglyceride transfer protein) expression, which inhibits the release of ApoB-100 [43]. MTTP, as a transporter of triglycerides, transfers triglycerides, phospholipids, and cholesterol to ApoB-100 in lipidation. ApoB-100 would be degraded if not subjected to lipidation. Therefore, insulin likely degrades ApoB-100 through the action of MTTP [44]. Clinically, ApoB-100 is a well-established marker of the atherogenic particle number, and its reduction is considered a strong predictor of decreased cardiovascular risk. The observed decrease in ApoB-100 levels is clinically significant compared to reference values [45].

We also found reduced ApoJ levels in the TG and TSG compared to the SG and CG. An increase in adipocyte-derived ApoJ in the circulation is a marker of IR [5]. A recent study reported that consuming broccoli florets or broccoli stalks increased AMPK and PPARα levels in mice [40]. PPARα levels are associated with increases in LRP2 expression, which belongs to the low-density lipoprotein receptor (LDLR) protein family. Furthermore, PPARα agonists induce significant increases in *LRP2* mRNA and protein expression. LRP2 is an endocytic cell surface receptor that belongs to the LDL receptor family [46] and, as a potential receptor for ApoJ, plays a crucial role in patients with T2DM. As a result, if muscle LRP2 is increased, ApoJ levels decrease in the serum [47]. However, since we did not assess AMPK, PPARα, or LRP2 levels, these findings remain speculative and should be interpreted as hypotheses for future research. Additionally, adipocytes are increasingly recognized as essential sites for the secretion of ApoJ. Combined training decreases intra-abdominal fat and ApoJ levels more effectively than food restriction [38]. Our findings in obese males support previous findings that decreases in circulating ApoJ levels induced by exercise are associated with improvements in IR in T2DM [24]. A prior study demonstrated that ApoJ impairs insulin signaling by decreasing Akt phosphorylation and upregulating genes related to gluconeogenesis, indicating that enhanced insulin sensitivity may be linked to lower ApoJ concentrations [5,47]. Although reference ranges for ApoJ are less well-established clinically, elevated ApoJ has been associated with IR and metabolic dysfunction. Therefore, the reduction observed in ApoJ levels suggests a potentially beneficial adaptive response. This may have clinical implications for improving insulin sensitivity in patients with T2DM [11]. In this context, it is plausible that the reduction in ApoJ observed in our study may be due to reduced adiposity, improved insulin sensitivity, or a combination of both.

Our study also demonstrates decreases in insulin and HOMA-IR levels in the SG, TG, and TSG, with the most significant improvements observed in the training groups. Combined training appears to be more effective in enhancing insulin and glucose uptake in individuals with T2DM, possibly due to the distinct mechanisms of combined training [48,49].

Our findings also demonstrate improvements in the lipid profiles in the experimental groups, with significant differences in HDL-C and LDL-C levels between the TSG and CG. Broccoli sprout supplementation lowers plasma LDL-C concentrations by modulating cellular and tissue redox balance, enhancing AMPK signaling, and inhibiting the phosphoinositide 3-kinase (PI3K) pathway [50]. Moreover, aerobic exercise and weight loss reduce blood cholesterol, LDL-C, triglycerides, and HDL-C [51].

There was weight loss in the TG and TSG groups after 12 weeks, while body mass did not differ between the CG and SG groups. Additionally, Murashima et al. (2004) reported that consuming fresh broccoli (100 g/day) for one week decreased TC and LDL-C while significantly increasing HDL-C in twelve healthy subjects [52]. Furthermore, the consumption of broccoli sprout powder by patients with T2DM has been reported to improve their lipid profiles [33], consistent with our results. Moreover, combined training (aerobic and resistance exercise) improves lipid profiles in individuals with T2DM [20]. Increasing insulin sensitivity and improving insulin signaling may be a mechanism for changes in lipid profiles following combined training [53]. We hypothesized that combining exercise with broccoli sprout supplementation would result in greater improvements in apolipoprotein levels compared to either intervention alone. However, except for ApoA-I, we found that the TSG exhibited greater changes in ApoB-100 and ApoJ levels compared to the SG and CG, but not the TG. Interestingly, however, when the predefined contrasts were performed, we found that the combined group elicited significantly greater improvements in all apolipoprotein levels compared to the following groups: (1) CG, (2) SG, and (3) TG, as well as the comparison of the CG, TG, and SG.

Taken together, consuming broccoli sprouts and engaging in combined training can synergistically benefit circulating ApoB-100, ApoJ, glucose, insulin, and HOMA-IR levels, beyond that of supplementation or training alone. Although the statistical analysis did not demonstrate significant differences between the TSG and TG, the percentage changes in key variables were greater in the TSG. This trend suggests that combining training and broccoli sprout supplementation may modulate apolipoprotein levels through distinct biological pathways, potentially resulting in synergistic effects.

Moreover, the robust contrast analysis, taking into consideration the grand means of the specified contrasts, highlighted the superiority of the combined intervention group. Nevertheless, a definitive conclusion regarding a synergistic interaction cannot be drawn without further studies with larger sample sizes and mechanistic investigations to determine whether these interventions exert synergistic effects and elucidate the underlying biological mechanisms.

Study Limitations

Our study cannot be generalized, as young men and women were excluded from patient recruitment. Additionally, we did not monitor dietary intake and energy expenditure, which can potentially have significant impacts on various physiological outcomes. This lack of dietary control may have introduced inter-individual variability in metabolic responses, particularly in glucose- and lipid-related parameters. We did not measure muscle mass or the percentage and distribution of body fat. Additionally, some effect sizes in our study were not very robust, possibly due to the small sample size (n = 11) in each group. This small sample size may have reduced the statistical power and increased the risk of Type II error, potentially masking subtle but clinically meaningful effects. Future studies with larger sample sizes are recommended to confirm these results. Moreover, the SFN content of the broccoli sprout supplement was not independently verified in our laboratory. It was solely based on the manufacturer's information, which may limit the precision of our interpretation regarding its bioactivity. Lastly, our study included a homogenous group of individuals diagnosed with T2DM, which limits our interpretations as this condition is phenotypically heterogeneous. Future research should aim to include women, younger individuals, and other age groups to enhance the generalizability and external validity of the findings.

One limitation of this study is the absence of prior registration in a public clinical trial registry. Although the study design fulfills the criteria for a randomized controlled trial, registration was not completed before participant enrollment due to limited awareness of international registration requirements at the time. We acknowledge this limitation and are committed to ensuring prospective registration of all future clinical trials in accordance with ICMJE and WHO standards.

5. Conclusions

This study highlights the efficacy of combining structured exercise training with broccoli sprout supplementation as a multifaceted strategy to improve metabolic and cardiovascular biomarkers in men with T2DM. The intervention led to significant improvements in ApoA-I, ApoB-100, ApoJ, insulin, glucose, HOMA-IR, and HDL-C, with training emerging as the dominant contributor to these effects. While supplementation alone showed moderate benefits, its combination with exercise amplified the overall impact, particularly on apolipoprotein and insulin resistance markers. From a practical standpoint, these findings support the integration of supervised aerobic and resistance training into standard diabetes care, with broccoli sprout supplementation serving as a safe and accessible adjunct. Clinicians and exercise professionals may consider recommending this dual-modality approach to enhance lipid metabolism, glycemic control, and cardiovascular risk profiles in patients with T2DM. Future research should explore its applicability across diverse populations and investigate the underlying molecular mechanisms driving these improvements. Importantly, in cases where implementing both interventions is not feasible, exercise should be prioritized due to its broader and more robust impact across metabolic and lipoprotein outcomes.

Author Contributions: M.D., A.S. and H.Z. designed the study. M.D., M.G. and A.S. conducted the study. M.D., F.Z. and R.E.H. analyzed the obtained data. M.D., M.G. and F.Z. wrote the first draft of the manuscript. M.D., R.E.H., I.L., A.C.H., N.L.B., H.İ.C. and H.Z. read and revised the manuscript. All authors have read and agreed to the published version of the manuscript.

Funding: This research received no external funding.

Institutional Review Board Statement: This study was approved by the Ethics Committee of the Sport Sciences Research Institute, Tehran, Iran (Ethics code: IR.SSRC.REC.1401.142, 19 February 2023) and was conducted using the most recent version of the Declaration of Helsinki.

Informed Consent Statement: Informed consent was obtained from all subjects involved in the study.

Data Availability Statement: The datasets generated and analyzed for this study are available from the corresponding authors upon request due to the privacy of the participants.

Acknowledgments: The authors thank all the volunteers for their enthusiastic participation in this study. Special thanks are due to Cain C. T. Clark and Juan Del Coso for their valuable assistance with the statistical analysis.

Conflicts of Interest: The authors declare that they have no conflicts of interest.

References

1. Zhang, S.; Sun, S.; Wei, X.; Zhang, M.; Chen, Y.; Mao, X.; Chen, G.; Liu, C. Short-term moderate caloric restriction in a high-fat diet alleviates obesity via AMPK/SIRT1 signaling in white adipocytes and liver. *Food Nutr. Res.* **2022**, *66*, 10-29219. [CrossRef]
2. Gao, L.; Zhang, Y.; Wang, X.; Dong, H. Association of apolipoproteins A1 and B with type 2 diabetes and fasting blood glucose: A cross-sectional study. *BMC Endocr. Disord.* **2021**, *21*, 59. [CrossRef]
3. Wolkowicz, P.; White, C.R.; Anantharamaiah, G. Apolipoprotein mimetic peptides: An emerging therapy against diabetic inflammation and dyslipidemia. *Biomolecules* **2021**, *11*, 627. [CrossRef] [PubMed]
4. Croyal, M.; Wargny, M.; Chemello, K.; Chevalier, C.; Blanchard, V.; Bigot-Corbel, E.; Lambert, G.; Le May, C.; Hadjadj, S.; Cariou, B. Plasma apolipoprotein concentrations and incident diabetes in subjects with prediabetes. *Cardiovasc. Diabetol.* **2022**, *21*, 21. [CrossRef] [PubMed]
5. Wittwer, J.; Bradley, D. Clusterin and its role in insulin resistance and the cardiometabolic syndrome. *Front. Immunol.* **2021**, *12*, 612496. [CrossRef]
6. Fritzen, A.; Domingo-Espin, J.; Lundsgaard, A.; Kleinert, M.; Israelsen, I.; Carl, C. ApoA-1 improves glucose tolerance by increasing glucose uptake into heart and skeletal muscle independently of AMPKa2. *Mol. Metab.* **2020**, *35*, 2021. [CrossRef] [PubMed]
7. Mooradian, A.D.; Haas, M.J.; Wong, N.C. Transcriptional control of apolipoprotein AI gene expression in diabetes. *Diabetes* **2004**, *53*, 513–520. [CrossRef]
8. Behbodikhah, J.; Ahmed, S.; Elyasi, A.; Kasselman, L.J.; De Leon, J.; Glass, A.D.; Reiss, A.B. Apolipoprotein B and Cardiovascular Disease: Biomarker and Potential Therapeutic Target. *Metabolites* **2021**, *11*, 690. [CrossRef] [PubMed]
9. Haas, M.E.; Attie, A.D.; Biddinger, S.B. The regulation of ApoB metabolism by insulin. *Trends Endocrinol. Metab.* **2013**, *24*, 391–397. [CrossRef]
10. Rodriguez-Rivera, C.; Garcia, M.M.; Molina-Álvarez, M.; González-Martín, C.; Goicoechea, C. Clusterin: Always protecting. Synthesis, function and potential issues. *Biomed. Pharmacother.* **2021**, *134*, 111174. [CrossRef]

11. Seo, J.A.; Kang, M.-C.; Ciaraldi, T.P.; Kim, S.S.; Park, K.S.; Choe, C.; Hwang, W.M.; Lim, D.M.; Farr, O.; Mantzoros, C.; et al. Circulating ApoJ is closely associated with insulin resistance in human subjects. *Metabolism* **2018**, *78*, 155–166. [CrossRef] [PubMed]
12. Sgrò, P.; Emerenziani, G.P.; Antinozzi, C.; Sacchetti, M.; Di Luigi, L. Exercise as a drug for glucose management and prevention in type 2 diabetes mellitus. *Curr. Opin. Pharmacol.* **2021**, *59*, 95–102. [CrossRef] [PubMed]
13. Supriya, R.; Delfan, M.; Saeidi, A.; Samaie, S.S.; Al Kiyumi, M.H.; Escobar, K.A.; Laher, I.; Heinrich, K.M.; Weiss, K.; Knechtle, B.; et al. Spirulina Supplementation with High-Intensity Interval Training Decreases Adipokines Levels and Cardiovascular Risk Factors in Men with Obesity. *Nutrients* **2023**, *15*, 4891. [CrossRef]
14. Rahman, M.M.; Islam, M.R.; Shohag, S.; Hossain, M.E.; Rahaman, M.S.; Islam, F.; Ahmed, M.; Mitra, S.; Khandaker, M.U.; Idris, A.M.; et al. The multifunctional role of herbal products in the management of diabetes and obesity: A comprehensive review. *Molecules* **2022**, *27*, 1713. [CrossRef]
15. Maiyoh, G.K.; Kuh, J.E.; Casaschi, A.; Theriault, A.G. Cruciferous indole-3-carbinol inhibits apolipoprotein B secretion in HepG2 cells. *J. Nutr.* **2007**, *137*, 2185–2189. [CrossRef]
16. Mirmiran, P.; Bahadoran, Z.; Hosseinpanah, F.; Keyzad, A.; Azizi, F. Effects of broccoli sprout with high sulforaphane concentration on inflammatory markers in type 2 diabetic patients: A randomized double-blind placebo-controlled clinical trial. *J. Funct. Foods* **2012**, *4*, 837–841. [CrossRef]
17. Bahadoran, Z.; Mirmiran, P.; Azizi, F. Potential efficacy of broccoli sprouts as a unique supplement for management of type 2 diabetes and its complications. *J. Med. Food* **2013**, *16*, 375–382. [CrossRef]
18. Ruhee, R.T.; Suzuki, K. The integrative role of sulforaphane in preventing inflammation, oxidative stress and fatigue: A review of a potential protective phytochemical. *Antioxidants* **2020**, *9*, 521. [CrossRef]
19. Harty, P.S.; Cottet, M.L.; Malloy, J.K.; Kerksick, C.M. Nutritional and supplementation strategies to prevent and attenuate exercise-induced muscle damage: A brief review. *Sports Med.-Open* **2019**, *5*, 1. [CrossRef]
20. Terauchi, Y.; Takada, T.; Yoshida, S. A randomized controlled trial of a structured program combining aerobic and resistance exercise for adults with type 2 diabetes in Japan. *Diabetol. Int.* **2022**, *13*, 75–84. [CrossRef] [PubMed]
21. Zhao, X.; He, Q.; Zeng, Y.; Cheng, L. Effectiveness of combined exercise in people with type 2 diabetes and concurrent overweight/obesity: A systematic review and meta-analysis. *BMJ Open* **2021**, *11*, e046252. [CrossRef] [PubMed]
22. Jorge, M.L.M.P.; de Oliveira, V.N.; Resende, N.M.; Paraiso, L.F.; Calixto, A.; Diniz, A.L.D.; Resende, E.S.; Ropelle, E.R.; Carvalheira, J.B.; Espindola, F.S.; et al. The effects of aerobic, resistance, and combined exercise on metabolic control, inflammatory markers, adipocytokines, and muscle insulin signaling in patients with type 2 diabetes mellitus. *Metabolism* **2011**, *60*, 1244–1252. [CrossRef]
23. Cradock, K.A.; ÓLaighin, G.; Finucane, F.M.; Gainforth, H.L.; Quinlan, L.R.; Ginis, K.A.M. Behaviour change techniques targeting both diet and physical activity in type 2 diabetes: A systematic review and meta-analysis. *Int. J. Behav. Nutr. Phys. Act.* **2017**, *14*, 18. [CrossRef]
24. Jeon, Y.K.; Kim, S.S.; Kim, J.H.; Kim, H.J.; Park, J.J.; Cho, Y.S.; Joung, S.H.; Kim, J.R.; Kim, B.H.; Song, S.H.; et al. Combined aerobic and resistance exercise training reduces circulating apolipoprotein J levels and improves insulin resistance in postmenopausal diabetic women. *Diabetes Metab. J.* **2020**, *44*, 103–112. [CrossRef]
25. Bennetsen, S.L.; Feineis, C.S.; Legaard, G.E.; Lyngbæk, M.P.; Karstoft, K.; Ried-Larsen, M. The impact of physical activity on glycemic variability assessed by continuous glucose monitoring in patients with type 2 diabetes mellitus: A systematic review. *Front. Endocrinol.* **2020**, *11*, 486. [CrossRef]
26. Jin, Y.; Arroo, R.R. Application of dietary supplements in the prevention of type 2 diabetes-related cardiovascular complications. *Phytochem. Rev.* **2021**, *20*, 181–209. [CrossRef]
27. Meuffels, F.M.; Isenmann, E.; Strube, M.; Lesch, A.; Oberste, M.; Brinkmann, C. Exercise Interventions Combined with Dietary Supplements in Type 2 Diabetes Mellitus Patients—A Systematic Review of Relevant Health Outcomes. *Front. Nutr.* **2022**, *9*, 817724. [CrossRef]
28. Nathanson, V. Revising the declaration of Helsinki. *Br. Med. J. Publ. Group* **2013**, *346*, f2837. [CrossRef]
29. Pescatello, L.S. *ACSM's Guidelines for Exercise Testing and Prescription*; Lippincott Williams & Wilkins: New York, NY, USA, 2014.
30. Saeidi, A.; Soltani, M.; Daraei, A.; Nohbaradar, H.; Haghighi, M.M.; Khosravi, N.; Johnson, K.E.; Laher, I.; Hackney, A.C.; VanDusseldorp, T.A.; et al. The effects of aerobic-resistance training and broccoli supplementation on plasma dectin-1 and insulin resistance in males with type 2 diabetes. *Nutrients* **2021**, *13*, 3144. [CrossRef]
31. Brzycki, M. Strength testing—Predicting a one-rep max from reps-to-fatigue. *J. Phys. Educ. Recreat. Danc.* **1993**, *64*, 88–90. [CrossRef]
32. Mendes, R.; Sousa, N.; Almeida, A.; Subtil, P.; Guedes-Marques, F.; Reis, V.M.; Themudo-Barata, J.L. Exercise prescription for patients with type 2 diabetes—A synthesis of international recommendations: Narrative review. *Br. J. Sports Med.* **2016**, *50*, 1379–1381. [CrossRef] [PubMed]

33. Mirmiran, P.; Mohtadinia, J.; Hedayati, M.; Shakeri, N. Effects of broccoli sprout powder on fasting serum glucose and lipid profiles in type 2 diabetic patients. *Iran. J. Endocrinol. Metab.* **2011**, *13*, 18–25.
34. Bahadoran, Z.; Mirmiran, P.; Hosseinpanah, F.; Hedayati, M.; Hosseinpour-Niazi, S.; Azizi, F. Broccoli sprouts reduce oxidative stress in type 2 diabetes: A randomized double-blind clinical trial. *Eur. J. Clin. Nutr.* **2011**, *65*, 972–977. [CrossRef]
35. Wallace, T.M.; Levy, J.C.; Matthews, D.R. Use and abuse of HOMA modeling. *Diabetes Care* **2004**, *27*, 1487–1495. [CrossRef]
36. Delfan, M.; Radkia, F.; Juybari, R.A.; Daneshyar, S.; Willems, M.E.; Saeidi, A.; Hackney, A.C.; Laher, I.; Zouhal, H. Unveiling the effects of interval resistance training and chlorella vulgaris supplementation on Meteorin-like protein and oxidative stress in obese men. *Curr. Dev. Nutr.* **2024**, *8*, 104428. [CrossRef] [PubMed]
37. Hopkins, W.; Marshall, S.; Batterham, A.; Hanin, J. Progressive statistics for studies in sports medicine and exercise science. *Med.+ Sci. Sports+ Exerc.* **2009**, *41*, 3. [CrossRef] [PubMed]
38. Park, S.-K.; Park, J.-H.; Kwon, Y.-C.; Kim, H.-S.; Yoon, M.-S.; Park, H.-T. The effect of combined aerobic and resistance exercise training on abdominal fat in obese middle-aged women. *J. Physiol. Anthropol. Appl. Hum. Sci.* **2003**, *22*, 129–135. [CrossRef]
39. Yonesi, F.; Rashidlamir, A.; Khajei, R.; Yazdi, A.B. The Effect of Combined Training Courses on the Expression of ABCG4 Gene and Interleukin-4 Plasma Level in Middle-Aged Men Undergoing Coronary Artery Bypass Grafting. *Int. J. Basic Sci. Med.* **2020**, *5*, 147–154. [CrossRef]
40. Zandani, G.; Kaftori-Sandler, N.; Sela, N.; Nyska, A.; Madar, Z. Dietary broccoli improves markers associated with glucose and lipid metabolism through modulation of gut microbiota in mice. *Nutrition* **2021**, *90*, 111240. [CrossRef]
41. Peters, J.M.; Hennuyer, N.; Staels, B.; Fruchart, J.-C.; Fievet, C.; Gonzalez, F.J.; Auwerx, J. Alterations in lipoprotein metabolism in peroxisome proliferator-activated receptor α-deficient mice. *J. Biol. Chem.* **1997**, *272*, 27307–27312. [CrossRef]
42. Walldius, G.; Jungner, I. The apoB/apoA-I ratio: A strong, new risk factor for cardiovascular disease and a target for lipid-lowering therapy–a review of the evidence. *J. Intern. Med.* **2006**, *259*, 493–519. [CrossRef]
43. Gilbert, M. Role of skeletal muscle lipids in the pathogenesis of insulin resistance of obesity and type 2 diabetes. *J. Diabetes Investig.* **2021**, *12*, 1934–1941. [CrossRef]
44. Rabizadeh, S.; Rajab, A.; Mechanick, J.I.; Moosaie, F.; Rahimi, Y.; Nakhjavani, M.; Esteghamati, A. LDL/apo B ratio predict coronary heart disease in Type 2 diabetes independent of ASCVD risk score: A case-cohort study. *Nutr. Metab. Cardiovasc. Dis.* **2021**, *31*, 1477–1485. [CrossRef]
45. Sniderman, A.D.; Thanassoulis, G.; Glavinovic, T.; Navar, A.M.; Pencina, M.; Catapano, A.; Ference, B.A. Apolipoprotein B particles and cardiovascular disease: A narrative review. *JAMA Cardiol.* **2019**, *4*, 1287–1295. [CrossRef]
46. Marzolo, M.-P.; Farfán, P. New insights into the roles of megalin/LRP2 and the regulation of its functional expression. *Biol. Res.* **2011**, *44*, 89–105. [CrossRef] [PubMed]
47. Seo, J.A.; Kang, M.-C.; Yang, W.-M.; Hwang, W.M.; Kim, S.S.; Hong, S.H.; Heo, J.-I.; Vijyakumar, A.; de Moura, L.P.; Uner, A.; et al. Apolipoprotein J is a hepatokine regulating muscle glucose metabolism and insulin sensitivity. *Nat. Commun.* **2020**, *11*, 2024. [CrossRef] [PubMed]
48. Magalhães, J.P.; Santos, D.A.; Correia, I.R.; Hetherington-Rauth, M.; Ribeiro, R.; Raposo, J.F.; Matos, A.; Bicho, M.D.; Sardinha, L.B. Impact of combined training with different exercise intensities on inflammatory and lipid markers in type 2 diabetes: A secondary analysis from a 1-year randomized controlled trial. *Cardiovasc. Diabetol.* **2020**, *19*, 169. [CrossRef]
49. Zouhal, H.; Zare-Kookandeh, N.; Haghighi, M.M.; Daraei, A.; de Sousa, M.; Soltani, M.; Ben Abderrahman, A.; Tijani, J.M.; Hackney, A.C.; Laher, I.; et al. Physical activity and adipokine levels in individuals with type 2 diabetes: A literature review and practical applications. *Rev. Endocr. Metab. Disord.* **2021**, *22*, 987–1011. [CrossRef]
50. Armah, C.N.; Derdemezis, C.; Traka, M.H.; Dainty, J.R.; Doleman, J.F.; Saha, S.; Leung, W.; Potter, J.F.; Lovegrove, J.A.; Mithen, R.F. Diet rich in high glucoraphanin broccoli reduces plasma LDL cholesterol: Evidence from randomised controlled trials. *Mol. Nutr. Food Res.* **2015**, *59*, 918–926. [CrossRef] [PubMed]
51. Gordon, B.; Chen, S.; Durstine, J.L. The effects of exercise training on the traditional lipid profile and beyond. *Curr. Sports Med. Rep.* **2014**, *13*, 253–259. [CrossRef]
52. Murashima, M.; Watanabe, S.; Zhuo, X.G.; Uehara, M.; Kurashige, A. Phase 1 study of multiple biomarkers for metabolism and oxidative stress after one-week intake of broccoli sprouts. *Biofactors* **2004**, *22*, 271–275. [CrossRef] [PubMed]
53. Amaro, A.B.; Curco, A.S.; Garcia, E.; Julve, J.; Rives, J.; Benitez, S.; Cortes, V.L. Apolipoprotein and LRP1-based peptides as new therapeutic tools in atherosclerosis. *J. Clin. Med.* **2021**, *10*, 3571. [CrossRef] [PubMed]

nutrients

MDPI

Article

Effect of Dealcoholized Muscadine Wine on the Development of Spontaneous Colitis and Gut Microbiome in IL-10$^{-/-}$ Mice

Hao Li and Liwei Gu *

Food Science and Human Nutrition Department, Institute of Food and Agriculture Sciences, University of Florida, Gainesville, FL 32611, USA
* Correspondence: lgu@ufl.edu

Abstract: Background/Objectives: Colitis is a chronic condition affecting millions worldwide. Purple muscadine wine polyphenols have a unique composition and possible disease-preventive properties. This study aims to determine how dealcoholized muscadine wine (DMW) affects the development of colitis and gut microbiome in IL-10$^{-/-}$ mice, compared to wild types (WT). **Methods**: Six-week-old male IL-10$^{-/-}$ and WT C57BL/6 mice were fed either a DMW-supplemented diet (4.8% v/w) or a control diet based on AIN-93M for 154 days. Colitis severity was evaluated by disease activity, intestinal permeability, gene expression of cytokines and tight junction proteins in the colon, and inflammatory cytokines in the serum. Fecal samples were collected for gut microbiome profiling via 16S rRNA gene sequencing. **Results**: DMW contained predominantly anthocyanins and a significant amount of ellagic acid. IL-10$^{-/-}$ mice developed mild colitis as indicated by the disease activity index. DMW × gene interactions decreased intestinal permeability, colonic mRNA levels of IL-1β, and serum TNF-α in the IL-10$^{-/-}$ mice. DMW suppressed the colonic mRNA levels of IL-6, enhanced the gene expression of ZO-1, but did not influence the mRNA level of TNF-α or occludin. While DMW did not alter α-diversity of the gut microbiome, it significantly influenced β-diversity in the WT mice. DMW significantly reduced the relative abundances of *Akkermansia* in the IL-10$^{-/-}$ and WT mice. DMW and DMW×gene interaction decreased the relative abundance of *Parasutterella* only in IL-10$^{-/-}$ mice. **Conclusions**: These results suggested that polyphenols from DMW interacted with genes to moderately alleviate the development of colitis in IL-10$^{-/-}$ mice and could be a useful dietary strategy for IBD prevention.

Keywords: IL-10$^{-/-}$ mice; dealcoholized muscadine wine; colitis; gut microbiome; diet-gene interactions

1. Introduction

Inflammatory bowel diseases (IBD), consisting of Crohn's disease and ulcerative colitis, are a group of chronic and recurring inflammatory conditions in the colon and intestine. The prevalence of IBD grows steadily in early industrialized countries, while its incidence increases in newly industrialized regions since 2000 [1]. Common symptoms of IBD include abdominal pain, diarrhea, fever, fatigue, and blood in the stool. IBD increases the risk of colorectal cancer by 2–3 fold [2].

Many studies have suggested that polyphenols are effective in preventing the development and managing the symptoms of IBD. For example, hydroxytyrosol inhibited the TLR4/NF-κB signaling pathway, reduced colon expression of IL-6 and TNF-α, and increased the abundance of *Bacteroidota* in mice with DSS-induced acute colitis [3]. Resveratrol decreased the gene expression of IL-1β, TNF-α, and IL-6, but increased the expression of IL-10 in DSS-treated mice by inhibiting the JAK2/STAT3 pathway [4]. Polyphenol ligustroside preserved the structural integrity of the colon tissue and affected both the α- and β-diversities of gut microbiome, compared to DSS-treated colitis mice [5].

Muscadine grapes (*Vitis rotundifolia*) originate from the south-central and southeastern United States. Muscadine grapes or wines contain six anthocyanins, all in the form of 3,5-diglucosides. In contrast, common grapes contain primarily anthocyanins in 3-glucoside forms. They also contain other polyphenols, including ellagitannins, ellagic acid, myricetin, quercetin, epicatechin, and catechin, but with a low content of resveratrol [6]. High levels of ellagitannins and ellagic acid are also unique to muscadine grapes [7]. Muscadine grapes are characterized by thick, tough skin and large seeds. Partially due to the lack of seedless cultivars, over 90% of muscadine grapes are made into wine.

It was reported that muscadine grape extracts decreased the superoxide level in neutrophils of rats treated with phorbol myristate acetate. The levels of IL-1β, IL-6 and TNF-α were reduced in peripheral blood mononuclear cells stimulated by lipopolysaccharides. Muscadine grape skin extracts were also found to mitigate the paw edema in carrageenan-stimulated rats [8]. In addition, muscadine skin or seed extracts prohibited edema and decreased the myeloperoxidase activity in mice ears irritated by tetradecanoylphorbol acetate [9]. Muscadine wine polyphenols were shown to prevent weight loss and colon shortening, downregulate the NF-κB pathway and secretion of IL-1β, IL-6, and TNF-α in the colon of mice with DSS-induced colitis [6].

Many studies have demonstrated the effect of polyphenols on chemically induced colitis in mice. However, there are few studies investigating the effect of polyphenols on the colitis developed in genetically susceptible mice. IL-10$^{-/-}$ mice have been widely used to investigate IBD because they develop colitis spontaneously [10]. After the onset of colitis, IL-10$^{-/-}$ mice have a higher secretion of inflammatory cytokines than wild-type mice, including TNF-α, IL-1β, IL-6, and IFN-γ [11]. Previous studies demonstrated that muscadine wine polyphenols restored the gut dysbiosis in DSS-treated mice [12]. However, it is unknown whether muscadine wine has similar effects in IL-10$^{-/-}$ mice. Nutrigenomics and nutrigenetics reveal the complex and bidirectional interactions between diet and genes and a vital role of such interactions in health and disease. Diets influence gene expression via epigenetic modification, transcription factor activation, and microRNA regulation. Genetic differences, such as single-nucleotide polymorphisms, enzyme function variability, and taste preference, affect how individuals metabolize and respond to nutrients [13]. Most of the previous research focused on the diet, while the interaction between diet and genes was ignored. Therefore, this study aimed to test the hypothesis that a diet supplemented with DMW interacts with genes to alleviate IBD in IL-10$^{-/-}$ mice. Dealcoholized wine has been extensively used to study the nutritional properties of wine polyphenols in humans and rodents without the interference of alcohol. The non-alcoholic wine is also gaining popularity among consumers in recent years [14].

2. Materials and Methods

2.1. Materials

Muscadine wine (Lakeridge Winery, Clermont, FL, USA) was condensed to 10% of the original volume under partial vacuum to prepare dealcoholized muscadine wine. Standards of phytochemicals (anthocyanins, ellagic acid, myricetin, quercetin, and kaempferol) and FITC-dextran (4 KD) were provided by MilliporeSigma, Inc. (Burlington, MA, USA).

2.2. HPLC Analysis of Dealcoholized Muscadine Wine

To quantify anthocyanins, DMW was dispersed in methanol: water: formic acid (50:49:1, *v*/*v*/*v*). The filtered solution was injected onto an HPLC with ZORBAX C18

Column (5 μm, 4.6 × 250 mm, Agilent Technologies, Santa Clara, CA, USA). The mobile phase consisted of 5% formic acid (phase A) and 100% methanol (phase B). The linear gradient was 0–10 min, 5–15% B; 10–30 min, 15–30% B; 30–45 min, 30% B; 47 min, 70% B. The flow rate and detection wavelength were 0.8 mL/min and 520 nm, respectively. DMW was hydrolyzed before non-anthocyanins were analyzed on HPLC. One mL of DMW was mixed with 3 mL of 50% methanol and 0.45 mL of 37% (*w*/*w*) HCl. The mixture was placed in a water bath at 90 °C for 80 min. After that, the final volume of the mixture was adjusted to 5 mL with 50% methanol. The diluted and filtered solution was injected into an Agilent ZORBAX C18 Column (5 μm, 4.6 × 250 mm). Mobile phases included 0.5% formic acid in water (phase A) and acetonitrile (phase B). The linear gradient was 0–5 min, 10–30% B; 10 min, 40% B; 20 min, 50% B; 23 min, 70% B; 25 min, 10% B. The flow rate and detection wavelength were 1.0 mL/min and 360 nm, respectively.

2.3. Proximate Analysis of DMW and Diet Formulation

The total fiber and total protein in DMW were analyzed according to AOAC 991.43 and AOAC 991.20.I, respectively, at Mérieux NutriScience Inc. (Gainesville, FL, USA). Ash was analyzed in a furnace based on AOAC 942.15. Moisture was analyzed after DMW was dried in an oven at 105 °C for 3 h. Fat content in DMW was assessed using the chloroform-methanol method [15]. Sugar content was assessed on an Agilent HPLC with a refractive index detector. Sugars were separated on a Luna NH2 column (5 μm, 250 × 4.6 mm, Phenomenex, Torrance, CA, USA). The column was eluted with 75% aqueous acetonitrile at a flow rate of 0.8 mL/min.

An AIN-93M control diet and an AIN-93M diet supplemented with DMW were prepared by Research Diets, Inc. (New Brunswick, NJ, USA). DMW was added at 4.8% (*v*/*w*). The composition of the diets is shown in Supplemental Table S1.

2.4. Animal Care and Experimental Design

The Institutional Animal Care and Use Committee at the University of Florida reviewed and approved the protocol. IL-10$^{-/-}$ C57BL/6 mice and their wild-type counterparts (male, six weeks old) were provided by Jackson Lab (Bar Harbor, ME, USA). They were housed three per cage and acclimated on the AIN-93M control diet for one week. After that, twenty-four IL-10$^{-/-}$ mice were randomly separated into two groups of equal size. One group was given an AIN-93M control diet, while the other group was given the AIN-93M diet supplemented with 4.8% DMW. The same protocol was repeated on the twenty-four WT mice (Table S2). The grouping of mice was not blinded to the researchers. The number of mice in each group was comparable to a published study [16]. Feeding lasted for 154 days (22 weeks). Body weight, food intake, stool consistency, and rectal bleeding were recorded twice a week. Disease activity index (DAI) was calculated based on reduced weight gain, stool consistency, and rectal bleeding, according to a published method with modifications [17]. The reduced weight gain was calculated as the difference between 100% and the ratio of individual mouse weight over the average weight of WT mice on the control diet on the same feeding day. The reduced weight gain was used because mice in this 22-week study had no weight loss, which is typical only in the DSS-induced acute colitis mouse models [17].

For assessment of intestinal permeability on day 142, mice were deprived of food for 6 h before they were gavaged with FITC-dextran (44 mg/100 g weight). After 4 h, blood was sampled from a facial vein and separated into serum. The fluorescence intensity of diluted serum was measured using 485-nm excitation and 585-nm emission.

Mice were euthanized on day 154, and blood was collected by cardiac puncture, and the colon was removed. This study did not control the location of mouse cages and the sequence of measurements.

2.5. Quantitative Reverse Transcription PCR (RT-qPCR)

Mouse colon RNA was extracted using RNAzol® RT (Molecular Research Center, Inc., Cincinnati, OH, USA) and reverse-transcribed with iScript cDNA Synthesis kit (Bio-Rad Laboratories, Inc., Hercules, CA, USA). The primers are listed in Supplemental Table S3. The plates containing primers, cDNA, SYBR Green supermix (Bio-Rad Laboratories, Inc., USA), and nuclease-free water were sealed and centrifuged at 3000× g for 3 min. Real-Time PCR Detection System (Bio-Rad Laboratories, Inc., Hercules, CA, USA) was used to amplify the genes. GAPDH served as a reference gene, and the relative gene expressions were calculated using the $2^{-\Delta\Delta Ct}$ method.

2.6. Analysis of Serum IL-6, IL-1β and TNF-α

Serum IL-6, IL-1β, and TNF-α on day 154 were analyzed using ELISA kits according to the protocols provided by the manufacturers (Invitrogen, Carlsbad, CA, USA).

2.7. Gut Microbiome Analysis

Fecal samples from individual mice were collected the day before euthanasia and stored at −80 °C. The bacterial DNA was extracted using the QIAamp Fast DNA Stool Mini Kit (Qiagen, Venlo, The Netherlands). The 16S ribosomal RNA genes (V3-4 region) were amplified. The clean sequences were compared with those in a database (silva-132-99-nb-classifier.qza). Qiime2 scripts written in Linux were used to filter and clean sequences, merge paired-end sequences, and generate taxonomy, rooted-tree, and OTU tables.

2.8. Statistical Analysis

Data are expressed as mean ± standard deviation. Parametric data were analyzed with generalized linear regression two-way ANOVA. Non-parametric data (α-diversity and bacterial abundance) were analyzed using aligned rank transform two-way ANOVA. Two-way ANOVA was selected as a statistical method because this study had a two-factor (diet and gene) and two-level design (+ and −). If a significant effect of diet, gene, or diet × gene interaction was detected, post-hoc contrasts were performed for group comparisons. The p-values for multiple group comparisons were adjusted using the Benjamini-Hochberg procedure. Analyses were performed in R (Version 4.4.2). PERMANOVA and its pairwise tests (adonis2) were used to assess beta diversity.

3. Results and Discussion

3.1. DMW Contained Anthocyanins, Ellagic Acid, and Flavonols

The most abundant anthocyanins in DMW were delphinidin-3,5-diglucoside (1008.3 μg/mL) and cyanidin 3,5-diglucoside (1000.5 μg/mL), followed by peonidin 3,5-diglucoside (Table 1). The total content of anthocyanins was 3454.8 μg/mL. DMW also contained a significant amount of ellagic acid (348.9 μg/mL) but a small amount of myricetin (106.1 μg/mL) and quercetin (17.7 μg/mL) (Chromatograms in Supplemental Figure S1). The polyphenol profile of DMW was comparable to a published paper [12]. In this study, the dose of anthocyanins for mice was 16.56 mg/(kg·d). Based on body surface area [18], the human equivalent dose of muscadine wine and anthocyanins was 234 mL and 81 mg, respectively, for a person weighing 60 kg.

Table 1. Contents of polyphenols in DMW.

Polyphenols	Concentration (μg/mL)
Delphinidin-3,5-diglucoside	1008.3 ± 62.7
Cyanidin 3,5-diglucoside	1000.5 ± 62.2
Petunidin 3,5-diglucoside	562.3 ± 36.7
Pelargonidin 3,5-diglucoside	49.9 ± 1.8
Peonidin 3,5-diglucoside	590.3 ± 39.6
Malvidin 3,5-diglucoside	243.5 ± 15.5
Total anthocyanins	3454.8 ± 217.9
Myricetin	106.1 ± 18.3
Quercetin	17.7 ± 2.5
Kaempeferol	3.7 ± 0.7
Ellagic acid	348.9 ± 16.9
Total other polyphenols	476.4 ± 36.5

Data are mean ± SD of triplicate tests.

3.2. DMW Significantly Affected Body Weight but Not DAI

Both DMW ($p = 0.047$) and gene ($p < 0.01$) significantly affected body weight at day 154 (Figure 1A). DMW had greater impact on the body weight gain in IL-10$^{-/-}$ mice ($p = 0.052$) than in WT mice ($p = 0.37$). IL-10$^{-/-}$ mice had lower body weight than WT mice in the DMW feeding groups ($p = 0.01$), which was consistent with the spontaneous development of colitis in IL-10$^{-/-}$ mice. The impact of DMW on body weight was similar to the result by Kang et al., who found that a diet with 1% Goji Berry for 10 weeks did not alter the body weight of IL-10$^{-/-}$ mice [19].

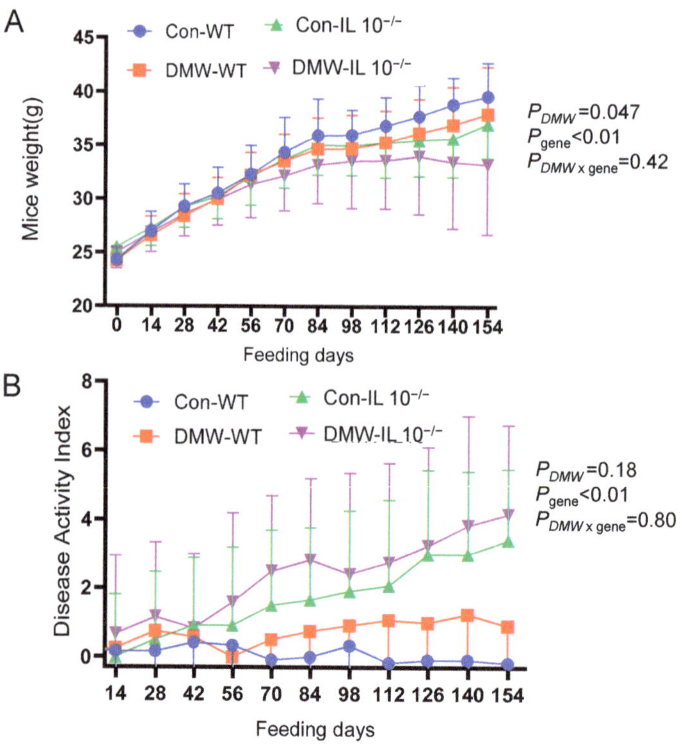

Figure 1. DMW and gene affected body weight (**A**) and Disease Activity Index (**B**) of wild-type (WT) and IL-10$^{-/-}$ mice fed control or DMW-supplemented diet. $n = 12$ mice per group. p-Values of two-way ANOVA were shown for day 154.

The symptoms and severity of colitis were assessed using DAI, which is a combined score of reduced weight gain, stool consistency, and rectal bleeding. The maximum score for each of the three symptoms was 4. Therefore, mice with extremely severe colitis receive a maximum DAI of 12. The WT mice showed no sign of colitis throughout the feeding period of 22 weeks. The DAI in IL-10$^{-/-}$ mice gradually increased from zero to about 4.1 after 22 weeks of feeding (Figure 1B). The DAI scores were primarily due to reduced weight gain and soft stool. Severe diarrhea or rectal bleeding was not observed. DAI was significantly affected by gene ($p < 0.01$) but not by diet ($p = 0.18$) or diet x gene interaction ($p = 0.80$). A previous study fed C57BL/6 IL-10$^{-/-}$ mice a control diet for 10 weeks and reported an average DAI of 6.5, which was much higher than the value in this study. The onset and severity of colitis in IL-10$^{-/-}$ mice depend on both the genetic background of the mice and the environmental microbiome. The C57BL/6 IL-10$^{-/-}$ mice typically develop milder and delayed colitis compared to mice of other strains, such as the 29/SvEv or BALB/c mice [10]. It was observed that colitis symptoms can be absent in C57BL/6 IL-10$^{-/-}$ mice in some animal facilities due to the lack of some environmental microbiome [20]. The very mild colitis observed in this study suggested the environmental microbiome in the animal facility did not favor the development of severe colitis. This study did not use antibiotics to accelerate the onset and severity of colitis because antibiotics were known to disrupt the gut microbiome composition [21].

Previous studies using the DSS-induced acute colitis model have shown that anthocyanins reduce DAI in mice [6,22]. DSS-treated mice are characterized by body weight loss of up to 15%, diarrhea, and rectal bleeding after three days. However, these severe symptoms were absent in this study, which may have limited the impact of DMW on DAI. Replacing weight loss with reduced weight gain in the calculation of DAI may also affect its response to diet. Nevertheless, these results suggested that DMW had limited effects on IL-10-deficient mice, an observation shared by a published study that showed the limited effect of dietary curcumin [23]. In vitro studies suggested that the anti-inflammatory activities of curcumin were attenuated in IL-10-deficient mice because part of its full activity depends on IL-10 [23].

3.3. *DMW Interacted with Gene to Reduce Intestinal Permeability in IL-10$^{-/-}$ Mice*

IBD patients have high intestinal permeability, which mainly results from a defective mucosal barrier and exacerbates intestinal inflammation [24]. The intestinal permeability of mice was significantly affected by gene and DMW $\times$ gene interaction (Figure 2). DMW interacted with the gene to decrease the intestinal permeability in IL-10$^{-/-}$ mice but did not alter the intestinal permeability in WT mice. The result partially agreed with a published study, which found that grape seed extract for 12 weeks reduced gut permeability in IL-10-deficient mice with mild colitis [25].

Polyphenols have been shown to interact with the presence and absence of the IL-10 gene through multiple mechanisms. For example, epigallocatechin gallate has been found to modulate IL-10 mRNA and protein levels in mice under inflammatory conditions [26]. IL-10 and its receptors regulate immune response mainly through the JAK-STAT signaling pathway [27]. Several polyphenols have been found to directly affect their activities. For instance, hesperidin in combination with cinnamaldehyde significantly decreased p-JAK2 and p-STAT3 and significantly increased the expression of SOCS3 protein in ulcerative colitis [28]. In addition, polyphenols and IL-10 can influence each other's activities through the gut microbiome because both are known to interact with gut microbiota reciprocally [29]. Since IL-10 is essential for anti-inflammatory signaling and immune homeostasis, its absence is expected to diminish or alter the biological effects of dietary polyphenol interventions such as DMW.

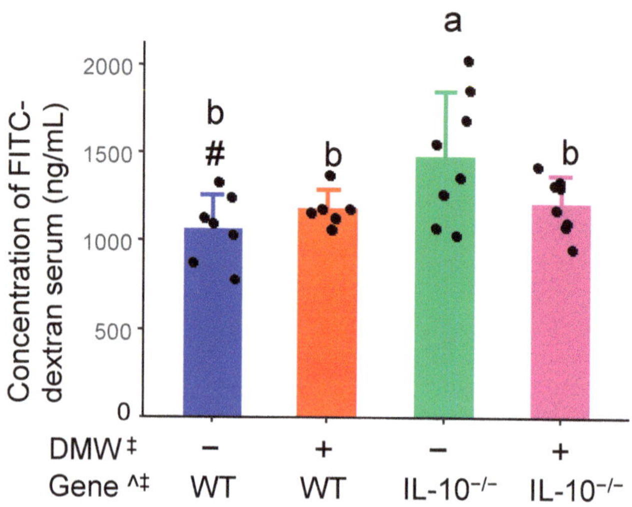

Figure 2. DMW interacted with gene to decrease intestinal permeability (FITC-dextran level on day 142) in IL-10$^{-/-}$ mice (n = 6–8). ^ significant effect by gene; ‡ significant effect of DMW × gene interaction; # significant genetic difference in the same dietary group. Data were square-transformed before the analysis. Letters on the columns indicate significant all-pairs-wise differences when there is a significant effect of DMW × gene interaction.

3.4. DMW, Gene, and Their Interactions Differentially Affect Gene Expression of Cytokines and Tight Junction Proteins

IL-6, IL-1β, and TNF-α are key pro-inflammatory cytokines involved in the initiation and progression of colitis. DMW and DMW × gene interaction significantly reduced IL-6 and IL-1β mRNA in the colon of IL-10$^{-/-}$ mice, respectively, but not in WT mice (Figure 3A,B). IL-10$^{-/-}$ mice had higher TNF-α than WT mice, but DMW had no impact in either group (Figure 3C). The reduction in mRNA expression of IL-6 and IL-1β in the colon has been consistently observed in mice with induced colitis, including purple-fleshed potatoes, black rice anthocyanin-rich extract, and raspberry anthocyanin-rich fractions [22,30,31]. The lack of DMW's effect on mRNA level of TNF-α is likely because TNF-α is an early response cytokine regulated via different signaling cascades than IL-6 or IL-1β [32].

The integrity of the epithelial barrier is maintained by tight junction proteins, including ZO-1 and occludin [33]. DMW significantly enhanced the colonic gene expression of ZO-1 in IL-10$^{-/-}$ mice compared to the control diet, but not in WT mice (Figure 3D). The gene expression of occludin in IL-10$^{-/-}$ mice was significantly lower than that in WT mice. However, it was not affected by DMW in either the WT or IL-10$^{-/-}$ mice (Figure 3E). The observation on ZO-1 agreed with a previous study showing that mulberry anthocyanins restored the expression of intestinal tight junction protein ZO-1 [34]. Red wine polyphenols are known to increase mRNA of ZO-1 in HT-29 colon cells [35]. ZO-1 acts as a scaffold protein that connects transmembrane proteins (like claudins and occludins) to the actin cytoskeleton. This helps to form and stabilize tight junctions between cells. The increased ZO-1 mRNA in the colon helps to explain the decreased intestinal permeability in the IL-10$^{-/-}$ mice fed a DMW-supplemented diet.

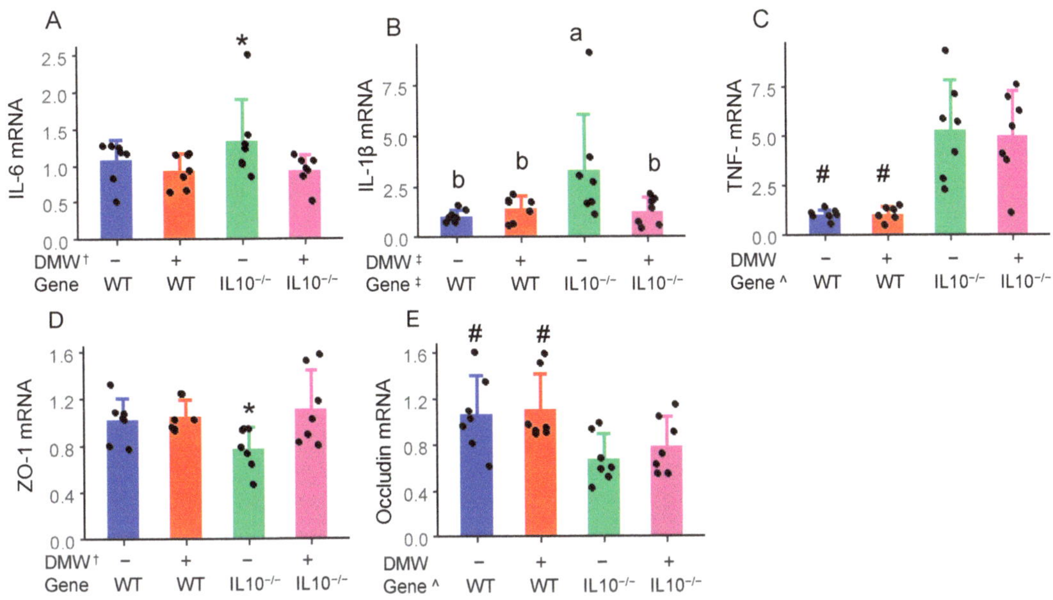

Figure 3. DMW, gene, and their interactions differentially affected relative mRNA levels of IL-6 (**A**), IL-1β (**B**), TNF-α (**C**), ZO-1 (**D**), and occludin (**E**) in the colon of mice ($n = 7$). † significant effect by DMW; ^ significant effect by gene; ‡ significant effect of DMW × gene interaction. * Significant dietary difference in the same genotype. # significant genetic differences in the same diet group. Letters on the columns indicate significant all-pairs-wise differences when there is a significant effect of DMW × gene interaction.

3.5. DMW × Gene Interaction Reduced the Serum TNF-α in IL-10$^{-/-}$ Mice

The mRNA of inflammatory cytokines in the colon reflects a localized early stage of immune response, while the serum levels of IL-6, IL-1β, and TNF-α are indicators of systemic inflammation. This is because serum cytokines are produced by the entire immune system, including those from the colon. Although DMW and DMW × gene interaction affected mRNA of IL-6 and IL-1β in the colon, their serum levels were not impacted (Figure 4A,B), suggesting the localized effect of DMW on IL-6 and IL-1β was stronger in the colon than its systemic activities. Anthocyanins and ellagic acid are known to have extremely low absorption rates, as indicated by their low contents in systemic circulation after oral ingestion. A vast majority of them enter the colon to exert a localized effect [36]. IL-10$^{-/-}$ mice had a higher serum level of TNF-α than WT mice due to genetic impact (Figure 4C), which was consistent with TNF-α mRNA in the colon. Although DMW alone did not affect serum TNF-α ($p = 0.06$), DMW × gene interaction significantly decreased the serum content of TNF-α in IL-10$^{-/-}$ mice but not in WT mice. Serum TNF-α appeared to be more responsive to dietary DMW, likely due to its role as a master cytokine in the pathogenesis of IBD and its status as a primary target for therapeutic intervention. The systemic anti-inflammatory activity of DMW was consistent with previous research, which reported that black rice extract and blackcurrant reduced serum levels of IL-1β, TNF-α, and IL-6 in mice with DSS-induced colitis [37,38].

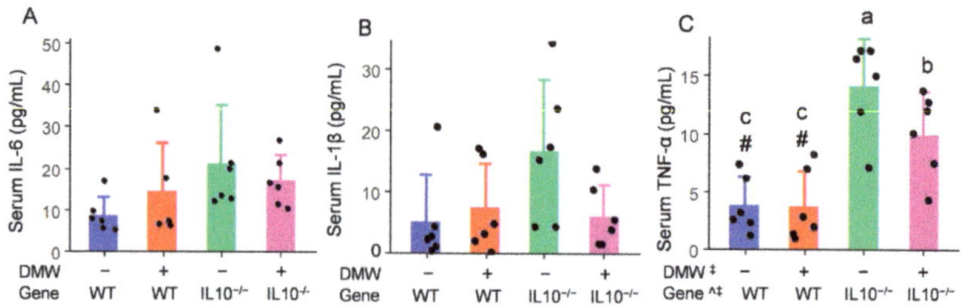

Figure 4. DMW × gene interaction did not affect serum levels of IL-6 (**A**) and IL-1β (**B**), but reduced TNF-α (**C**) in IL-10$^{-/-}$ mice (n = 6). ^ significant effect by gene; ‡ significant effect of DMW × gene interaction. # significant genetic differences in the same diet group. Data were square-transformed before the analysis. Letters on the columns indicate significant all-pairs-wise differences when there was a significant effect of DMW × gene interaction.

3.6. *DMW Did Not Affect α-Diversity but Altered the Beta-Diversity of the Gut Microbiome*

DMW or gene did not affect α-diversity among all four groups (Figure 5A,B). Observed OTU is calculated based on the richness of species, and Shannon is a balanced index based on both the richness and evenness of species. A similar study also found that 8 weeks of pomegranate extract did not affect the Shannon index of the cecum of IL-10$^{-/-}$ mice [39]. IL-10$^{-/-}$ mice in this study developed very mild colitis after 22 weeks of feeding, most likely due to an unfavorable environmental microbiome. This may have blunted the impact of the gene on α-diversity.

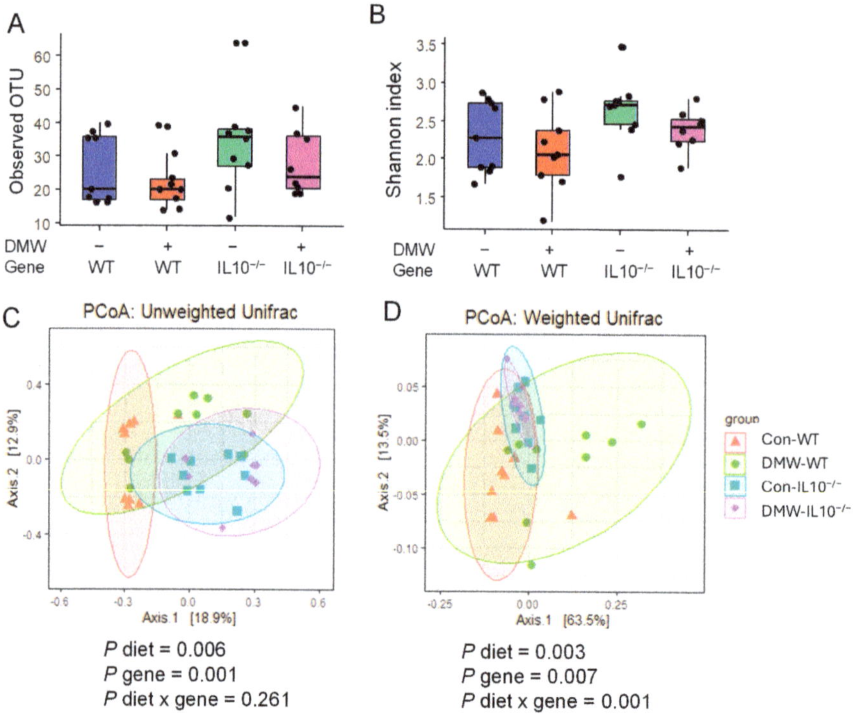

Figure 5. DMW or gene did not change the α-diversity of gut microbiome measured by observed OTU (**A**) or Shannon index (**B**); both DMW and gene altered bacterial β-diversity based on PCoA plots of unweighted UniFrac distance (**C**) and weighted UniFrac distance (**D**) (n = 8–9). The p-values for β-diversity were from PERMANOVA tests.

Both diet and gene significantly affected the β-diversity of gut microbiomes based on the PCoA plot of unweighted and weighted UniFrac distances and PERMANOVA tests (Figure 5C,D). Significant diet x gene interaction was only observed in weighted UniFrac distances, but not in unweighted UniFrac distances. Pairwise comparison showed that DMW significantly altered β-diversity in the WT mice but not in the IL-$10^{-/-}$ mice (Tables S4 and S5). These results agreed with a similar study that reported that pomegranate extract did not alter beta-diversity in IL-$10^{-/-}$ mice [39]. Both unweighted and weighted UniFrac are phylogenetic methods of comparing microbial communities. Unweighted UniFrac detects compositional change according to the presence and absence of taxa, while the weighted UniFrac detects structural change according to the relative abundance of taxa. Unweighted UniFrac is more sensitive to rare taxa than weighted UniFrac distance [40]. The altered β-diversity in IL-$10^{-/-}$ mice compared to WT mice may have reduced the gut microbiome's responsiveness to DMW in the diet.

3.7. DMW and DMW × Gene Interaction Altered the Relative Abundance of Some Gut Microbes

The relative abundance of four gut microbes at the genus level is depicted in Figure 6. DMW did not affect the abundance of *Bacteroides* and *Anaeroplasma*, whereas only the gene had significant impacts (Figure 6A,B). WT mice had a higher abundance of *Bacteroides* than IL-$10^{-/-}$ mice, while the opposite was observed for *Anaeroplasma*. *Bacteroides* are known to modulate immune function and ferment complex polysaccharides to produce SCFA [41], which was the possible reason for their higher relative abundance in WT mice. *Anaeroplasma* was an opportunistic pathogen which has been reported to induce diverse immune responses in human diseases such as colon cancer [42], which was the possible reason that there was a higher relative abundance of them in IL-$10^{-/-}$ mice than in WT mice.

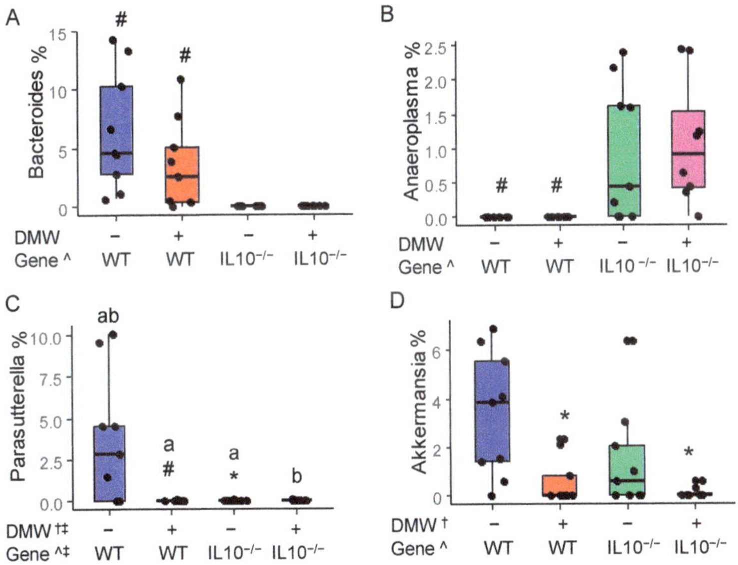

Figure 6. DMW, gene, and their interactions altered the relative abundance of gut microbiome at the genus level for (**A**) *Bacteroides*, (**B**) *Anaeroplasma*, (**C**) *Parasutterella*, and (**D**) *Akkermansia*. † significant effect by DMW; ^ significant effect by genotype; ‡ significant effect of DMW × gene interaction; * significant dietary difference in the same genotype; # significant genetic difference in the same diet group. Letters on the columns indicate significant all-pairs-wise differences when there is a significant effect of DMW × gene interaction.

The abundance of *Parasutterella* was affected by DMW, gene, and their interaction. *Parasutterella* was a potential pathogen because they are involved in bile acid metabolism and are associated with inflammatory bowel diseases [43]. DMW significantly reduced the abundance of *Parasutterella* in IL-$10^{-/-}$ mice (Figure 6C), which may provide benefits to alleviate colitis.

DMW reduced the relative abundance of *Akkermansia* in both WT and IL-$10^{-/-}$ mice. IL-$10^{-/-}$ mice had a lower abundance of *Akkermansia* than the WT mice (Figure 6D). Previous studies also found a lower abundance of *Akkermansia* in IL-$10^{-/-}$ mice and suggested that *Akkermansia* correlates negatively with gut inflammation [44,45]. *Akkermansia* are mucin-degrading bacteria in the phylum of *Verrucomicrobia* colonizing the intestinal mucosa of humans and rodents. An optimal level of *Akkermansia* is critical for gut health because a lower abundance may impair mucus renewal and compromise the gut barrier [46]. However, a higher abundance can lead to over-degradation and thinning of the mucus layer. The activity of DMW in IL$10^{-/-}$ mice appeared to be similar to NLRP6 [44], which was shown to protect IL$10^{-/-}$ mice from colitis by limiting colonization of *Akkermansia*.

3.8. Spearman Correlation Between mRNA and Significantly Changed Gut Microbiota

Bacteroides negatively correlated with colon IL-1β and TNF-α mRNA, which was consistent with its lower abundance in IL-$10^{-/-}$ mice compared to WT mice, in contrast to higher colon mRNA of IL-1β and TNF-α in IL-$10^{-/-}$ mice (Figure 7). *Bacteroides* correlated positively with occludin because both had a lower amount in IL$10^{-/-}$ mice than in WT mice. *Bacteroides* isolates were found to inhibit the IL-1β-triggered inflammatory response in CFTR$^{-/-}$ Caco-2 intestinal epithelial cells [47]. Another study found that the administration of *Bacteroides fragilis* inhibited the gene expression of inflammatory cytokines (TNF-α, IL-1β, IL-6) but enhanced the gene expression of tight junction proteins (ZO-1, occludin, claudin-1) [48]. This suggests that *Bacteroides* may be a potential probiotic for treating colitis. *Anaeroplasma* positively correlated with TNF-α because both had higher levels in IL$10^{-/-}$ Mice than in WT mice, suggesting *Anaeroplasma* may have contributed to immune activation. *Akkermansia* positively correlated with IL-6. The impact of *Akkermansia* on inflammatory cytokine IL-6 depends on the biological context. *Akkermansia* was found to increase transcriptional levels of IL-6 in the colon in mice treated with Azoxymethane/DSS and antibiotics [49], whereas IL-6 was reduced by *Akkermansia* in mice with DSS-induced colitis [50].

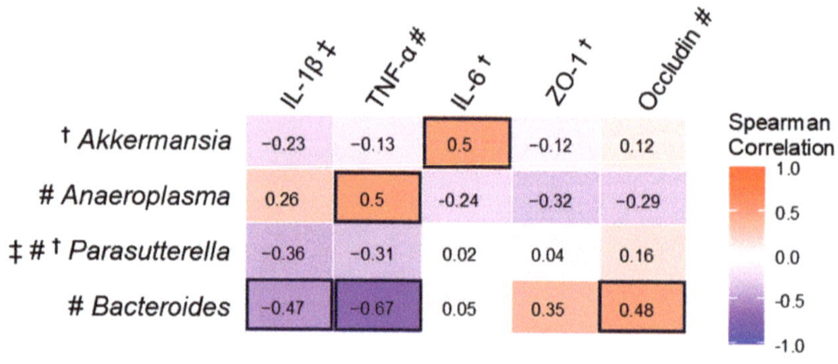

Figure 7. Gut microbiome at the genus level correlated with relative mRNA levels of cytokines and tight junction proteins in the colon. † significantly affected by DMW; # significantly affected by gene; ‡ significantly affected by DMW × gene interaction. Rectangles with dark outlines indicate significant correlations. Numbers in the rectangles are the correlation coefficients.

The dose of DMW used in this study was equivalent to 1.5 glasses of wine for a 60-kg adult, which is twice the daily amount estimated for regular wine drinkers (0.5–0.7 glasses of wine per day). However, the obstacles of high dose and alcohol content can be solved by non-alcoholic wines, which have gained popularity among consumers in recent years. Such a trend will help to translate these preclinical results to the human population.

The IL-10$^{-/-}$ C57BL/6 mice in this study developed very mild colitis after 22 weeks of feeding, which may have limited the bioactivities of DMW; this remains a limitation of this study. The 16S rRNA sequencing resolved the gut microbiome to the genus level. The lack of abundance at the species level or functional data was another limitation of this study. Other limitations included not considering the cage effect for β-diversity analysis, lack of histological data, and possible genetic compensation for the lost IL-10 function in the knockout mice. It should also be noted that the significant statistical effects of DMW × gene interaction should not be misunderstood as biological signaling.

4. Conclusions

This study was among the few that investigated how chronic intake of polyphenols impacts colitis development in genetically susceptible mice compared to wild-type counterparts. Results showed that DMW and DMW × gene interaction reduced intestinal permeability, gene expression of inflammatory cytokines, and serum TNF-α, and enhanced the gene expression of tight junction proteins (ZO-1) in IL-10$^{-/-}$ mice. DMW significantly reduced the relative abundances of *Parasutterella* and *Akkermansia* in the IL-10$^{-/-}$ mice. These results suggested that polyphenols from DMW moderately alleviated the development of colitis in IL-10$^{-/-}$ mice and could be a useful dietary strategy for IBD prevention. Results in this study should be verified in a future study using mouse strains that are more susceptible to colitis development, such as the 29/SvEv or BALB/c mice. Modulation of the gut microbiome should be verified using whole-genome sequencing.

Supplementary Materials: The following supporting information can be downloaded at: https://www.mdpi.com/article/10.3390/nu17142327/s1, Table S1. Nutrition composition of the control diet, DMW, and diet with 4.8% (*w*/*v*) DMW. Table S2: Experimental design and mouse grouping. Table S3. Genes and primers for RT-qPCR. Table S4 Pairwise-PERMANOVA results based on unweighted UniFrac distance. Table S5 Pairwise-PERMANOVA results based on weighted UniFrac distance. Figure S1: HPLC chromatogram of anthocyanins (A) and other polyphenols (B) in DMW using 520 nm and 360 nm detection, respectively. Peaks 1, 2, 3, 4, 5 and 6 in panel A are delphinidin-3,5-diglucoside, cyanidin-3,5-diglucoside, petunidin-3,5-diglucoside, pelargonidin-3,5-diglucoside, peonidin-3,5-diglucoside and malvidin-3,5-diglucoside, respectively. Peaks 7, 8, 9 and 10 in panel B are ellagic acid, myricetin, quercetin, and kaempferol, respectively.

Author Contributions: H.L.: Investigation, data curation, formal analysis, writing—original draft. L.G.: conceptualization, supervision, formal analysis, writing—review and editing. All authors have read and agreed to the published version of the manuscript.

Funding: This research was funded by a grant from the National Institute of Food and Agriculture (No: 2019-67017-29366).

Institutional Review Board Statement: Experiments on mice were approved by the Institutional Animal Care and Use Committee of the University of Florida (Protocol: 201910540, date of approval: 6 March 2019).

Informed Consent Statement: Not applicable.

Data Availability Statement: The original contributions presented in the study are included in the article/Supplementary Material; further inquiries can be directed to the corresponding author.

Conflicts of Interest: There are no conflicts of interest.

Abbreviations

DAI	Disease activity index
DMW	Dealcoholized muscadine wine
DSS	Dextran sulfate sodium
FITC	Fluorescein isothiocyanate
IBD	Inflammatory bowel diseases
WT	Wild type

References

1. Hracs, L.; Windsor, J.W.; Gorospe, J.; Cummings, M.; Coward, S.; Buie, M.J.; Quan, J.; Goddard, Q.; Caplan, L.; Markovinović, A.; et al. Global IBD Visualization of Epidemiology Studies in the 21st Century (GIVES-21) Research Group Global evolution of inflammatory bowel disease across epidemiologic stages. *Nature* **2025**, *642*, 458–466. [CrossRef] [PubMed]
2. Fanizza, J.; Bencardino, S.; Allocca, M.; Furfaro, F.; Zilli, A.; Parigi, T.L.; Fiorino, G.; Peyrin-Biroulet, L.; Danese, S.; D'Amico, F. Inflammatory bowel disease and colorectal cancer. *Cancers* **2024**, *16*, 2943. [CrossRef] [PubMed]
3. Tang, J.; Zhang, M.; Wang, J.; Zhang, H.; Wang, Z.; Lei, Z.; Wang, C.; Chen, W. Hydroxytyrosol Ameliorates Colon Inflammation: Mechanistic Insights into Anti-Inflammatory Effects, Inhibition of the TLR4/NF-κB Signaling Pathway, Gut Microbiota Modulation, and Liver Protection. *Foods* **2025**, *14*, 1270. [CrossRef] [PubMed]
4. Yaqin, Z.; Kehan, W.; Yi, Z.; Naijian, W.; Wei, Q.; Fei, M. Resveratrol alleviates inflammatory bowel disease by inhibiting JAK2/STAT3 pathway activity via the reduction of O-GlcNAcylation of STAT3 in intestinal epithelial cells. *Toxicol. Appl. Pharmacol.* **2024**, *484*, 116882. [CrossRef] [PubMed]
5. Gao, R.; Ren, Y.; Xue, P.; Sheng, Y.; Yang, Q.; Dai, Y.; Zhang, X.; Lin, Z.; Liu, T.; Geng, Y.; et al. Protective Effect of the Polyphenol Ligustroside on Colitis Induced with Dextran Sulfate Sodium in Mice. *Nutrients* **2024**, *16*, 522. [CrossRef] [PubMed]
6. Li, R.; Kim, M.-H.; Sandhu, A.K.; Gao, C.; Gu, L. Muscadine grape (Vitis rotundifolia) or wine phytochemicals reduce intestinal inflammation in mice with dextran sulfate sodium-induced colitis. *J. Agric. Food Chem.* **2017**, *65*, 769–776. [CrossRef] [PubMed]
7. Pastrana-Bonilla, E.; Akoh, C.C.; Sellappan, S.; Krewer, G. Phenolic content and antioxidant capacity of muscadine grapes. *J. Agric. Food Chem.* **2003**, *51*, 5497–5503. [CrossRef] [PubMed]
8. Greenspan, P.; Bauer, J.D.; Pollock, S.H.; Gangemi, J.D.; Mayer, E.P.; Ghaffar, A.; Hargrove, J.L.; Hartle, D.K. Antiinflammatory properties of the muscadine grape (Vitis rotundifolia). *J. Agric. Food Chem.* **2005**, *53*, 8481–8484. [CrossRef] [PubMed]
9. Bralley, E.E.; Hargrove, J.L.; Greenspan, P.; Hartle, D.K. Topical anti-inflammatory activities of Vitis rotundifolia (muscadine grape) extracts in the tetradecanoylphorbol acetate model of ear inflammation. *J. Med. Food* **2007**, *10*, 636–642. [CrossRef] [PubMed]
10. Keubler, L.M.; Buettner, M.; Häger, C.; Bleich, A. A Multihit Model: Colitis Lessons from the Interleukin-10-deficient Mouse. *Inflamm. Bowel Dis.* **2015**, *21*, 1967–1975. [CrossRef] [PubMed]
11. Wang, H.; Xue, Y.; Zhang, H.; Huang, Y.; Yang, G.; Du, M.; Zhu, M.-J. Dietary grape seed extract ameliorates symptoms of inflammatory bowel disease in IL10-deficient mice. *Mol. Nutr. Food Res.* **2013**, *57*, 2253–2257. [CrossRef] [PubMed]
12. Li, R.; Wang, G.P.; Whitlock, J.A.; Zhao, S.; Yagiz, Y.; Gu, L. Muscadine grapes (Vitis rotundifolia) and dealcoholized muscadine wine alleviated symptoms of colitis and protected against dysbiosis in mice exposed to dextran sulfate sodium. *J. Funct. Foods* **2020**, *65*, 103746. [CrossRef]
13. Mishra, U.N.; Jena, D.; Sahu, C.; Devi, R.; Kumar, R.; Jena, R.; Irondi, E.A.; Rout, S.; Tiwari, R.K.; Lal, M.K.; et al. Nutrigenomics: An inimitable interaction amid genomics, nutrition and health. *Innov. Food Sci. Emerg. Technol.* **2022**, *82*, 103196. [CrossRef]
14. Shaw, C.L.; Dolan, R.; Corsi, A.M.; Goodman, S.; Pearson, W. Exploring the barriers and triggers towards the adoption of low- and no-alcohol (NOLO) wines. *Food Qual. Prefer.* **2023**, *110*, 104932. [CrossRef]
15. Shin, J.-M.; Hwang, Y.-O.; Tu, O.-J.; Jo, H.-B.; Kim, J.-H.; Chae, Y.-Z.; Rhu, K.-H.; Park, S.-K. Comparison of different methods to quantify fat classes in bakery products. *Food Chem.* **2013**, *136*, 703–709. [CrossRef] [PubMed]
16. Hurtubise, R.; Audiger, C.; Dominguez-Punaro, M.C.; Chabot-Roy, G.; Chognard, G.; Raymond-Marchand, L.; Coderre, L.; Chemtob, S.; Michnick, S.W.; Rioux, J.D.; et al. Induced and spontaneous colitis mouse models reveal complex interactions between IL-10 and IL-12/IL-23 pathways. *Cytokine* **2019**, *121*, 154738. [CrossRef] [PubMed]
17. Okayasu, I.; Hatakeyama, S.; Yamada, M.; Ohkusa, T.; Inagaki, Y.; Nakaya, R. A novel method in the induction of reliable experimental acute and chronic ulcerative colitis in mice. *Gastroenterology* **1990**, *98*, 694–702. [CrossRef] [PubMed]
18. Nair, A.B.; Jacob, S. A simple practice guide for dose conversion between animals and human. *J. Basic Clin. Pharm.* **2016**, *7*, 27–31. [CrossRef] [PubMed]
19. Kang, Y.; Yang, G.; Zhang, S.; Ross, C.F.; Zhu, M.-J. Goji Berry Modulates Gut Microbiota and Alleviates Colitis in IL-10-Deficient Mice. *Mol. Nutr. Food Res.* **2018**, *62*, e1800535. [CrossRef] [PubMed]

20. Yang, I.; Eibach, D.; Kops, F.; Brenneke, B.; Woltemate, S.; Schulze, J.; Bleich, A.; Gruber, A.D.; Muthupalani, S.; Fox, J.G.; et al. Intestinal microbiota composition of interleukin-10 deficient C57BL/6J mice and susceptibility to Helicobacter hepaticus-induced colitis. *PLoS ONE* **2013**, *8*, e70783. [CrossRef] [PubMed]
21. Li, S.; Jin, Y.; Fu, W.; Cox, A.D.; Lee, D.; Reddivari, L. Intermittent antibiotic treatment accelerated the development of colitis in IL-10 knockout mice. *Biomed. Pharmacother.* **2022**, *146*, 112486. [CrossRef] [PubMed]
22. Zhao, L.; Zhang, Y.; Liu, G.; Hao, S.; Wang, C.; Wang, Y. Black rice anthocyanin-rich extract and rosmarinic acid, alone and in combination, protect against DSS-induced colitis in mice. *Food Funct.* **2018**, *9*, 2796–2808. [CrossRef] [PubMed]
23. Larmonier, C.B.; Uno, J.K.; Lee, K.-M.; Karrasch, T.; Laubitz, D.; Thurston, R.; Midura-Kiela, M.T.; Ghishan, F.K.; Sartor, R.B.; Jobin, C.; et al. Limited effects of dietary curcumin on Th-1 driven colitis in IL-10 deficient mice suggest an IL-10-dependent mechanism of protection. *Am. J. Physiol. Gastrointest. Liver Physiol.* **2008**, *295*, G1079–G1091. [CrossRef] [PubMed]
24. Zhao, Z.; Liu, X.; Zhang, R.; Ke, R.; Zhang, S.; Chen, Y. Intestinal barrier in inflammatory bowel disease: Mechanisms and treatment. *J. Transl. Gastroenterol.* **2025**. [CrossRef]
25. Yang, G.; Xue, Y.; Zhang, H.; Du, M.; Zhu, M.-J. Favourable effects of grape seed extract on intestinal epithelial differentiation and barrier function in IL10-deficient mice. *Br. J. Nutr.* **2015**, *114*, 15–23. [CrossRef] [PubMed]
26. Yang, N.; Shang, Y.-X. Epigallocatechin gallate ameliorates airway inflammation by regulating Treg/Th17 imbalance in an asthmatic mouse model. *Int. Immunopharmacol.* **2019**, *72*, 422–428. [CrossRef] [PubMed]
27. Yin, Q.; Wang, L.; Yu, H.; Chen, D.; Zhu, W.; Sun, C. Pharmacological Effects of Polyphenol Phytochemicals on the JAK-STAT Signaling Pathway. *Front. Pharmacol.* **2021**, *12*, 716672. [CrossRef] [PubMed]
28. Elhennawy, M.G.; Abdelaleem, E.A.; Zaki, A.A.; Mohamed, W.R. Cinnamaldehyde and hesperetin attenuate TNBS-induced ulcerative colitis in rats through modulation of the JAk2/STAT3/SOCS3 pathway. *J. Biochem. Mol. Toxicol.* **2021**, *35*, e22730. [CrossRef] [PubMed]
29. Han, D.; Wu, Y.; Lu, D.; Pang, J.; Hu, J.; Zhang, X.; Wang, Z.; Zhang, G.; Wang, J. Polyphenol-rich diet mediates interplay between macrophage-neutrophil and gut microbiota to alleviate intestinal inflammation. *Cell Death Dis.* **2023**, *14*, 656. [CrossRef] [PubMed]
30. Li, L.; Wang, L.; Wu, Z.; Yao, L.; Wu, Y.; Huang, L.; Liu, K.; Zhou, X.; Gou, D. Anthocyanin-rich fractions from red raspberries attenuate inflammation in both RAW264.7 macrophages and a mouse model of colitis. *Sci. Rep.* **2014**, *4*, 6234. [CrossRef] [PubMed]
31. Li, S.; Wang, T.; Wu, B.; Fu, W.; Xu, B.; Pamuru, R.R.; Kennett, M.; Vanamala, J.K.P.; Reddivari, L. Anthocyanin-containing purple potatoes ameliorate DSS-induced colitis in mice. *J. Nutr. Biochem.* **2021**, *93*, 108616. [CrossRef] [PubMed]
32. Turner, N.A.; Mughal, R.S.; Warburton, P.; O'Regan, D.J.; Ball, S.G.; Porter, K.E. Mechanism of TNFalpha-induced IL-1alpha, IL-1beta and IL-6 expression in human cardiac fibroblasts: Effects of statins and thiazolidinediones. *Cardiovasc. Res.* **2007**, *76*, 81–90. [CrossRef] [PubMed]
33. Lee, B.; Moon, K.M.; Kim, C.Y. Tight Junction in the Intestinal Epithelium: Its Association with Diseases and Regulation by Phytochemicals. *J. Immunol. Res.* **2018**, *2018*, 2645465. [CrossRef] [PubMed]
34. Mo, J.; Ni, J.; Zhang, M.; Xu, Y.; Li, Y.; Karim, N.; Chen, W. Mulberry Anthocyanins Ameliorate DSS-Induced Ulcerative Colitis by Improving Intestinal Barrier Function and Modulating Gut Microbiota. *Antioxidants* **2022**, *11*, 1674. [CrossRef] [PubMed]
35. Nunes, C.; Freitas, V.; Almeida, L.; Laranjinha, J. Red wine extract preserves tight junctions in intestinal epithelial cells under inflammatory conditions: Implications for intestinal inflammation. *Food Funct.* **2019**, *10*, 1364–1374. [CrossRef] [PubMed]
36. Li, H.; Christman, L.M.; Li, R.; Gu, L. Synergic interactions between polyphenols and gut microbiota in mitigating inflammatory bowel diseases. *Food Funct.* **2020**, *11*, 4878–4891. [CrossRef] [PubMed]
37. Li, Y.; Yuan, F.; He, X.; Fu, S.; Fan, B. Anthocyanin extract from black rice attenuates chronic inflammation in DSS-induced colitis mouse model by modulating the gut microbiota. *Open Chem.* **2023**, *21*, 20220288. [CrossRef]
38. Moon, H.-J.; Cha, Y.-S.; Kim, K.-A. Blackcurrant Alleviates Dextran Sulfate Sodium (DSS)-Induced Colitis in Mice. *Foods* **2023**, *12*, 1073. [CrossRef] [PubMed]
39. Yang, J.; Germano, P.M.; Oh, S.; Wang, S.; Wang, J.; Lee, R.; Paige, H.; Yang, S.; Henning, S.M.; Zhong, J.; et al. Pomegranate Extract Improves Colitis in IL-10 Knockout Mice Fed a High Fat High Sucrose Diet. *Mol. Nutr. Food Res.* **2022**, *66*, e2100730. [CrossRef] [PubMed]
40. Lozupone, C.; Knight, R. UniFrac: A new phylogenetic method for comparing microbial communities. *Appl. Environ. Microbiol.* **2005**, *71*, 8228–8235. [CrossRef] [PubMed]
41. Zafar, H.; Saier, M.H. Gut *Bacteroides* species in health and disease. *Gut Microbes* **2021**, *13*, 1–20. [CrossRef] [PubMed]
42. Chen, Q.; He, Z.; Zhuo, Y.; Li, S.; Yang, W.; Hu, L.; Zhong, H. Rubidium chloride modulated the fecal microbiota community in mice. *BMC Microbiol.* **2021**, *21*, 46. [CrossRef] [PubMed]
43. Wan, P.; Peng, Y.; Chen, G.; Xie, M.; Dai, Z.; Huang, K.; Dong, W.; Zeng, X.; Sun, Y. Modulation of gut microbiota by Ilex kudingcha improves dextran sulfate sodium-induced colitis. *Food Res. Int.* **2019**, *126*, 108595. [CrossRef] [PubMed]

44. Seregin, S.S.; Golovchenko, N.; Schaf, B.; Chen, J.; Pudlo, N.A.; Mitchell, J.; Baxter, N.T.; Zhao, L.; Schloss, P.D.; Martens, E.C.; et al. NLRP6 Protects Il10-/- Mice from Colitis by Limiting Colonization of Akkermansia muciniphila. *Cell Rep.* **2017**, *19*, 733–745. [CrossRef] [PubMed]
45. López-Cauce, B.; Puerto, M.; García, J.J.; Ponce-Alonso, M.; Becerra-Aparicio, F.; Del Campo, R.; Peligros, I.; Fernández-Aceñero, M.J.; Gómez-Navarro, Y.; Lara, J.M.; et al. Akkermansia deficiency and mucin depletion are implicated in intestinal barrier dysfunction as earlier event in the development of inflammation in interleukin-10-deficient mice. *Front. Microbiol.* **2022**, *13*, 1083884. [CrossRef] [PubMed]
46. Everard, A.; Belzer, C.; Geurts, L.; Ouwerkerk, J.P.; Druart, C.; Bindels, L.B.; Guiot, Y.; Derrien, M.; Muccioli, G.G.; Delzenne, N.M.; et al. Cross-talk between Akkermansia muciniphila and intestinal epithelium controls diet-induced obesity. *Proc. Natl. Acad. Sci. USA* **2013**, *110*, 9066–9071. [CrossRef] [PubMed]
47. Price, C.E.; Valls, R.A.; Ramsey, A.R.; Loeven, N.A.; Jones, J.T.; Barrack, K.E.; Schwartzman, J.D.; Royce, D.B.; Cramer, R.A.; Madan, J.C.; et al. Intestinal Bacteroides modulates inflammation, systemic cytokines, and microbial ecology via propionate in a mouse model of cystic fibrosis. *MBio* **2024**, *15*, e0314423. [CrossRef] [PubMed]
48. He, Q.; Niu, M.; Bi, J.; Du, N.; Liu, S.; Yang, K.; Li, H.; Yao, J.; Du, Y.; Duan, Y. Protective effects of a new generation of probiotic Bacteroides fragilis against colitis in vivo and in vitro. *Sci. Rep.* **2023**, *13*, 15842. [CrossRef] [PubMed]
49. Wang, K.; Wu, W.; Wang, Q.; Yang, L.; Bian, X.; Jiang, X.; Lv, L.; Yan, R.; Xia, J.; Han, S.; et al. The negative effect of Akkermansia muciniphila-mediated post-antibiotic reconstitution of the gut microbiota on the development of colitis-associated colorectal cancer in mice. *Front. Microbiol.* **2022**, *13*, 932047. [CrossRef] [PubMed]
50. Zhang, H.; Pan, Y.; Jiang, Y.; Chen, M.; Ma, X.; Yu, X.; Ren, D.; Jiang, B. Akkermansia muciniphila ONE effectively ameliorates dextran sulfate sodium (DSS)-induced ulcerative colitis in mice. *Npj Sci. Food* **2024**, *8*, 97. [CrossRef] [PubMed]

nutrients

MDPI

Article

Artemisiae Iwayomogii Herba Protects Dopaminergic Neurons Against 1-Methyl-4-phenylpyridinium/1-methyl-4-phenyl-1,2,3,6-tetrahydropyridine Neurotoxicity in Models of Parkinson's Disease

Hanbyeol Lee [1,†], In Gyoung Ju [2,†], Jin Hee Kim [1], Yujin Choi [1], Seungmin Lee [1], Hi-Joon Park [3,4] and Myung Sook Oh [1,2,*]

1 Department of Biomedical and Pharmaceutical Sciences, Graduate School, Kyung Hee University, Seoul 02447, Republic of Korea
2 Department of Oriental Pharmaceutical Science and Kyung Hee East-West Pharmaceutical Research Institute, College of Pharmacy, Kyung Hee University, Seoul 02447, Republic of Korea
3 Department of Science in Korean Medicine, College of Korean Medicine, Kyung Hee University, Seoul 02447, Republic of Korea; acufind@khu.ac.kr
4 Acupuncture and Meridian Science Research Center (AMSRC), Kyung Hee University, Seoul 02447, Republic of Korea
* Correspondence: msohok@khu.ac.kr; Tel.: +82-2-961-9436; Fax: +82-2-963-9436
† These authors contributed equally to this work.

Abstract: Background/Objectives: Parkinson's disease (PD) is a common neurodegenerative disease characterized by motor symptoms caused by the loss of dopaminergic neurons. While the pathophysiology of PD is still not fully understood, it is recognized that oxidative stress plays a major role in its progression. Previous studies have shown that the aerial parts of *Artemisia iwayomogi* Kitamura (AIK) possess medicinal properties, including antioxidant activity. This study aimed to investigate whether AIK can alleviate neuronal loss and motor symptoms in a PD model and to explore its therapeutic mechanisms. **Methods:** For the in vitro study, PC12 cells were treated with AIK and 1-methyl-4-phenylpyridinium (MPP^+). For the in vivo study, C57BL/6J mice were orally administered AIK for 12 days; they received intraperitoneal injections of 1-methyl-4-phenyl-1,2,3,6-tetrahydropyridine (MPTP) for 5 consecutive days, starting on the 8th day of AIK administration. **Results:** AIK treatment to PC12 cells in the presence of MPP^+ enhanced the phosphorylation of the protein kinase B/glycogen synthase kinase-3β signaling pathway, which is a crucial regulator of nuclear factor erythroid 2-related factor 2 (Nrf2) translocation. Additionally, AIK treatment increased cell survival and induced an antioxidant response involving heme oxygenase-1, via increasing the level of Nrf2 in the nucleus. In an MPTP-induced mouse model of PD, AIK administration activated Nrf2 in dopaminergic neurons and prevented the loss of dopaminergic neurons in the brain, which in turn alleviated motor dysfunction. **Conclusions:** Collectively, these findings suggest that AIK is a potential botanical candidate for PD treatment by protecting dopaminergic neurons through antioxidant activity.

Keywords: Parkinson's disease; *Artemisia iwayomogi*; nuclear factor erythroid 2-related factor 2; heme oxygenase-1

1. Introduction

Parkinson's disease (PD) is the second most common neurodegenerative disorder. Typically, PD develops after age 60, with incidence increasing with age [1]. Motor symptoms such as bradykinesia and postural instability are indicative of PD [2]. PD has key pathological features of progressive loss of dopaminergic neurons in the substantia nigra pars compacta (SNpc) and the formation of Lewy bodies [3]. The standard treatment for PD is dopamine replacement therapy (DRT), which supplements depleted dopamine levels. Levodopa (L-DOPA), a precursor of dopamine, is commonly used with dopamine agonists and monoamine oxidase B inhibitors [4]. However, DRT does not have a positive impact on disease progression, and there is currently no disease-modifying therapy available to slow or halt disease progression [5].

The pathogenesis of PD is thought to involve a multifaceted pathophysiological process, with several key pathogenic factors identified to date, including mitochondrial dysfunction, oxidative stress, and neuroinflammation [6]. Environmental and genetic variables cause mitochondrial malfunction, which raises reactive oxygen species (ROS) and worsens oxidative stress [7]. An imbalance between the capacity of the body to detoxify reactive chemicals and the generation of ROS results in oxidative stress, which seriously damages cellular structures [8].

In the PD brain, increased ROS buildup has been shown in numerous studies to be a significant factor in inflammation and dopaminergic neuronal death, which further accelerates neurodegenerative processes [9–11]. The SN is widely recognized to be especially susceptible to oxidative stress as it contains a high density of dopaminergic neurons [12]. Thus, oxidative stress has been recognized as a main mechanism for the death of dopaminergic neurons in PD [6]. Therefore, strategies aimed at controlling oxidative stress-induced cellular damage are crucial for preventing neurodegeneration.

Artemisia iwayomogi Kitamura (AIK) is a plant in the Compositae family that is distributed throughout Korea and commonly known as "Hanin-jin" or "Dowijigi" [13]. The aerial parts of AIK have been used in traditional medicine for the treatment of various liver diseases [14]. The various biological functions of AIK have been proven through numerous studies. Aqueous extracts of AIK have been shown to suppress mast-cell-mediated allergic reactions [15] and exhibit hepatoprotective activity against carbon tetrachloride-induced liver fibrosis in rats [16]. In other studies, polyphenolic extracts of AIK were shown to inhibit the expression of pro-inflammatory mediators induced by lipopolysaccharide (LPS) and to attenuate high-fat-diet-induced hypertriglyceridemia in mice [17,18]. Additionally, it has been demonstrated that the scopoletin that was separated from AIK possesses cellular antioxidant, reduction, and superoxide radical scavenging activities [19]. However, whether AIK can regulate the oxidative stress that causes neurological diseases and improve PD has yet to be investigated.

This study was conducted to investigate the potential ameliorative effects of AIK on PD in both in vitro and in vivo models. We examined how AIK treatment affects the defense mechanisms against oxidative stress in PC12 cells under 1-methyl-4-phenylpyridinium (MPP^+)-induced PD conditions. We also assessed whether AIK administration alleviates the behavioral and histological changes in PD in an animal model induced by 1-methyl-4-phenyl-1,2,3,6-tetrahydropyridine (MPTP).

2. Materials and Methods

2.1. Materials

2,2-azinobis-(3-ethyl-benzthiazolin-6-sulphonic acid) (ABTS), 2,2-diphenyl-1-picrylhydrazyl (DPPH), MPP^+ iodide, 3-(4,5-dimethylthiazol-2-yl)-2,5-diphenyl-2H-tetrazolium bromide (MTT), MPTP, L-DOPA, and benserazide hydrochloride were purchased from Sigma-Aldrich (St. Louis, MO, USA). Rabbit anti-protein kinase B (Akt, #9272), anti-phospho-Akt (Ser473, #4060), anti-glycogen synthase kinase-3β (GSK3β, #12456), and phospho-GSK3β (Ser9, #5558) antibodies were obtained from Cell Signaling Technology (Danvers, MA, USA).

Mouse anti-proliferating cell nuclear antigen (PCNA, 610665) was purchased from BD Biosciences (Bergen County, NJ, USA). Mouse horseradish peroxidase (HRP)-conjugated β-actin antibody (sc-47778) was purchased from Santa Cruz Biotechnology (Temecula, CA, USA). Anti-rabbit HRP secondary antibody (ADI-SAB-300) and rabbit anti-heme oxygenase-1 (HO-1, ADI-SPA-895) antibody were acquired from Enzo Life Science, Inc. (Farmingdale, NY, USA). Rabbit anti-nuclear factor erythroid 2-related factor 2 (Nrf2) antibody (AB31163) was purchased from Abcam (Cambridge, UK). Rabbit anti-tyrosine hydroxylase (TH, AB152) antibody, rat anti-dopamine transporter (DAT, MAB369) antibody, and 3,3′-diaminobenzidine (DAB) were purchased from Merck Millipore (Burlington, MA, USA). Mouse anti-TH antibody (MA1-24654) and radio-immunoprecipitation assay lysis buffer (RIPA) was purchased from Thermo Fisher Scientific (Waltham, MA, USA). Biotinylated anti-rabbit immunoglobulin G (IgG) antibody (BA-1000), biotinylated anti-rat IgG antibody (BA-4000), avidin–biotin complex (ABC), anti-rabbit DyLight 594 (DI-1594), and anti-mouse DyLight 488 (DI-2488) were purchased from Vector Labs (Burlingame, CA, USA).

2.2. Preparation and Standardization of AIK Extract

AIK was purchased from Naemomedah (Kwangmyoungdang Medicinal Herbs, Ulsan, Republic of Korea). AIK was prepared following previously reported methods. In brief, AIK was extracted with 70% ethanol for 3 h using reflux extraction. The extract was filtered, evaporated, and lyophilized into a powder. AIK was dissolved in the vehicle before each experiment. AIK was standardized based on scopoletin and isochlorogenic acid B using ultra-performance liquid chromatography–mass spectrometry, in our previous study [20].

2.3. ABTS Radical Cation Scavenging Assay

One day before the experiment, 2.6 mM potassium persulfate was added to 7.4 mM ABTS solution in dark conditions. The absorbance was measured at 732 nm with a microplate reader (Sunnyvale, CA, USA) after the incubation of the pre-made ABTS solution with various concentrations of AIK for 5 min. We used an extract of *Scutellaria baicalensis* Georgi root (SB) as a positive control to assess the potency of AIK, as SB is well-known for its outstanding radical scavenging activities [21,22]. The concentration required to scavenge 50% of the ABTS cation is known as the half-maximal inhibitory concentration (IC_{50}), and it was used to express the antioxidant capacity. The cation scavenging capacity of ABTS was determined using the following equation:

$$ABTS\ cation\ scavenging\ activity\ (\%) = (Control - Sample)/Control \times 100.$$

2.4. DPPH Radical Scavenging Assay

A microplate reader was used to detect absorbance at 517 nm after a 0.2 mM DPPH ethanolic solution was combined with different concentrations of AIK and left in the dark for 30 min. SB was used as a positive control. IC_{50} values were used to express the antioxidant capacity against the DPPH radical. The following equation was used to determine the DPPH radical scavenging capacity:

$$\text{DPPH radical scavenging activity } (\%) = \{\text{Control} - (\text{Sample} - \text{Blank})\}/\text{Control} \times 100$$

2.5. Cell Culture and Drug Treatment

PC12 rat pheochromocytoma cells were cultured in Roswell Park Memorial Institute 1640 medium supplemented with 10% fetal bovine serum and 1% penicillin–streptomycin. The cells were incubated at 37 °C under a humidified atmosphere containing 5% CO_2. The cells were seeded at a density of 3.0×10^5 cells/mL in 96-well plates or 1.0×10^6 cells/well in 6-well plates. After seeding, the cells were allowed to adhere for an additional 24 h. Prior to MPP^+ treatment, the cells were pre-exposed to various concentrations of AIK for 1 h, followed by treatment with equal volumes of vehicle for both the control (CON) and MPP^+-treated groups. Subsequently, the cells were treated with or without 1 mM MPP^+ for 48 h for MTT assays or 4 h for Western blot analysis.

2.6. Measurement of Cell Viability

The MTT assay was used to evaluate cell viability. Briefly, 1 mg/mL of MTT was added to the cells and incubated for 3 h at 37 °C. Following the dimethyl sulfoxide dilution of the MTT formazan, the absorbance was measured at 570 nm using a microplate reader.

2.7. Western Blotting

Samples were harvested and lysed using RIPA buffer supplemented with protease and phosphatase inhibitors for whole-cell lysis. For the isolation of cytoplasmic and nuclear fractions, the collected cells were rinsed with phosphate-buffered saline (PBS) and subsequently resuspended in lysis buffer (10 mM HEPES [pH 7.9], 50 mM KCl, 1 mM EDTA, 1 mM DTT, and protease–phosphatase inhibitor cocktail). The suspension was then placed on ice for 3 min, followed by the addition of 0.075% IGEPAL CA-630. After mixing thoroughly, the samples were subjected to centrifugation at 15,000 rpm for 4 min, yielding the cytoplasmic fraction in the supernatant. The nuclear pellet was resuspended in nuclear extraction buffer (20 mM HEPES [pH 8.0], 400 mM NaCl, 1 mM EDTA, 1 mM EGTA, 1 mM DTT, and protease phosphatase inhibitor cocktail). The samples were then incubated on ice for 10 min, vortexed for 10 s, and centrifuged at 15,000 rpm for 10 min. The resulting supernatant was collected as the nuclear fraction. The resulting supernatant was used as the nuclear fraction. All protein samples were stored in a deep freezer at − 80 °C.

The Bradford protein assay was used to quantify protein concentration. After being denatured, cell lysates were separated using sodium dodecyl sulfate-polyacrylamide gel electrophoresis. Following the transfer of proteins onto polyvinylidene fluoride membranes, the membranes were blocked for 1 h using 5% bovine serum albumin. Primary antibodies were applied to the membranes overnight at 4 °C. Membranes containing bound primary antibodies were applied to secondary antibodies, and the reaction was allowed to proceed at room temperature for 1 h. The immunoreactive bands were located using the enhanced chemiluminescence reagent. The band intensity was viewed using the Image Lab (Bio-Rad Laboratories, Hercules, CA, USA) and quantified using ImageJ 1.38x (National Institutes of Health, Bethesda, MD, USA).

2.8. Animals and Drug Treatment

Seven-week-old male C57BL/6J mice were purchased from Daehan Biolink (Eumseong, Republic of Korea). The mice were kept in a room with consistent humidity (60 ± 10%), light/dark cycles lasting 12 h, and a temperature of 23 ± 1 °C. Food and water were freely available to the animals. Every animal study was conducted in accordance with the National Institutes of Health's "Guide for the Care and Use of Laboratory Animals, 8th edition" (2011) and authorized by "Animal Care and Use Guidelines" of Kyung Hee University (Seoul, Republic of Korea, approval number: KHSASP-18-167; approved on 16 January 2019).

The mice were randomly divided into six groups: (1) NOR group (normal mice; intraperitoneally injected saline plus intraorally administered vehicle, $n = 8$); (2) MPTP group (intraperitoneally injected MPTP plus intraorally administered vehicle, $n = 10$); (3) MPTP + AIK 30 group (intraperitoneally injected MPTP plus intraorally administered AIK 30 mg/kg/day, $n = 8$); (4) MPTP + AIK 100 group (intraperitoneally injected MPTP plus intraorally administered AIK 100 mg/kg/day, $n = 7$); (5) MPTP + AIK 300 group (intraperitoneally injected MPTP plus intraorally administered AIK 300 mg/kg/day, $n = 8$); (6) MPTP + L-DOPA group (intraperitoneally injected MPTP plus intraorally administered L-DOPA 80 mg/kg/day with Benserazide 20 mg/kg/day, $n = 8$). The dosage of AIK was determined based on prior reports [20,23]. AIK, L-DOPA, and Benserazide were dissolved in vehicle (2% Tween 80) and were administered intraorally once per day for 12 days. MPTP was dissolved in saline and intraperitoneally injected at 30 mg/kg/day for 5 consecutive days from the 8th day of AIK administration. The time scheme of experimental procedures was shown in the Supplementary Information (Figure S1).

2.9. Rotarod Test

The rotarod test was performed 8 days after the last injection of MPTP. Mice were trained 1 day prior to the test. The apparatus used in the experiment had a spindle with a 3 cm diameter and was divided into five compartments. Training was performed at a constant speed of 10 rpm, and testing was performed at 11 rpm for 3 min. The time taken for each mouse to fall off the spindle for the first time and the total number of falls were measured.

2.10. Preparation of Brain Tissues

Tribromoethanol (312.5 mg/kg, *i.p.*) was used to administer anesthesia to each mouse 8 days after the last MPTP injection. The animals were then fixed with 4% paraformaldehyde in 0.1 M phosphate buffer after being transcardially perfused with 0.05 M PBS. Then, the brains of the mice were collected, post-fixed overnight in 4% PFA, and immersed in a solution containing 30% sucrose in PBS until they were dehydrated at 4 °C. Then, 25 μm thick coronal sections were created using a cryostat (Leica Microsystems Inc., Nussloch, Germany) and kept at 4 °C in a cryoprotectant solution (25% ethylene glycol, 25% glycerol, 0.05 M phosphate buffer).

2.11. Immunohistochemistry and Immunofluorescence

Brain sections were rinsed with PBS and treated with 1% hydrogen peroxide in 0.05 M PBS for 15 min. Following incubation, the sections underwent PBS wash before being exposed to anti-TH or anti-DAT antibody, which were dissolved in 0.3% Triton X-100 and incubated overnight at 4 °C. Next, the sections were treated with biotinylated anti-rabbit or anti-rat IgG antibody for 1 h, followed by ABC solution for 1 h at room temperature. Then, DAB was added to 0.05 M Tris buffer to improve staining visibility. Following several PBS washes, histomount media were used to mount the sections. Images were obtained with an optical bright-field microscope (Olympus Microscope System BX51; Olympus, Tokyo, Japan). Optical densities of TH- and DAT-positive areas were measured using the Image J software [National Institutes of Health (Bethesda, MD, USA)]. TH-immunopositive cells were quantified by stereological quantification. Data are shown as percentages of the NOR group values.

In order to obtain fluorescence images, brain sections were placed in anti-Nrf2 antibody overnight at 4 °C and then incubated with anti-rabbit Alexa 594 for 1 h at room temperature. The sections were rinsed with PBS, treated with anti-TH antibody for a whole night at 4 °C, then incubated with anti-mouse DyLight 488 for 1 h at room temperature. The sections were stained for 1 h with 4′,6-diamidino-2-phenylindole (DAPI) and then placed on an anti-fade fluorescent mounting medium. A Nanoscope Systems K1-Fluo confocal microscope (Nanoscope Systems, Daejeon, Republic of Korea) was used to take pictures.

2.12. Statistical Analysis

To calculate all statistical parameters, GraphPad Prism 8.0 software (Graphpad Software, San Diego, CA, USA) was used. The results were presented as the mean ± standard error of the mean (S.E.M.) and examined using one-way analysis of variance (ANOVA) followed by Dunnett's post hoc test. p values below 0.05 were regarded as statistically significant differences.

3. Results

3.1. Effects of AIK on Free Radical Scavenging Activities

The antioxidant activity of AIK was assessed by measuring its capacity to scavenge ABTS and DPPH radicals. In these experiments, SB, which has been reported to have potent antioxidant activity, was used as a positive control [22]. AIK exhibited dose-dependent scavenging activity against radicals in both assays. AIK showed IC_{50} values (μg/mL) of 32.95 and 25.14 for ABTS and DPPH radicals, respectively, which were comparable to those of the SB extract (Figure 1).

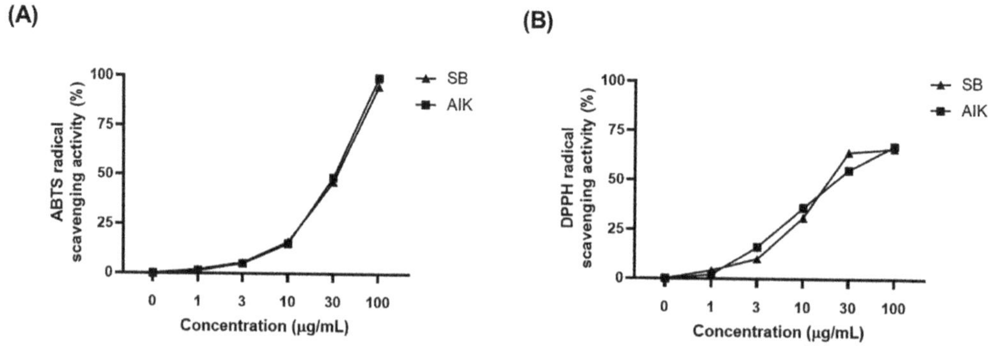

Figure 1. AIK possesses free radical scavenging activity. (**A**) ABTS radical cation and (**B**) DPPH free radical scavenging activities at concentrations of 1–100 μg/mL.

3.2. Effects of AIK on MPP^+-Induced Cytotoxicity in PC12 Cells

To determine the protective effect of AIK, we assessed the survival of PC12 cells after AIK treatment, with or without MPP^+ treatment. The cells were treated with different concentrations of AIK for 1 h before being exposed to MPP^+ for 48 h, after which we assessed the viability of the cells. The results showed that AIK alone had no significant effect on cell viability within the 10–100 μg/mL range. Treatment with 1 mM MPP^+ led to a considerable decrease in cell viability when compared to the CON group; however, pre-treatment with AIK was shown to significantly increase cell viability compared to the MPP^+-treated group (Figure 2).

3.3. Effects of AIK on Akt/GSK3β/Nrf2 Signaling Pathway in PC12 Cells

To explore how AIK protected PC12 cells, we analyzed whether it affected antioxidant factors. The phosphorylation of Akt/GSK3β is known to facilitate Nrf2 translocation [24]. To investigate whether AIK treatment affected the activation of the Akt/GSK3β signaling pathway, Western blot analysis was performed. Although the CON and MPP^+-treated group did not differ significantly, AIK pre-treatment markedly raised the phosphorylation levels of Akt (ser473) in comparison to the MPP^+-treatment group (Figure 3B). Treatment with MPP^+ reduced the GSK3β (ser9) phosphorylation, whereas treatment with AIK tended to increase levels (Figure 3C).

We then measured cytoplasmic and nuclear Nrf2 expression levels to assess the effect of AIK on the translocation of Nrf2. The AIK-treated group exhibited markedly elevated nuclear Nrf2 protein levels, whereas cytoplasmic Nrf2 levels were notably lower in the AIK-treated group compared to the MPP^+-treated group (Figure 3E,F). The movement of

Nrf2 from the cytoplasm to the nucleus plays a role in regulating HO-1 expression [25]. The MPP$^+$-treated group showed a marked decrease in HO-1 protein expression relative to the CON group, whereas the HO-1 protein levels in the AIK-treated group were considerably restored to levels similar to those of the CON group (Figure 3G).

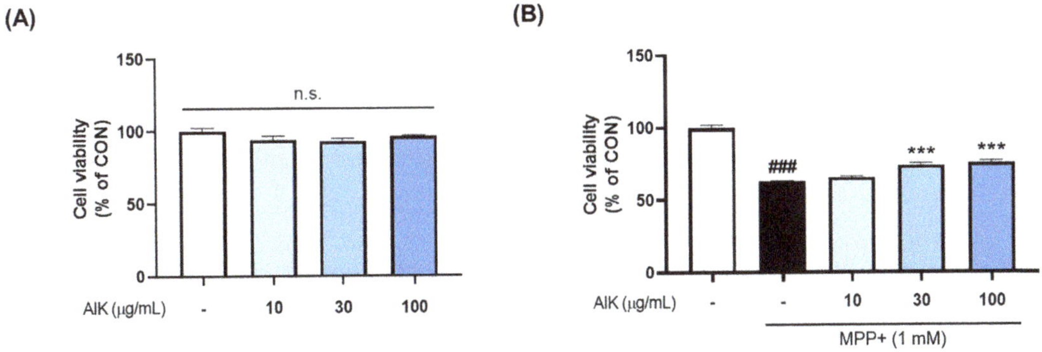

Figure 2. AIK treatment protects PC12 cells from MPP$^+$-induced cytotoxicity. (**A**) After PC12 cells were stabilized, they were treated with various concentrations of AIK, and cell viability was measured 48 h later. (**B**) Various concentrations of AIK were treated for 1 h and then incubated with 1 mM MPP$^+$ for an additional 48 h. Values are indicated as the mean ± S.E.M. Data were analyzed by one-way ANOVA, followed by Dunnett's multiple-comparison test. ### $p < 0.001$ compared to the CON group; *** $p < 0.001$ compared to the MPP$^+$ treated group. n.s.; not significant.

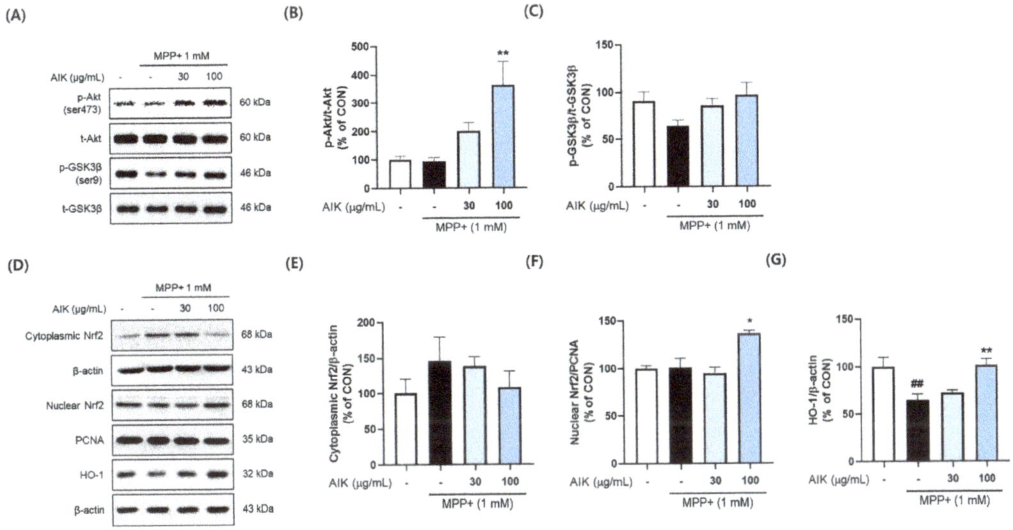

Figure 3. AIK treatment stimulates the Akt/GSK3β/Nrf2 signaling pathway to induce the expression of HO-1 in PC12 cells. Cells were treated with AIK at concentrations of 30 and 100 μg/mL and then incubated with 1 mM of MPP$^+$ for 4 h. (**A**) Representative band images and the quantifications of (**B**) p-Akt normalized to t-Akt and (**C**) GSK3β normalized to t-GSK3β. (**D**) Representative band images and quantifications of (**E**) cytoplasmic Nrf2, (**F**) nuclear Nrf2, and (**G**) HO-1. Cytoplasmic Nrf2 and HO-1 were normalized to β-actin, and nuclear Nrf2 was normalized to PCNA. Values are indicated as the mean ± S.E.M. Data were analyzed by one-way ANOVA, followed by Dunnett's multiple-comparison test. ## $p < 0.01$ compared to the control group; ** $p < 0.01$ and * $p < 0.05$ compared to the MPP$^+$-treated group.

3.4. Effects of AIK on the Nuclear Translocation of Nrf2 in Dopaminergic Neurons in Mice with MPTP-Induced PD

We used double immunofluorescence staining against TH and Nrf2 to examine whether AIK affected Nrf2 translocation in the SNpc of mice with PD. There was no discernible difference in Nrf2 translocation between the MPTP and NOR groups. In contrast to the MPTP group, Nrf2 translocation was increased in the AIK-treated groups. The MPTP + L-DOPA group and the MPTP group did not differ in their Nrf2 translocation (Figure 4).

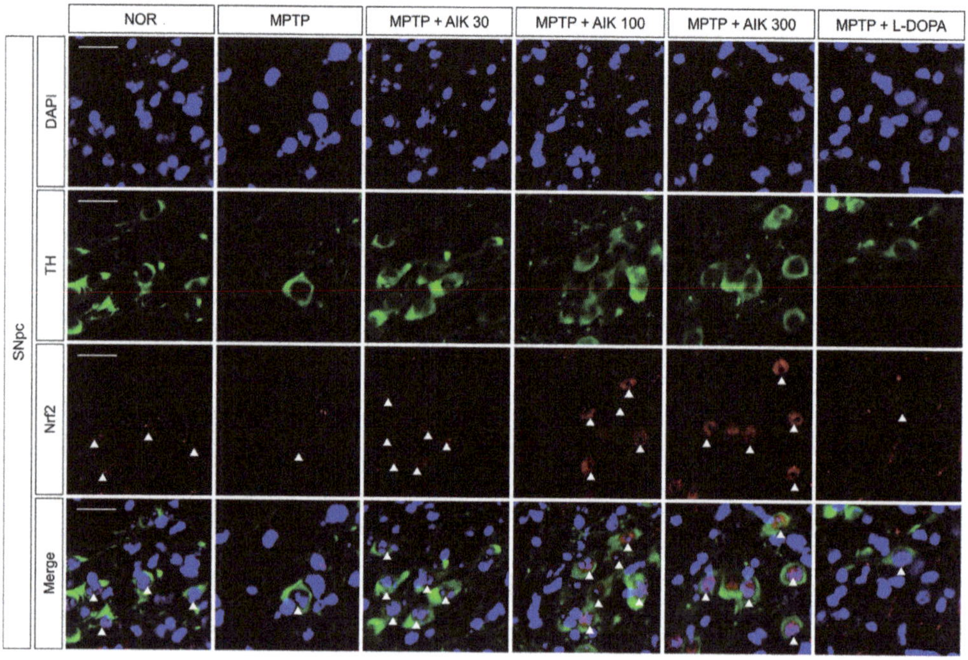

Figure 4. AIK administration induces the translocation of Nrf2 to the nucleus of dopaminergic neurons in the SNpc of MPTP-induced PD mice. Representative images of Nrf2 translocated to the nucleus of TH-positive dopaminergic neurons in SNpc are shown. Scale bar = 50 μm (n = 7–10 per group). The presence of Nrf2 in the nucleus of dopaminergic neurons was indicated by white arrows.

3.5. Effects of AIK on Dopaminergic Neuronal Loss in Mice with MPTP-Induced PD

Immunohistochemistry for TH and DAT, which are markers of dopaminergic neurons, was performed in order to evaluate the protective effects of AIK on nigrostriatal dopaminergic neuronal loss. When TH-positive cells in the SNpc were quantified, the MPTP group had a significantly lower number of dopaminergic neurons than the NOR group. The TH-positive cell count was significantly higher in the MPTP + AIK 300 group than in the MPTP group. Additionally, the striatum (ST) of the MPTP group contained noticeably fewer TH- and DAT-positive fibers than those of the NOR group. However, compared to the MPTP group, we discovered that the MPTP + AIK 300 group had markedly more TH- and DAT-positive fibers. Treatment with L-DOPA had no effect on the survival of dopaminergic cells (Figure 5).

3.6. Effects of AIK on Behavioral Impairment in Mice with MPTP-Induced PD

The rotarod test was used to determine whether AIK improves motor dysfunction in mice with MPTP-induced PD. The MPTP group showed shorter latency times until falling, compared to the NOR group, and recorded significantly higher frequencies of falls. However, the time spent on the rotarod spindle was relatively longer in the AIK-treated group than the MPTP group, and the falling frequency was significantly lower. Latency times were significantly increased, while the number of falls was significantly reduced in the MPTP + L-DOPA group compared with the MPTP group (Figure 6).

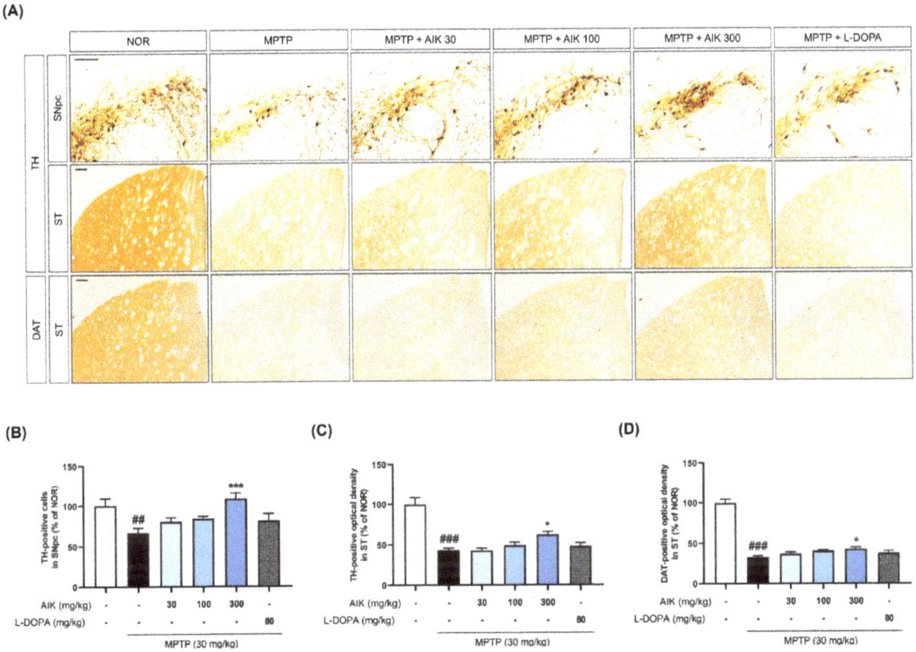

Figure 5. AIK administration protects dopaminergic neurons in the SNpc and ST of MPTP-induced PD mouse brain. (**A**) Dopaminergic neurons were visualized using immunohistochemistry. (**B**) The numbers of TH-positive cells in the SNpc were counted, and the optical density of (**C**) TH- and (**D**) DAT-positive fibers was measured in the ST. Scale bar = 200 μm (n = 7–10 per group). Values are indicated as the mean ± S.E.M. Data were analyzed by one-way ANOVA, followed by Dunnett's multiple-comparison test. ## $p < 0.01$ and ### $p < 0.001$ compared to the NOR group; * $p < 0.05$ and *** $p < 0.001$ compared to the MPTP group.

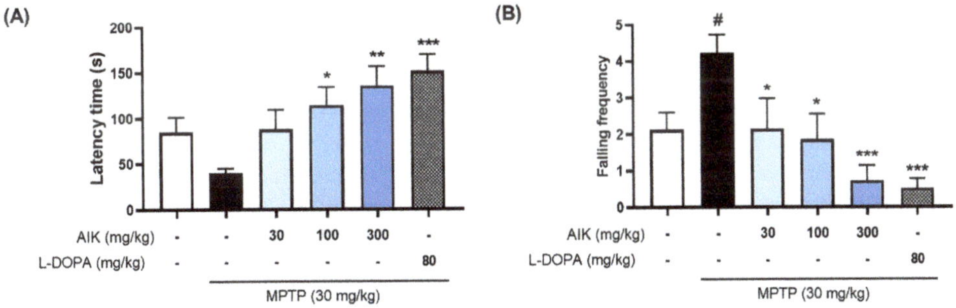

Figure 6. AIK administration ameliorates motor deficits in MPTP-induced PD mice. (**A**) Latency time to the first fall and (**B**) the frequency of falls during 3 min in the rotarod test were recorded (n = 7–10 per group). Values are indicated as the mean ± S.E.M. Data were analyzed by one-way ANOVA, followed by Dunnett's multiple-comparison test. # $p < 0.05$ compared to the NOR group; * $p < 0.05$, ** $p < 0.01$, *** $p < 0.001$ compared to the MPTP group.

4. Discussion

This study demonstrated that AIK had a mitigating effect on dopaminergic neuronal damage and motor impairments. AIK exhibited potent ABTS and DPPH radical scavenging activities. Furthermore, experiments in PC12 cells stimulated with MPP^+ showed that pre-treatment with AIK prevented cell death and significantly upregulated HO-1 levels through the activation of the Akt/GSK3β /Nrf2 pathway. In addition, the administration of AIK in mice with MPTP-induced PD activated the Nrf2 system in dopaminergic neurons, thereby protecting these neurons and subsequently improving behavioral impairments.

MPTP is a widely used neurotoxin that induces oxidative stress, leading to dopaminergic neuronal degeneration in the brains of animals. Upon injection into mice, MPTP crosses the blood–brain barrier and is metabolized to MPP^+, the active neurotoxic form, within astrocytes [26]. The overaccumulation of MPP^+ in the synaptic vesicles of dopaminergic neurons inhibits mitochondrial electron transport chain complex I, resulting in ROS generation and ultimately causing cellular damage and apoptosis. Simultaneously, it activates microglia, triggering the release of pro-inflammatory cytokines [27]. In this study, we utilized MPP^+ in vitro, which directly induces neurotoxicity in neuronal cells, and demonstrated that AIK is a potential neuroprotective agent. The results obtained from our in vivo study using MPTP as a toxin confirmed the therapeutic efficacy of AIK in combating PD, as evidenced by the restoration of motor function and neuronal survival.

Oxidative stress, primarily caused by the accumulation of ROS, is one of the major pathogenic mechanisms in MPTP-induced PD, and it is counteracted by defense mechanisms activated through the Nrf2-mediated pathway [28]. The regulation of ROS is primarily mediated by Nrf2 and its downstream mediator, HO-1. As a key regulatory protein, Nrf2 controls how cells react to environmental stimuli that cause oxidative stress. By stimulating the expression of several antioxidant enzymes, such as HO-1, which controls ROS levels to avoid excessive accumulation, Nrf2 shields cells from harm caused by ROS [29,30]. Oxidative damage is closely linked to the activation of cell death signaling pathways. The activation of the Akt/GSK3β signaling pathway under oxidative conditions is known to promote the nuclear translocation of Nrf2, thereby contributing to the regulation of neuronal survival or death [31]. Kelch-like ECH-associated protein 1 (Keap1) and Nrf2 coexist in the cytoplasm under normal physiological settings. On the other hand, Nrf2 separates from Keap1 during stimulation and binds to DNA sites in the nucleus called antioxidant response elements (AREs) [32]. Nrf2 translocated to the nucleus is converted into a heterodimer form with the Maf protein, and this heterodimer binds to the antioxidant response element to induce the expression of genes that protect the cell. Nrf2-mediated expression of antioxidant factors restores the redox imbalance and induces a response to cellular damage and inflammation [33,34].

HO-1 is a key antioxidant enzyme induced by this process. It is upregulated upon exposure to oxidative stimuli and protects neuronal cells through its role in heme group degradation and the subsequent yield of biliverdin, carbon monoxide, and free iron. In addition to reducing oxidative damage, the compounds generated by HO-1 have been shown to have anti-inflammatory properties by scavenging ROS [35]. Biliverdin reductase (BVR) transforms the biliverdin generated during heme breakdown by HO-1 into bilirubin, a potent antioxidant. Continuous ROS clearance is made possible by bilirubin's 1:1 stoichiometry of scavenging ROS, oxidizing to biliverdin, which is then reduced to bilirubin by BVR [36,37]. Extensive studies have demonstrated that HO-1 plays a role in protecting neuronal cells from oxidative stress. Wang et al. reported that the Nrf2/HO-1 pathway mediates neuroprotective effects through the mitochondrial apoptotic pathway and the alleviation of neuroinflammation [38]. Jin et al. demonstrated that *Acanthopanax senticosus* (Rupr. & Maxim.) Harms inhibited neuroinflammation and protected neuronal cells against glutamate-induced toxicity through the regulation of HO-1 signaling [39]. Morroni et al. reported that caffeic acid phenethyl ester attenuated amyloid-β peptide-induced neuronal apoptosis and neuroinflammation through the activation of the Nrf2/HO-1 pathway in a mouse model of Alzheimer's disease [40]. In a similar context, we found that AIK activated the Akt/Nrf2 pathway and upregulated the expression of HO-1 in PC12 cells stimulated with MPP^+, suggesting that AIK confers protection against oxidative stress.

The intricate relationship between inflammation and oxidative stress has been demonstrated in numerous studies. ROS released from damaged mitochondria exacerbate oxidative stress by activating various inflammatory pathways [41]. Specifically, inflammatory responses are induced by activated astrocytes and microglia, leading to neurodegeneration and cell death in PD [42]. In our previous study, we confirmed the anti-inflammatory effects of AIK on LPS-induced inflammation [20]. AIK inhibited nuclear factor kappa-light-chain-enhancer of activated B cells and mitogen-activated protein kinase-mediated pro-inflammatory pathways in LPS-stimulated BV2 microglial cells and suppressed the activation of microglia and the nucleotide-binding oligomerization domain, leucine-rich repeat, and pyrin domain-containing protein 3 inflammasome in LPS-injected mice [20]. Another study discovered that scopoletin, a major component of AIK, enhances antioxidant signaling via increased nuclear translocation of Nrf2 and offers neuroprotection against rotenone-induced neurotoxicity in SH-SY5Y cells [43]. Additional findings from this investigation demonstrated that AIK reduced neuroinflammation in the MPTP-induced PD mice's SN and ST (Figures S2 and S3). Taken together, data from previous studies and the current study suggest that AIK is a promising therapeutic agent that modulates neuroinflammation and protects neuronal cells, leading to integrative and effective treatment of PD.

5. Conclusions

In conclusion, we demonstrated that AIK exerted neuroprotective effects on dopaminergic neurons by promoting antioxidant signaling and ameliorating motor impairment and neuroinflammation. These results suggest that AIK is a promising therapeutic approach to prevent or treat the progression of PD.

Supplementary Materials: The following supporting information can be downloaded at: https://www.mdpi.com/article/10.3390/nu17101672/s1. Figure S1. The time scheme of experimental procedures. Figure S2: AIK administration inhibits the activation of microglia in the brain of MPTP-induced mice. Figure S3: AIK administration inhibits the activation of astrocytes in the brain of MPTP-induced PD mice.

Author Contributions: Conceptualization, I.G.J. and M.S.O.; methodology, I.G.J.; validation, H.L. and I.G.J.; investigation, H.L. and I.G.J.; writing—original draft, H.L.; writing—review and editing, H.L., I.G.J., J.H.K., Y.C., and S.L.; visualization, H.L.; supervision, M.S.O.; project administration, M.S.O.; funding acquisition, H.-J.P. and M.S.O. All authors have read and agreed to the published version of the manuscript.

Funding: This research was supported by grants from the National Research Foundation of Korea, funded by the Korean government (grant number 2022M3A9B6017813) and a grant of the Korea Health Technology R&D Project through the Korea Health Industry Development Institute (KHIDI), funded by the Ministry of Health and Welfare, Republic of Korea (grand number: RS-2023-KH139287).

Institutional Review Board Statement: This study was conducted according to the Guide for the Care and Use of Laboratory Animals, 8th edition (National Institutes of Health, 2011) and approved by the Animal Care and Use Guidelines of Kyung Hee University (Seoul, Republic of Korea; approval number: KHSASP-18-167; approved on 16 January 2019).

Informed Consent Statement: Not applicable.

Data Availability Statement: Data are contained within the article or Supplementary Material.

Conflicts of Interest: The authors declare no conflicts of interest.

Abbreviations

ABC	avidin–biotin complex
ABTS	2,2-azinobis-(3-ethyl-benzthiazolin-6-sulphonic acid)
AIK	aerial parts of *Artemisia iwayomogi* Kitamura
Akt	protein kinase B
ANOVA	analysis of variance
AREs	antioxidant response elements
BVR	biliverdin reductase
CON	control
DAB	3,3′-diaminobenzidine
DAPI	4′,6-diamidino-2-phenylindole
DAT	dopamine transporter
DPPH	2,2-diphenyl-1-picrylhydrazyl
DRT	dopamine replacement therapy
GSK3β	glycogen synthase kinase-3β
HO-1	heme oxygenase-1
HRP	horseradish peroxidase
IC_{50} values	half-maximal inhibitory concentration
IgG	immunoglobulin G
Keap1	Kelch-like ECH-associated protein 1
L-DOPA	levodopa
LPS	lipopolysaccharide
MPP+	1-methyl-4-phenylpyridinium
MPTP	1-methyl-4-phenyl-1,2,3,6-tetrahydropyridine
MTT	3-(4,5-dimethylthiazol-2-yl)-2,5-diphenyl-2H-tetrazolium bromide
Nrf2	nuclear factor erythroid 2-related factor 2
PBS	phosphate-buffered saline
PCNA	proliferating cell nuclear antigen
PDRIPA	Parkinson's diseaseradio-immunoprecipitation assay lysis buffer
ROS	reactive oxygen species
SB	*Scutellaria baicalensis* Georgi root
S.E.M	standard error of the mean
SN	substantia nigra
SNpc	substantia nigra pars compacta
ST	striatum
TH	tyrosine hydroxylase

References

1. Ramesh, S.; Arachchige, A. Depletion of dopamine in Parkinson's disease and relevant therapeutic options: A review of the literature. *AIMS Neurosci.* **2023**, *10*, 200–231. [CrossRef] [PubMed]
2. Moustafa, A.A.; Chakravarthy, S.; Phillips, J.R.; Gupta, A.; Keri, S.; Polner, B.; Frank, M.J.; Jahanshahi, M. Motor symptoms in Parkinson's disease: A unified framework. *Neurosci. Biobehav. Rev.* **2016**, *68*, 727–740. [CrossRef] [PubMed]
3. Wang, J.; Dai, L.; Chen, S.; Zhang, Z.; Fang, X.; Zhang, Z. Protein-protein interactions regulating alpha-synuclein pathology. *Trends Neurosci.* **2024**, *47*, 209–226. [CrossRef] [PubMed]
4. Ferrazzoli, D.; Carter, A.; Ustun, F.S.; Palamara, G.; Ortelli, P.; Maestri, R.; Yucel, M.; Frazzitta, G. Dopamine Replacement Therapy, Learning and Reward Prediction in Parkinson's Disease: Implications for Rehabilitation. *Front. Behav. Neurosci.* **2016**, *10*, 121. [CrossRef]
5. Dawson, V.L.; Dawson, T.M. Promising disease-modifying therapies for Parkinson's disease. *Sci. Transl. Med.* **2019**, *11*, eaba1659. [CrossRef]

6. Aryal, S.; Skinner, T.; Bridges, B.; Weber, J.T. The Pathology of Parkinson's Disease and Potential Benefit of Dietary Polyphenols. *Molecules* **2020**, *25*, 4382. [CrossRef]
7. Moon, H.E.; Paek, S.H. Mitochondrial Dysfunction in Parkinson's Disease. *Exp. Neurobiol.* **2015**, *24*, 103–116. [CrossRef]
8. Dias, V.; Junn, E.; Mouradian, M.M. The role of oxidative stress in Parkinson's disease. *J. Parkinsons Dis.* **2013**, *3*, 461–491. [CrossRef]
9. Fabisiak, T.; Patel, M. Crosstalk between neuroinflammation and oxidative stress in epilepsy. *Front. Cell Dev. Biol.* **2022**, *10*, 976953. [CrossRef]
10. Guo, J.D.; Zhao, X.; Li, Y.; Li, G.R.; Liu, X.L. Damage to dopaminergic neurons by oxidative stress in Parkinson's disease (Review). *Int. J. Mol. Med.* **2018**, *41*, 1817–1825. [CrossRef]
11. Salim, S. Oxidative Stress and the Central Nervous System. *J. Pharmacol. Exp. Ther.* **2017**, *360*, 201–205. [CrossRef] [PubMed]
12. Loeffler, D.A.; DeMaggio, A.J.; Juneau, P.L.; Havaich, M.K.; LeWitt, P.A. Effects of enhanced striatal dopamine turnover in vivo on glutathione oxidation. *Clin. Neuropharmacol.* **1994**, *17*, 370–379. [CrossRef] [PubMed]
13. Abad, M.J.; Bedoya, L.M.; Apaza, L.; Bermejo, P. The *artemisia* L. Genus: A review of bioactive essential oils. *Molecules* **2012**, *17*, 2542–2566. [CrossRef] [PubMed]
14. Ryu, S.H.; Jo, H.; Kim, J.W.; Youn, H.J.; Kim, K.B. Four-Week Repeated Oral Toxicity Study of AIP1, a Water-soluble Carbohydrate Fraction from Artemisia iwayomogi in Mice. *Toxicol. Res.* **2011**, *27*, 261–267. [CrossRef]
15. Shin, T.Y.; Park, J.S.; Kim, S.H. *Artemisia iwayomogi* inhibits immediate-type allergic reaction and inflammatory cytokine secretion. *Immunopharmacol. Immunotoxicol.* **2006**, *28*, 421–430. [CrossRef]
16. Park, E.J.; Nan, J.X.; Kim, J.Y.; Kang, H.C.; Choi, J.H.; Lee, S.J.; Lee, B.H.; Kim, S.J.; Lee, J.H.; Kim, Y.C.; et al. The ethanol-soluble part of a hot-water extract from Artemisia iwayomogi inhibits liver fibrosis induced by carbon tetrachloride in rats. *J. Pharm. Pharmacol.* **2000**, *52*, 875–881. [CrossRef]
17. Kim, S.M.; Vetrivel, P.; Kim, H.H.; Ha, S.E.; Saralamma, V.V.G.; Kim, G.S. *Artemisia iwayomogi* (Dowijigi) inhibits lipopolysaccharide-induced inflammation in RAW264.7 macrophages by suppressing the NF-kappaB signaling pathway. *Exp. Ther. Med.* **2020**, *19*, 2161–2170. [CrossRef]
18. Lee, J.; Narayan, V.P.; Hong, E.Y.; Whang, W.K.; Park, T. *Artemisia iwayomogi* Extract Attenuates High-Fat Diet-Induced Hypertriglyceridemia in Mice: Potential Involvement of the Adiponectin-AMPK Pathway and Very Low Density Lipoprotein Assembly in the Liver. *Int. J. Mol. Sci.* **2017**, *18*, 1762. [CrossRef]
19. Lee, S.H.; Ding, Y.; Yan, X.T.; Kim, Y.H.; Jang, H.D. Scopoletin and scopolin isolated from Artemisia iwayomogi suppress differentiation of osteoclastic macrophage RAW 264.7 cells by scavenging reactive oxygen species. *J. Nat. Prod.* **2013**, *76*, 615–620. [CrossRef]
20. Ju, I.G.; Huh, E.; Kim, N.; Lee, S.; Choi, J.G.; Hong, J.; Oh, M.S. Artemisiae Iwayomogii Herba inhibits lipopolysaccharide-induced neuroinflammation by regulating NF-kappaB and MAPK signaling pathways. *Phytomedicine* **2021**, *84*, 153501. [CrossRef]
21. Gao, B.; Zhu, H.; Liu, Z.; He, X.; Sun, J.; Li, Y.; Wu, X.; Pehrsson, P.; Zhang, Y.; Yu, L. Chemical Compositions of *Scutellaria baicalensis* Georgi. (Huangqin) Extracts and Their Effects on ACE2 Binding of SARS-CoV-2 Spike Protein, ACE2 Activity, and Free Radicals. *Int. J. Mol. Sci.* **2024**, *25*, 2045. [CrossRef] [PubMed]
22. Kim, N.; Choi, J.G.; Park, S.; Lee, J.K.; Oh, M.S. Butterbur Leaves Attenuate Memory Impairment and Neuronal Cell Damage in Amyloid Beta-Induced Alzheimer's Disease Models. *Int. J. Mol. Sci.* **2018**, *19*, 1644. [CrossRef] [PubMed]
23. Ju, I.G.; Lee, S.; Im, H.; Kim, J.H.; Eo, H.; Oh, M.S. Artemisiae Iwayomogii Herba mitigates excessive neuroinflammation and Abeta accumulation by regulating the pro-inflammatory response and autophagy-lysosomal pathway in microglia in 5xFAD mouse model of Alzheimer's disease. *Geroscience* **2025**, *47*, 1957–1972. [CrossRef]
24. Zou, W.; Chen, C.; Zhong, Y.; An, J.; Zhang, X.; Yu, Y.; Yu, Z.; Fu, J. PI3K/Akt pathway mediates Nrf2/ARE activation in human L02 hepatocytes exposed to low-concentration HBCDs. *Environ. Sci. Technol.* **2013**, *47*, 12434–12440. [CrossRef]
25. Loboda, A.; Damulewicz, M.; Pyza, E.; Jozkowicz, A.; Dulak, J. Role of Nrf2/HO-1 system in development, oxidative stress response and diseases: An evolutionarily conserved mechanism. *Cell. Mol. Life Sci.* **2016**, *73*, 3221–3247. [CrossRef]
26. Mustapha, M.; Mat Taib, C.N. MPTP-induced mouse model of Parkinson's disease: A promising direction of therapeutic strategies. *Bosn. J. Basic Med. Sci.* **2021**, *21*, 422–433. [CrossRef]
27. Zawada, W.M.; Banninger, G.P.; Thornton, J.; Marriott, B.; Cantu, D.; Rachubinski, A.L.; Das, M.; Griffin, W.S.; Jones, S.M. Generation of reactive oxygen species in 1-methyl-4-phenylpyridinium (MPP+) treated dopaminergic neurons occurs as an NADPH oxidase-dependent two-wave cascade. *J. Neuroinflamm.* **2011**, *8*, 129. [CrossRef]
28. Liu, R.; Yang, J.; Li, Y.; Xie, J.; Wang, J. Heme oxygenase-1: The roles of both good and evil in neurodegenerative diseases. *J. Neurochem.* **2023**, *167*, 347–361. [CrossRef]
29. Chiang, S.K.; Chen, S.E.; Chang, L.C. The Role of HO-1 and Its Crosstalk with Oxidative Stress in Cancer Cell Survival. *Cells* **2021**, *10*, 2401. [CrossRef]
30. Upadhayay, S.; Mehan, S. Targeting Nrf2/HO-1 anti-oxidant signaling pathway in the progression of multiple sclerosis and influences on neurological dysfunctions. *Brain Disord.* **2021**, *3*, 100019. [CrossRef]

31. Rojo, A.I.; Sagarra, M.R.; Cuadrado, A. GSK-3beta down-regulates the transcription factor Nrf2 after oxidant damage: Relevance to exposure of neuronal cells to oxidative stress. *J. Neurochem.* **2008**, *105*, 192–202. [CrossRef] [PubMed]
32. Kim, J.H.; Kim, K.M.; Jeong, J.U.; Shin, J.H.; Shin, J.M.; Bang, K.T. Nrf2-Heme oxygenase-1 modulates autophagy and inhibits apoptosis triggered by elevated glucose levels in renal tubule cells. *Kidney Res. Clin. Pract.* **2019**, *38*, 318–325. [CrossRef] [PubMed]
33. Liu, C.; Li, Y.; Wang, X. TDAG51-Deficiency Podocytes are Protected from High-Glucose-Induced Damage Through Nrf2 Activation via the AKT-GSK-3beta Pathway. *Inflammation* **2022**, *45*, 1520–1533. [CrossRef]
34. Zhou, Z.; Li, H.; Bai, S.; Xu, Z.; Jiao, Y. Loss of serine/threonine protein kinase 25 in retinal ganglion cells ameliorates high glucose-elicited damage through regulation of the AKT-GSK-3beta/Nrf2 pathway. *Biochem. Biophys. Res. Commun.* **2022**, *600*, 87–93. [CrossRef]
35. Funes, S.C.; Rios, M.; Fernandez-Fierro, A.; Covian, C.; Bueno, S.M.; Riedel, C.A.; Mackern-Oberti, J.P.; Kalergis, A.M. Naturally Derived Heme-Oxygenase 1 Inducers and Their Therapeutic Application to Immune-Mediated Diseases. *Front. Immunol.* **2020**, *11*, 1467. [CrossRef]
36. Araujo, J.A.; Zhang, M.; Yin, F. Heme oxygenase-1, oxidation, inflammation, and atherosclerosis. *Front. Pharmacol.* **2012**, *3*, 119. [CrossRef]
37. Consoli, V.; Sorrenti, V.; Grosso, S.; Vanella, L. Heme Oxygenase-1 Signaling and Redox Homeostasis in Physiopathological Conditions. *Biomolecules* **2021**, *11*, 589. [CrossRef]
38. Wang, Z.; Guo, S.; Wang, J.; Shen, Y.; Zhang, J.; Wu, Q. Nrf2/HO-1 mediates the neuroprotective effect of mangiferin on early brain injury after subarachnoid hemorrhage by attenuating mitochondria-related apoptosis and neuroinflammation. *Sci. Rep.* **2017**, *7*, 11883. [CrossRef]
39. Jin, M.L.; Park, S.Y.; Kim, Y.H.; Park, G.; Lee, S.J. *Acanthopanax senticosus* exerts neuroprotective effects through HO-1 signaling in hippocampal and microglial cells. *Environ. Toxicol. Pharmacol.* **2013**, *35*, 335–346. [CrossRef]
40. Morroni, F.; Sita, G.; Graziosi, A.; Turrini, E.; Fimognari, C.; Tarozzi, A.; Hrelia, P. Neuroprotective Effect of Caffeic Acid Phenethyl Ester in A Mouse Model of Alzheimer's Disease Involves Nrf2/HO-1 Pathway. *Aging Dis.* **2018**, *9*, 605–622. [CrossRef]
41. Biswas, S.K. Does the Interdependence between Oxidative Stress and Inflammation Explain the Antioxidant Paradox? *Oxid. Med. Cell Longev.* **2016**, *2016*, 5698931. [CrossRef] [PubMed]
42. Kempuraj, D.; Thangavel, R.; Natteru, P.A.; Selvakumar, G.P.; Saeed, D.; Zahoor, H.; Zaheer, S.; Iyer, S.S.; Zaheer, A. Neuroinflammation Induces Neurodegeneration. *J. Neurol. Neurosurg. Spine* **2016**, *1*, 1003.
43. Kishore Kumar, S.N.; Deepthy, J.; Prema, V.; Ashokkumar, S.; Thangarajeswari, M.; Bhavani, R.D.; Saraswathi, U.; Yogesh Kanna, S.; Rajasekaran, N.S.; Kalaiselvi, P. Scopoletin Augments DJ1/Nrf2 Signalling and Prevents Protein Aggregation in Parkinson's disease. *bioRxiv* **2018**, 260521. [CrossRef]

nutrients

Article

Protective Effects of a Standardized Water Extract from the Stem of *Ipomoea batatas* L. Against High-Fat Diet-Induced Obesity

Chae-Won Lee [1,2,†], Ye Seul Yoon [3,†], Young-Seo Yoon [4], Kyung-Sook Chung [4], Mi-ju Kim [3], Geonha Park [5,6], Minsik Choi [5,7], Young-Pyo Jang [5,6,7,8,*] and Kyung-Tae Lee [1,2,*]

1 Department of Fundamental Pharmaceutical Science, Graduate School, Kyung Hee University, Seoul 02447, Republic of Korea; codnjs963@khu.ac.kr
2 Department of Pharmaceutical Biochemistry, College of Pharmacy, Kyung Hee University, Seoul 02447, Republic of Korea
3 Development Department, Dalim Biotech Co., Ltd., Wonju-si 26348, Gangwon-do, Republic of Korea; plan783@dalimpharm.co.kr (Y.S.Y.); miju0522@dalimpharm.co.kr (M.-j.K.)
4 BELABEL BIO. Inc., Gimhae-si 50969, Gyeongsangnam-do, Republic of Korea; shapira@naver.com (Y.-S.Y.); adella76@hanmail.net (K.-S.C.)
5 Division of Pharmacognosy, College of Pharmacy, Kyung Hee University, Seoul 02447, Republic of Korea; ginapark0326@khu.ac.kr (G.P.); alstlr7595@naver.com (M.C.)
6 Department of Oriental Pharmaceutical Sciences, College of Pharmacy, Kyung Hee University, Seoul 02447, Republic of Korea
7 Department of Biomedical and Pharmaceutical Sciences, Graduate School, Kyung Hee University, Seoul 02447, Republic of Korea
8 Department of Integrated Drug Development and Natural Products, Graduate School, Kyung Hee University, Seoul 02447, Republic of Korea
* Correspondence: ypjang@khu.ac.kr (Y.-P.J.); ktlee@khu.ac.kr (K.-T.L.); Tel.: +82-2-961-9421 (Y.-P.J.); +82-2-961-0860 (K.-T.L.)
† These authors contributed equally to this work.

Abstract: Background/Objectives: Obesity is a major health concern that can lead to various chronic diseases. Little is known about the anti-obesity effect of a standardized hot water extract from the stems of *Ipomoea batatas* (WIB). This study aimed to evaluate the therapeutic potential of WIB as a natural alternative to conventional anti-obesity treatments by assessing its effects on body weight, fat accumulation, and key metabolic biomarkers in a high-fat diet-induced obesity model. **Methods:** A high-fat diet (HFD) induced obesity in C57BL/6 mice. The mice were then treated orally with either orlistat (positive control) or WIB. Changes in body weight, food intake, and fat weight were measured, along with blood lipid profiles and adipokines. Western blot analyses were conducted to determine protein levels in each tissue. H&E staining in white adipose tissue and liver, and the gut microbiota composition were analyzed. **Results:** WIB treatment significantly reduced body weight and fat mass compared to the HFD group and demonstrated comparable effects to orlistat. WIB improved blood lipid profiles and adipokine levels. H&E staining revealed reduced fat accumulation in the white adipose tissue and liver. Also in those tissues, WIB restored expression levels of sterol regulatory element-binding protein-1 (SREBP-1) and CCAAT/enhancer-binding protein α (C/EBPα) and increased AMP-activated protein kinase (AMPK) phosphorylation. In brown adipose tissue, WIB enhanced AMPK phosphorylation and upregulated thermogenic-related proteins, including peroxisome proliferator-activated receptor-gamma coactivator-1α (PGC-1α), peroxisome proliferator-activated receptor α (PPARα), sirtuin 1 (SIRT1), uncoupling protein-1 (UCP-1), and cytochrome C oxidase subunit 4 (COX-IV). Analysis of gut microbiota revealed that WIB normalized β-diversity and reversed HFD-induced phyla imbalances (notably in *Bacteroidetes*, *Firmicutes*, and *Proteobacteria*). **Conclusions:** By reducing adiposity under the conditions tested in a murine model, improving metabolic markers, and favorably modulating gut microbiota, WIB demonstrates potential in mitigating obesity-related risks. These findings suggest that WIB may serve as a promising natural substance for the management of obesity. Further studies are warranted to confirm its efficacy and explore the potential underlying mechanisms in overweight or obese humans as a health supplement to help manage or prevent obesity.

Keywords: *Ipomoea batatas* L.; anti-obesity; AMP-activated protein kinase; white-adipose tissue; liver; lipogenesis; brown adipose tissue; thermogenesis; microbiota

1. Introduction

Globally, obesity is a major issue associated with several chronic ailments, such as heart disease, diabetes, and non-alcoholic fatty liver disease [1,2]. Because obesity is classified as a medical condition, appropriate treatment strategies should be implemented to mitigate obesity-associated health risks.

The relationship between obesity and adipose tissue is significant because adipose tissue plays a crucial role in the progression and development of obesity [3]. When a person eats too much food and has leftover caloric intake, excess energy is stored as fat in adipose tissue. Adipose tissue can be categorized into two primary types. White adipose tissue (WAT) functions as an energy reservoir. On the other hand, brown adipose tissue (BAT) contributes to energy consumption by generating heat [4]. Numerous studies and reviews have highlighted that adipose tissue acts as an active metabolic organ involved in systemic energy regulation and inflammation. Its dysfunction is closely associated with obesity and metabolic disorders [5,6]. Several transcription factors control lipogenesis. CCAAT/enhancer-binding protein alpha (C/EBPα) and sterol regulatory element-binding protein-1 (SREBP-1) are major transcription factors that regulate adipose lipid metabolism, with C/EBPα controlling adipocyte development and insulin sensitivity, and SREBP-1 regulating fatty acid and triglyceride synthesis in response to insulin [7]. The AMP-activated protein kinase (AMPK) has a crucial role in cellular energy balance and regulating adipocyte metabolism by controlling transcription factors, such as C/EBPα and SREBP-1, making it a stunning target of anti-obesity therapeutic strategies [8]. In BAT, AMPK and sirtuin 1 (SIRT1) activate peroxisome proliferator-activated receptor-gamma coactivator-1α (PGC-1α) by phosphorylation and deacetylation, respectively [9]. Activation of PGC-1α coactivates the peroxisome proliferator-activated receptor α (PPARα) and induces the expression of thermogenic genes like uncoupling protein 1 (UCP-1) [10]. Additionally, PGC-1α enhances the expression of cytochrome c oxidase IV (COX-IV) [11]. Because these signaling pathways are important for the regulation of thermogenesis, energy expenditure, and fat oxidation, BAT helps to counteract obesity and metabolic disorders [12].

The gut is an important organ for absorbing nutrients from digested foods, and the gut microbiota can influence this absorption process. *Proteobacteria*, *Firmicutes*, and *Bacteroidetes* are obesity-related bacterial phyla that affect energy regulation and fat storage [13,14]. In particular, studies have shown that obese individuals tend to have a higher ratio of *Firmicutes* to *Bacteroidetes* [15,16]. For these reasons, it is important to consider the restoration of the balance of gut microbes in obesity. Many studies have shown that intestinal microbiota participate in host energy metabolism through a range of metabolites and molecules, such as short-chain fatty acids (SCFAs), to fight obesity with bacteria [17,18]. Among these SCFAs, butyrate has been reported to serve as the main source of energy for intestinal epithelial cells, and it can improve fatty acid oxidation and reduce fat accumulation by regulating the AMPK signaling pathway [19].

In general, synthetic weight-loss drugs exhibit limited long-term efficacy, necessitating careful monitoring of the risk of adverse effects that may outweigh the therapeutic benefits in some individuals [20]. Orlistat was selected as the positive control drug in our animal experiments to compare its efficacy in reducing body weight and fat accumulation in obese animal models because it is a well-established anti-obesity medication that acts as a pancreatic lipase inhibitor and effectively reduces dietary fat absorption [21,22]. This selection allowed us to assess whether WIB exerts anti-obesity effects through mechanisms distinct from orlistat, thereby providing valuable insights into its potential therapeutic role. However, orlistat can cause adverse effects on the digestive system, including oily stools, flatulence, and increased bowel movement frequency [23]. The limitations of many synthetic weight-loss drugs imply growing interest in natural compounds with anti-obesity properties [24,25].

Sweet potatoes (*Ipomoea batatas*, Convolvulaceae) have been traditionally cultivated in many countries. Typically, only the tuber—the part most consumed—is utilized, while the stem is used only to a limited extent in countries like Korea. Consequently, the utilization of other parts of the sweet potato plants, such as the leaves and stems, remains restricted. Although several studies have demonstrated that the leaves and polyphenols of *I. batatas* showed anti-oxidant, anti-hyperglycemia, and anti-inflammatory effects, little is known about the anti-obesity effect from the stem of *I. batatas* [26–29]. Therefore, as a part of our ongoing screening program to evaluate the anti-obesity potential of natural products, we aimed to clarify the competence and molecular mechanisms underlying the anti-obesity properties of a standardized water extract from the stem of *Ipomoea batatas* L. (WIB) in a high-fat diet-induced mouse model.

2. Materials and Methods

2.1. Materials

The water used for the extraction was prepared using an ABBOTA NEO water purification system (UMC Science Co., Ilsan, Gyeonggi-do, Republic of Korea). HPLC-grade water, acetonitrile, and methanol were supplied by Fisher Scientific Korea (Seoul, Republic of Korea), and formic acid was purchased from Wako Pure Chemical Industries (Osaka, Japan). The substances used for preparing standard solutions, including L-tryptophan, neochlorogenic acid, chlorogenic acid, cryptochlorogenic acid, hyperoside, isoquercetin, isochlorogenic acid A, isochlorogenic acid B, and isochlorogenic acid C, were all supplied by ChemFaces (Wuhan, China), and caffeic acid was supplied by Sigma-Aldrich (Steinheim, Germany). JEOL's YOKUDELNA calibration kit (Tokyo, Japan) was used for the calibration of the ESI-TOF-MS chromatogram and spectra, and high-purity nitrogen gas from Shinyang Oxygen Co. (Seoul, Republic of Korea) was utilized for MS analysis. Orlistat (O4139) was purchased from Sigma-Aldrich (St. Louis, MO, USA). Diets (D12450B and D12492) were purchased from Research Diets Inc. (New Brunswick, NJ, USA). C/EBPα (8178), phospho-AMPKα (2531), AMPKα (2532), SIRT1 (9475), and COX-IV (4844) antibodies were purchased from Cell Signaling Technology (Danvers, MA, USA). PGC-1α (sc-518025), PPARα (sc-398394), UCP-1 (sc-293418), and β-actin (sc-81178) antibodies were obtained from Santa Cruz Biotechnology (Santa Cruz, CA, USA). The SREBP-1 (ab28481) antibody was purchased from Abcam (Cambridge, MA, USA).

2.2. WIB Preparation, Identification, and Standardization

Ipomoea batatas L. was cultivated in Yeoju (Republic of Korea) and was identified by Prof. Young Pyo Jang (Division of Pharmacognosy, College of Pharmacy, Kyung Hee University, Republic of Korea). A voucher specimen has been deposited in Darim Biotech (Seoul, Republic of Korea). The stems of *Ipomoea batatas* L. were washed, air-dried, and then oven-dried at 50 °C for 30 h to remove moisture. The dried stems were ground, and the fine powder obtained by passing through an 850 μm sieve was used. For extraction, 10 g of this fine powder was mixed with 300 mL of distilled water and refluxed at 100 °C for 2 h. The extract was then filtered, and the filtrate was freeze-dried to prepare the respective extracts. For UPLC-PDA analysis, the *Ipomoea batatas* L. stem extract powder was dissolved in HPLC-grade water at a concentration of 30 mg/mL and subjected to ultrasonic extraction for 10 min. The extract was then filtered through a 0.2 μm Polyvinylidene Fluoride (PVDF) syringe filter (Whatman International Ltd., Maidstone, Kent, UK) to obtain the hot water extract solution. Standard solutions were prepared by dissolving L-tryptophan, neochlorogenic acid, caffeic acid, chlorogenic acid, cryptochlorogenic acid, hyperoside, isoquercetin, isochlorogenic acid A, isochlorogenic acid B, and isochlorogenic acid C in methanol at a concentration of 1 mg/mL. For UPLC-PDA-ESI-TOF-MS analysis of the components in *Ipomoea batatas* L. stems, an Acquity™ H-class UPLC system with PDA and Empower 3 Software (version Service Release 1, Waters Corp., Milford, MA, USA) was used. Separation was achieved using a Kinetex® 1.7 μm EVO C18 100 Å 100 × 2.1 mm column and an EVO C18 guard column (Phenomenex, Torrance, CA, USA) with a flow rate of 0.3 mL/min. The column and autosampler temperatures were set at 25 °C and 20 °C, respectively. The injection volume was 2 μL, and the PDA detection wavelength was 254 nm. The mobile phase consisted of acetonitrile (A) and water (B) with 0.1% formic acid, and the gradient was as follows: A was maintained at 0% for 3 min, increased to 5% at 8 min, to 10% at 15 min, and finally to 25% at 35 min. For stabilization, A was increased to 95% at 40 min, held for 2 min, then decreased to 0% at 45 min and held for 5 min. The mass analysis of the extracts and standard solutions was performed using a JEOL Ltd. (Tokyo, Japan) JMS-T100TD (AccuTOF-TLC) with an electrospray ionization source. The mass range was 50 to 1000 m/z, and the positive mode conditions were as follows: orifice 1 voltage, 40 V; ring lens voltage, 15 V; orifice 2 voltage, 7 V; orifice 1 temperature, 80 °C; desolvation temperature, 250 °C; nitrogen gas flow for nebulizer and desolvation, 1 L/min and 3 L/min; needle electrode voltage, 2000 V; and peak voltage, 1000 V. Other conditions, including those for the negative mode, are detailed in Table S1.

2.3. Animals and Experimental Design

C57BL/6J mice (male, 5–6 weeks old, 21 ± 1 g) were obtained from Orient Bio Inc. (Seongnam, Republic of Korea). Mice were kept under standard conditions (light–dark cycle, 12 h; temperature, 22 ± 1 °C; humidity, 50 ± 10%) for a week. All procedures adhered to the Kyung Hee University Animal Care and Use Guidelines, and the experimental protocol was approved by the University's Experimentation Committee (KHSASP-22-215, Approval date: 22 July 2022). Mice were divided into 5 groups (n = 8) to examine the effect of WIB: vehicle-treated control (CON) group, HFD group for obesity, orlistat (20 mg/kg) group for positive control, and WIB (100 or 300 mg/kg) group. Each group was housed in a cage. The formula compositions of the diet are summarized in Table 1. Based on these diets, the CON group received a normal diet, while the rest of the group was fed a high-fat diet for 10 weeks to induce obesity. At the same time, each group received daily oral administration of vehicle, orlistat, or WIB using a zonde (8 cm, 15G, Duksan general science, Seoul, Republic of Korea). The weight of the mice and their food intake were measured once a week. At the end of the experiment, the mice were euthanized by 70% CO_2, and tissues were collected immediately after surgical sacrifice under sterile conditions. After dissection, the tissues were carefully excised and rinsed with PBS to remove any residual blood. They were subsequently stored in sterilized tubes at −80 °C until further analysis to ensure sample integrity.

Table 1. Formula composition of a normal and high-fat diet.

Comparative Profiles	Normal Diet		High-Fat Diet	
	g%	kcal%	g%	kcal%
Protein	19.2	20	26	20
Carbohydrate	67.3	70	26	20
Fat	4.3	10	35	60
Total		100		100
kcal/g	3.85		5.24	

2.4. Body Fat Composition Analysis

Before sacrifice, the body fat composition of each group was measured using dual-energy X-ray absorptiometry (DEXA) (InAlyzer, Medikors, Seongnam, Republic of Korea). The lean tissue, fat tissue, and differentiated tissue from lean to fat were exposed to blue, red, and green/yellow, respectively. The amount of fat in the tissue was determined and represented as grams.

2.5. H&E Staining Analysis

After sacrifice, WAT and liver obtained from the mice were fixed with 4% formaldehyde solution overnight. The fixed tissues were made into paraffin blocks, and the slices of paraffin blocks were stained with hematoxylin and eosin (H&E). The stained tissue sections were examined under a light microscope system (Cell Sense standard ver.1.9, Olympus corporation, Tokyo, Japan).

2.6. Protein Extraction and Western Blot Analysis

Total protein was extracted from adipose tissues and the liver with the protein extraction solution PRO-PREP (Intron Biotechnology, Seoul, Republic of Korea). The debris was removed by centrifuge at 4 °C for 30 min, and the supernatants were carefully transferred into a new tube. The protein concentration was quantified with the Bradford assay. A total of 30 μg of whole proteins were resolved by SDS-PAGE on 8–15% polyacrylamide gel and transferred electrically onto a PVDF membrane. The immunoblots were then incubated overnight with a 1:1000 diluted primary antibody at 4 °C, washed three times with TBS/T, incubated with a 1:2000 diluted secondary antibody for 2 h at room temperature, and washed three times again with TBS/T. The blots were finally developed using an ECL chemiluminescence substrate (Santa Cruz Biotechnology, Santa Cruz, CA, USA). The protein bands were visualized using Amersham Hyperfilm ECL (GE Healthcare Life Sciences, Chicago, IL, USA).

2.7. Biochemical Examination of Blood Plasma

During the sacrifice, blood samples were collected from a vein and stored in tubes coated with heparin. After collecting blood samples, they were centrifuged at 2500 rpm at room temperature for 10 min. The separated plasmas were stored at −80 °C. Plasma levels of total cholesterol (TC), triglycerides (TG), low-density lipoprotein (LDL), high-density lipoprotein (HDL), very-low-density lipoprotein (VLDL), GOT, GPT, BUN, insulin, leptin, and adiponectin were measured to evaluate common lipid parameters, hepatotoxicity, nephrotoxicity, and obesity-related hormonal status. Each parameter was analyzed using an AU480 chemistry analyzer (Beckman Coulter, Brea, CA, USA) from T&P Bio (Gwangju, Republic of Korea).

2.8. Genomic DNA (gDNA) Extraction and Microbiome Profiling

Total genomic DNA was extracted from the stool samples using a QIAamp® Fast DNA Stool Mini Kit (Qiagen, Hilden, Germany) according to the manufacturer's instructions. The V3–V4 regions of the bacterial 16S ribosomal RNA (rRNA) gene were amplified using barcode-indexed 515F and 806R primers. The 16S rRNA gene amplicons were detected by electrophoresis on 1.5% agarose gels, purified with a ProNex® Size-Selective Purification System (Promega, Madison, WI, USA), and quantified with a QuantiFluor® One dsDNA System (Promega, Madison, WI, USA). All samples were pooled in equivalent concentration for producing a sequencing library and the library was quantified at 2 nM using KAPA Library Quantification Kit Illumina® platforms (Roche, Basel, Switzerland). Finally, pyrosequencing was performed using an Illumina iSeq 100 platform (Illumina Inc., San Diego, CA, USA).

2.9. Statistical Analysis

Data are presented as mean ± standard error of the mean (SEM). One-way ANOVA with Duncan's test was used to assess differences between groups (SPSS, Chicago, IL, USA). $p < 0.05$ was regarded as representing statistical significance, and for multiple comparisons, statistical differences among the groups are indicated below using 'a, b, c, and d'.

3. Results

3.1. UPLC-PDA-ESI-TOF-MS for Identification of WIB Constituents

WIB (141.83 g) was obtained from 500 g of dried *I. batatas* stem powder, with a yield of 28.366%. UPLC-PDA-ESI-TOF-MS analysis successfully identified 11 key components of WIB. Figure 1 displays the characteristic chromatogram observed at 254 nm and UV spectrum of each peak. Table 2 outlines the essential information for each compound, including retention time (Rt) at 254 nm, precursor ions, mass-to-charge ratio (m/z), elemental composition, and mass differences (mmu). All compounds were confirmed through direct comparison with reference standard compounds, except for peak 6. This particular peak was tentatively identified as quercetin-3-*O*-β-D-sophoroside based on a review of the existing literature [30].

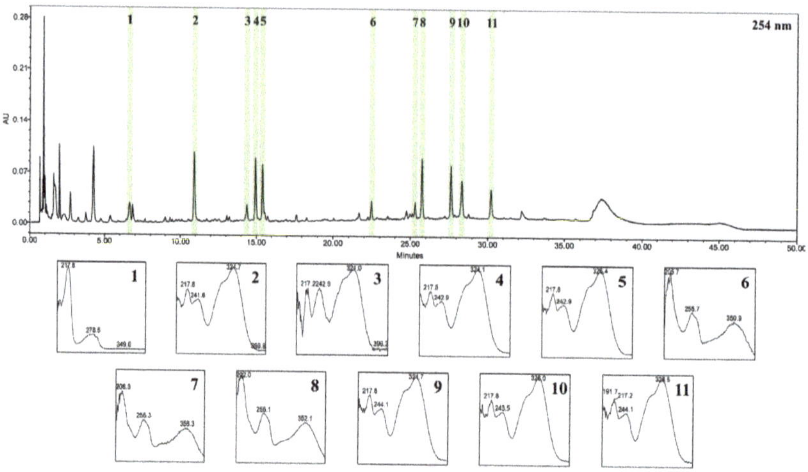

Figure 1. The UPLC-PDA chromatogram and peak-specific UV spectrum of identified WIB compounds; (**1**) L-tryptophan, (**2**) neochlorogenic acid, (**3**) caffeic acid, (**4**) chlorogenic acid, (**5**) cryptochlorogenic acid, (**6**) quercetin 3-O-β-D-sophoroside, (**7**) hyperoside, (**8**) isoquercetin, (**9**) isochlorogenic aicd B, (**10**) isochlorogenic acid A, (**11**) isochlorogenic acid C.

Table 2. Retention time (Rt), precursor ion, elemental composition, and mass difference in the identified peaks of WIB.

Peak No.	Rt (min)	Precursor Ion (*m*/*z*)	Elemental Composition (or Molecular Formula)	Mass Difference (mmu)	Identification
1	6.6	205.09655 $[M+H]^+$ 203.07701 $[M-H]^-$	$C_{11}H_{12}N_2O_2$	−1.16 −5.04	L-tryptophan [1]
2	10.8	355.10230 $[M+H]^+$ 377.08625 $[M+Na]^+$ 353.08623 $[M-H]^-$	$C_{16}H_{18}O_9$	−0.61 1.39 −1.03	Neochlorogenic acid [1]
3	14.	181.04995 $[M+H]^+$ 179.03368 $[M-H]^-$	$C_9H_8O_4$	−0.13 −0.75	Caffeic acid [1]
4	14.9	355.10254 $[M+H]^+$ 377.08614 $[M+Na]^+$ 353.08607 $[M-H]^-$	$C_{16}H_{18}O_9$	−0.36 1.29 −1.18	Chlorogenic acid [1]
5	15. 3	355.10254 $[M+H]^+$ 377.08647 $[M+Na]^+$ 353.08644 $[M-H]^-$	$C_{16}H_{18}O_9$	−0.36 1.62 −0.82	Cryptochlorogenic acid [1]
6	22.3	627.16048 $[M+H]^+$ 625.14879 $[M-H]^-$	$C_{27}H_{30}O_{17}$	4.35 8.31	Quercetin 3-*O*-*β*-D-sophoroside
7	25.1	465.10362 $[M+H]^+$ 463.08995 $[M-H]^-$	$C_{21}H_{20}O_{12}$	0.32 2.30	Hyperoside [1]
8	25.6	465.10496 $[M+H]^+$ 463.08931 $[M-H]^-$	$C_{21}H_{20}O_{12}$	1.66 1.66	Isoquercetin [1]
9	27.4	517.13593 $[M+H]^+$ 539.11944 $[M+Na]^+$ 515.12501 $[M-H]^-$	$C_{25}H_{24}O_{12}$	1.33 2.89 6.06	Isochlorogenic acid B [1]
10	28.1	517.13653 $[M+H]^+$ 539.11977 $[M+Na]^+$ 515.12431 $[M-H]^-$	$C_{25}H_{24}O_{12}$	1.93 3.23 5.36	Isochlorogenic acid A [1]
11	30.0	517.13486 $[M+H]^+$ 515.12623 $[M-H]^-$	$C_{25}H_{24}O_{12}$	0.26 7.28	Isochlorogenic acid C [1]

[1] Identified using reference standard compounds.

3.2. WIB Lessens the Body Weight Gain in HFD-Induced Mice

Five experimental groups were established to investigate the effect of WIB on the body weight of HFD-fed mice. Over a 10-week period, the HFD group exhibited a significant increase in body weight compared with the CON group. From the third week onward, the orlistat-administered group (positive control) and the WIB group exhibited lower body weights than the HFD group (Figure 2a). Especially, body weight on the final day of the experiment (HFD group: 42.72 ± 0.85 g vs. WIB 100 mg/kg group: 36.90 ± 1.20 g; WIB 300 mg/kg group: 36.67 ± 0.78 g) and body weight gain (HFD group: 22.21 ± 2.24 g vs. WIB 100 mg/kg group: 17.67 ± 3.17 g; WIB 300 mg/kg group: 17.71 ± 2.06 g) were elevated in HFD group and lessened by WIB treatment. Orlistat treatment significantly decreased body weight and weight gain, and a similar pattern was observed in the WIB (100 and 300 mg/kg) treatment groups (Figure 2b). Food intake was measured to determine whether there was a change in appetite. WIB treatment significantly decreased the amount of food intake compared to the vehicle-treated control and HFD group (Figure 2c).

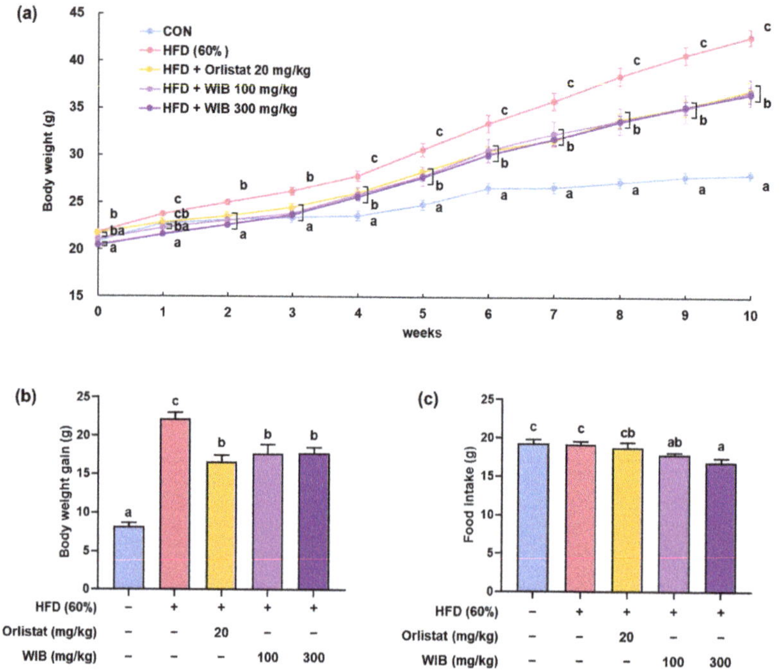

Figure 2. Repressive effects of WIB on body weight in HFD-induced obese mice. HFD-induced mice were administered the indicated doses of WIB (100 and 300 mg/kg) daily during the experiment. (**a**) Body weights, (**b**) total body weight gain for 10 weeks, and (**c**) food intake in 1 week (n = 8). Values are represented as the mean ± standard error of the mean (SEM). Values with different letters are significantly different, $p < 0.05$ (a < b < c).

3.3. WIB Modified the Fat Composition in HFD-Induced Mice

To comprehensively verify the inhibitory effects of WIB on fat accumulation without invasive assessments, we employed DEXA analysis. HFD caused mice to accumulate more fat than in the CON group, and WIB treatment reduced fat weight in the whole body (HFD group: 18.38 ± 0.86 g vs. WIB 100 mg/kg group: 14.86 ± 0.75 g; WIB 300 mg/kg group: 14.57 ± 0.90 g, $p < 0.05$) (Figure 3a,b). Among the various adipose tissue deposits, subcutaneous fat is the most susceptible to dietary modulation. Accordingly, we analyzed the accumulation of fat deposits in subcutaneous tissue, along with the mesenteric, gonadal, and renal tissue weights. Fat deposits gained by the HFD were significantly reduced by WIB treatment (Figure 3c–f). These results indicate that WIB-reduced fat accumulation in various body regions contributes to weight loss.

3.4. WIB Ameliorates the Lipid Parameters in Blood Plasma of HFD-Induced Mice

Obesity is associated with abnormal blood lipid levels. TC, TG, LDL, and VLDL levels were significantly higher in the HFD group than in the CON group (Table 3). The WIB 300 mg/kg and orlistat groups showed significantly reduced TG, LDL, and VLDL levels compared to the HFD group. Notably, WIB 100 mg/kg significantly decreased only LDL levels, while TG and VLDL levels showed a mild reduction without statistical significance. While only the orlistat group showed a statistically significant decrease in TC levels, the consistent, albeit non-significant, reduction observed in both WIB-treated groups suggests a potential lipid-lowering effect of WIB. Additionally, although HFD did not notably reduce HDL levels, orlistat treatment significantly increased HDL compared to the HFD group. A slight, non-significant increase in HDL levels was also observed in both WIB-treated groups.

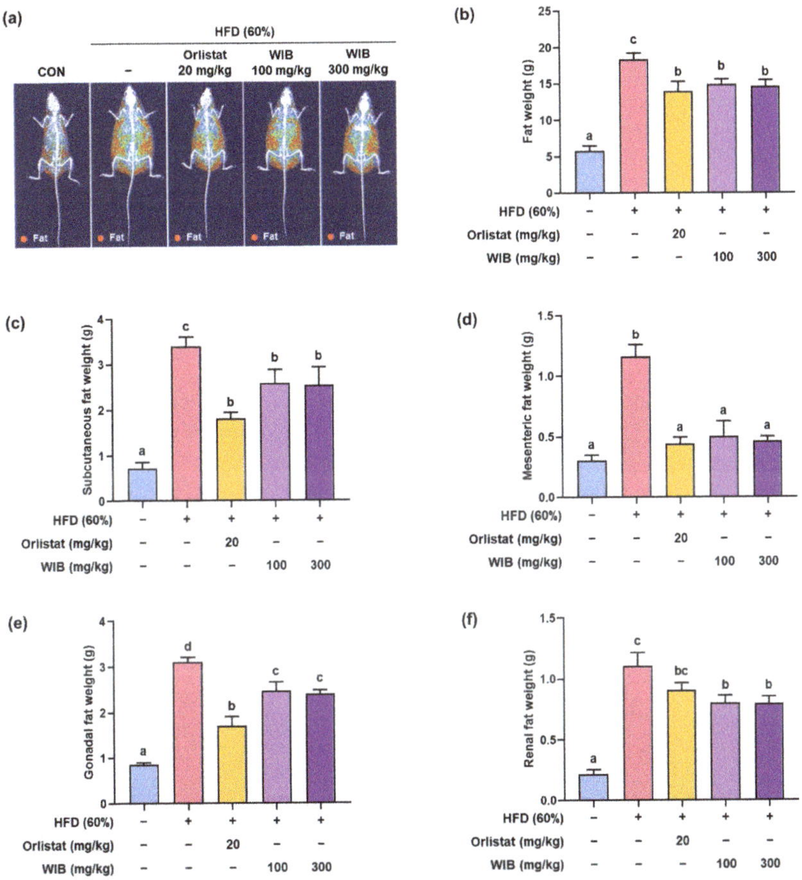

Figure 3. Effects of WIB on body composition and fat mass in HFD-induced obese mice. (**a**) Radiography images of fat tissues. (**b**) The fat weight in each group was measured through DEXA analysis. Fat was obtained from each tissue after sacrificing the mice, and their weights were measured. (**c–f**) Subcutaneous, mesenteric, gonadal, and renal fat weights. Values are represented as the mean ± SEM (DEXA analysis; $n = 3$, fat in tissue weight; $n = 5$). Values with different letters are significantly different, $p < 0.05$ (a < b < c < d).

Table 3. Effects of WIB on lipid parameters in HFD-induced obesity mice.

Variable (mg/dL)	CON	HFD	Orlistat (20 mg/kg)	WIB (100 mg/kg)	WIB (300 mg/kg)
TC	103.43 ± 14.88 [a]	158.71 ± 8.04 [c]	125.71 ± 37.84 [ab]	148.57 ± 23.14 [bc]	147.29 ± 10.73 [bc]
TG	52.86 ± 9.91 [a]	115.14 ± 15.60 [c]	66.57 ± 25.25 [ab]	86.43 ± 31.72 [bc]	68.00 ± 42.49 [ab]
LDL	9.71 ± 2.14 [a]	15.29 ± 1.25 [c]	11.57 ± 2.64 [ab]	12.86 ± 2.04 [b]	11.57 ± 2.23 [ab]
HDL	86.57 ± 5.91 [a]	91.14 ± 14.24 [a]	97.71 ± 13.83 [b]	96.00 ± 9.07 [ab]	99.57 ± 8.79 [ab]
VLDL	8.86 ± 1.65 [a]	18.29 ± 2.70 [c]	10.12 ± 2.29 [ab]	14.40 ± 5.29 [bc]	11.21 ± 6.93 [ab]

Values are represented as the mean ± SEM ($n = 8$). Values with different letters are significantly different, $p < 0.05$ (a < b < c).

3.5. WIB Refined the Obesity-Related Hormones in Blood Plasma of HFD-Induced Mice

Adipokines, such as leptin, adiponectin, and insulin, can influence lipid profile, lipolysis, and lipogenesis [31]. Compared with the CON group, the secretion of insulin and leptin in the HFD group was surpassed, and adiponectin was curtailed (Figure 4a–c). However, the altered leptin, adiponectin, and insulin levels were significantly normalized by WIB treatment.

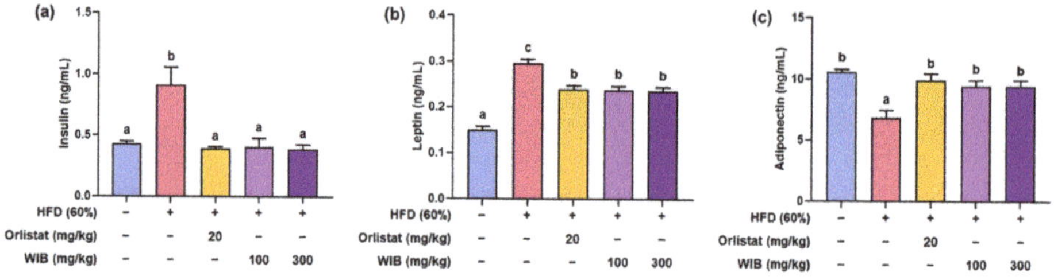

Figure 4. Effects of WIB on obesity-related hormones in HFD-induced obese mice. (**a–c**) Insulin, leptin, and adiponectin levels. Values are represented as the mean ± SEM (n = 5). Values with different letters are significantly different, $p < 0.05$ (a < b < c).

3.6. WIB Reduced Hypertrophy of Lipid Droplets and Lipogenesis in Subcutaneous Tissue of HFD-Induced Mice

Lipid parameters and adipocytes are closely linked because they play a central role in lipid storage [32]. To verify the effect of WIB on lipid accumulation in WAT, subcutaneous fat pads were visualized using H&E staining. The size of adipocytes was expanded in HFD mice and decreased significantly in orlistat and WIB-treated mice (HFD group: 139.18 ± 4.55 μm, WIB 100 mg/kg group: 84.74 ± 2.23 μm, $p < 0.05$, WIB 300 mg/kg group: 57.31 ± 2.82 μm, $p < 0.05$) (Figure 5a,b). Based on the histological analysis, phosphorylation of AMPKα and expression of C/EBPα and SREBP-1 were analyzed by Western blot (Figure 5c). Phosphorylation of AMPKα (Thr 172) was potently suppressed in the HFD group and significantly recovered by WIB treatment. However, WIB treatment did not alter the total AMPKα expression levels, indicating that only AMPKα phosphorylation was affected. In addition, WIB treatment significantly reduced the expression of C/EBPα and mature SREBP-1, which was notably increased in the HFD group.

3.7. WIB Prevents Lipid Accumulation in Liver Tissue of HFD-Induced Mice

Liver weight can indirectly indicate lipid accumulation in the hepatic tissues [33]. The weight of the liver increased in the HFD group and significantly decreased in orlistat or WIB treatment group (HFD group: 1.58 ± 0.06 g, WIB 100 mg/kg group: 1.12 ± 0.07 g, $p < 0.05$, WIB 300 mg/kg group: 1.05 ± 0.02 g, $p < 0.05$) (Figure 6a). To confirm whether the increase in liver weight was due to lipid accumulation, liver fat was visualized by H&E staining. The liver tissue of the HFD group showed fat accumulation, whereas the administration of orlistat or WIB prevented this amassment (Figure 6b). Based on the histological analysis and the liver weight, phosphorylation of AMPKα and expression of C/EBPα and SREBP-1 were analyzed by Western blot. In accordance with the findings observed in subcutaneous fat, WIB treatment recovered the HFD-induced downregulation of phosphorylated AMPKα (Thr 172) in the liver. The HFD group exhibited increased levels of C/EBPα, which were subsequently normalized by the WIB treatment. The precursor SREBP-1 showed reduced expression in the HFD group; however, its expression was restored upon WIB treatment (Figure 6c).

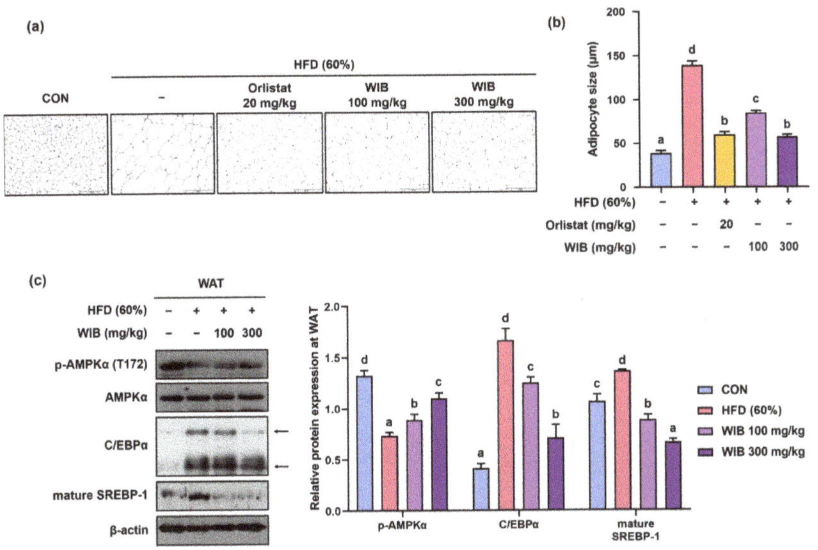

Figure 5. Effects of WIB on adipocyte size and lipogenesis in subcutaneous fat tissues of HFD-induced obese mice. (**a**) Histological analysis of subcutaneous fat tissue via H&E staining at ×20 magnification. (**b**) Representative diameters of adipocytes in the tissue. (**c**) Levels of p-AMPKα and lipogenic transcription factors were determined by Western blot analysis. Arrowed bands are the main band of that protein. Quantitative values for the Western blot of p-AMPKα to AMPKα, CEBP/α, and SREBP-1 are shown. β-Actin was used as an internal control. Values are represented as the mean ± SEM (adipocyte size; $n = 5$, density; $n = 3$). Values with different letters are significantly different, $p < 0.05$ (a < b < c < d).

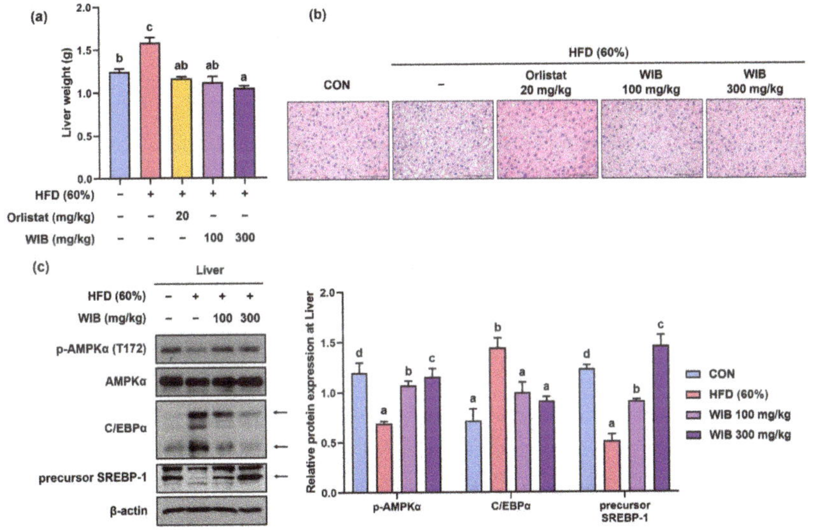

Figure 6. Effects of WIB on lipid accumulation in the liver tissues of HFD-induced obese mice. (**a**) Comparison of liver weights of each group. (**b**) The images of H&E-stained liver tissues at ×40 magnification. (**c**) Expression levels of p-AMPKα and lipogenic transcription factors were determined by Western blot analysis. Arrowed bands are the main band of that protein. Quantitative

values for the Western blot of p-AMPKα to AMPKα, CEBP/α, and SREBP-1 are shown. β-Actin was used as an internal control. Values are represented as the mean ± SEM (liver weight; n = 5, density; n = 3). Values with different letters are significantly different, $p < 0.05$ (a < b < c < d).

3.8. WIB Upregulates the Levels of Thermogenic-Related Proteins in BAT of HFD-Induced Mice

BAT is involved in thermogenesis by increasing energy expenditure via the utilization of stored fat [34]. Although no group attained statistically significant changes in BAT weight compared to the CON group, WIB treatment mildly increased BAT weight (Figure 7a). After the WIB treatment, the ratio of p-AMPKα/AMPKα was significantly elevated compared to the HFD group. The expression levels of key thermogenesis-related factors such as PGC-1α, PPARα, SIRT1, UCP-1, and COX-IV were significantly restored compared to those in the HFD group (Figure 7b).

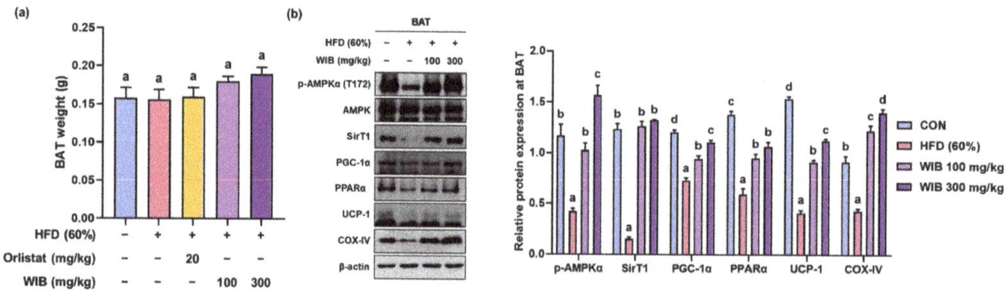

Figure 7. Effect of WIB on thermogenesis-related factors in the BAT of HFD-induced obese mice. (**a**) Weight of BAT in each group. (**b**) Expression levels of p-AMPKα, AMPKα, and thermogenesis-related proteins were determined by Western blot analysis. Quantitative values for Western blot are shown in graphs. β-Actin was used as an internal control. Values are represented as the mean ± SEM (BAT weight; n = 5, density; n = 3). Values with different letters are significantly different, $p < 0.05$ (a < b < c < d).

3.9. WIB Ameliorates the Dysbiosis by Regulating the Gut Microbiota Composition in HFD-Induced Mice

Obesity is often associated with unbalanced or disrupted gut microbiota, characterized by reduced microbial diversity and altered ratios of key bacterial groups [35]. This dysbiosis is associated with increased fat storage and metabolic disturbances [36]. Principal coordinate analysis (PCoA) plots based on β-diversity were used to examine the differences in the phylogenetic relationships of microbial communities. The plot indicated that the microbial community of the HFD group shifted from that of the CON group, whereas the WIB-treated groups were located at a distance from the HFD group, which was closer to that of the CON group (Figure 8a). Based on these results, the microbiome composition at the phylum level was analyzed for each group. Figure 8b shows that compared to the CON group, the phylum-level composition shifted in the HFD group, but was restored to resemble that of the CON group with WIB treatment. In the HFD group, *Bacteroidetes* levels decreased compared to those in the CON group but increased with WIB treatment (Figure 8c). Conversely, *Firmicutes* and *Proteobacteria* levels were upregulated in the HFD group compared to those in the CON group but downregulated with WIB treatment (Figure 8d,e). The F/B ratio was significantly higher in the HFD group than that in the CON group. However, WIB treatment ameliorated this increase relative to that observed in the HFD group (Figure 8f).

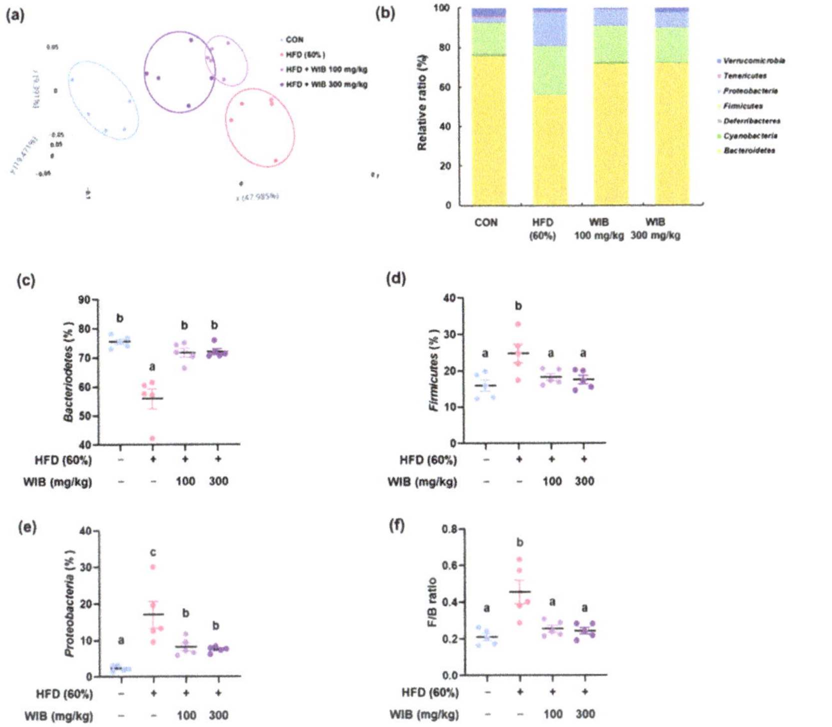

Figure 8. Regulatory effects of WIB on microbiota composition and colonization. (**a**) β-Diversity between groups was analyzed using a PCoA plot. (**b**) Phylum-level composition ratios in each group. (**c–f**) Relative ratios of *Bacteroidetes*, *Firmicutes*, and *Proteobacteria* and F/B ratio. Values are represented as the mean ± SEM (n = 5). Values with different letters are significantly different, $p < 0.05$ (a < b < c).

4. Discussion

Obesity is an excess body fat accumulation, which can cause several health problems related to hypertension, hyperlipidemia, atherosclerosis, and type 2 diabetes and can lead to heart attacks and strokes [37]. The well-known causes of obesity are genetic factors, high-calorie food intake, reduced physical activity, and psychological factors [38]. Currently, anti-obesity medications such as semaglutide offer satisfactory weight loss, but injections once a week may be less acceptable to patients. Additionally, its side effects include nausea, vomiting, and diarrhea, which may prevent patients from being consistent with the medication [39]. This indicates the demand for new agents that can alter metabolic processes with fewer side effects than pharmaceuticals [40]. Therefore, this study aimed to develop new functional food candidates for the prevention of obesity by leveraging the weight-reducing potential of standardized natural products. In this regard, we focused on the potential use of sweet potato stems, an edible natural resource, to develop functional materials aimed at reducing body fat.

Sweet potatoes are starchy root crops that are cultivated worldwide because of their nutritive value and taste [41]. Research on the stems of sweet potatoes has been less extensive than that on tubers. According to some studies, sweet potato leaves are known to contain high amounts of polyphenolic compounds such as flavonols, catechins, hydroxycinnamic acids, and hydroxybenzoic acids, as well as triterpenes, alkaloids, anthraquinones, and coumarins [42,43]. Each compound is known to have anti-oxidant, antidiabetic, and/or anti-inflammatory effects [44,45]. In particular, we identified quercetin 3-*O*-*β*-D-sophoroside as one of the constituents of WIB from sweet potato stems. Quercetin is well known for its anti-obesity effects; therefore, we hypothesized that WIB may possess anti-obesity properties [46]. To test this, we investigated the weight-reducing effects and molecular mechanisms of WIB in C57BL/6 mice fed HFD.

Fat accumulation accompanying obesity refers to the excessive storage of fat in the adipose tissue of the body [47]. First, we monitored overall weight changes to verify the inhibitory effects of WIB on fat accumulation. Despite the expectation that weight loss would be greater in the 300 mg/kg WIB group than in the 100 mg/kg WIB group, this decrease was similar in both groups. This is because, within the body, drugs can act non-linearly or become saturated above a certain concentration, leading to inconsistent increases in efficacy with increasing concentrations [42]. DEXA was used to measure the total fat distribution to quantify fat reduction. We analyzed fat weight reduction in various tissues to observe local effects. The findings illustrate how WIB contributes to the reduction in both total body fat and fat in specific tissues.

Blood analysis was conducted to analyze toxicity levels, lipid profiles, and hormone concentrations. Toxicity analysis revealed that WIB administration did not affect liver and kidney function, meaning that the observed weight loss in WIB was not caused by toxicity (Figure S1). Upregulated blood levels of TG, VLDL, and LDL occur when the liver stores excess fatty acids that cannot be efficiently processed or utilized [48,49]. As WIB restored normal level of TG, VLDL, and LDL, it is plausible that WIB ameliorates hepatic steatosis without adversely affecting liver function. There are many obesity-related hormones; however, only the key hormones, insulin, leptin, and adiponectin, were measured. Insulin regulates TG synthesis and lipogenesis in adipose tissue [50]. However, persistent HFD promotes insulin resistance, resulting in increased insulin secretion, but insulin becomes unable to perform its normal function [51]. Adiponectin can improve insulin sensitivity, and leptin reduces body weight and fat by inhibiting appetite [52]. Analysis of hormone levels revealed that HFD caused abnormal changes in insulin, leptin, and adiponectin levels, but these changes were recovered by WIB treatment. In particular, the reduced leptin secretion was reflected in a corresponding decrease in food intake. By restoring the hormone and blood lipid biomarkers linked to obesity, WIB is thought to decrease the development of metabolic syndrome and its associated chronic conditions.

Based on the widely accepted view that WAT secretes a diverse array of peptide and steroid hormones, including leptin, cytokines, and adiponectin, it is evident that obesity-induced adipokine dysregulation is closely linked to subcutaneous fat [53]. Alterations in the secretion profile of these adipokines from subcutaneous adipose tissue may significantly contribute to the development of metabolic disturbances. AMPK, a key cellular energy sensor, plays a regulatory role in protein, lipid, and glucose metabolism, and its activation downregulates SREBP-1 expression, thereby inhibiting lipogenesis [54,55]. SREBP-1 can regulate PPARγ, which in turn activates C/EBPα [56]. C/EBPα activates metabolic adipocyte genes, and SREBP-1 regulates lipogenesis [57]. WIB can inhibit fat accumulation by modulating the transcriptional level of lipogenesis through AMPK activation, exhibiting its potential against obesity.

Our bodies attempt to cope with excess caloric intake by burning fat [58]. BAT is essential for thermogenic activity and contributes to energy expenditure [59]. In BAT, AMPK also acts as a regulator of energy balance. BAT employs mitochondria for ATP synthesis and heat production, with UCP-1 playing a key role by uncoupling respiration from ATP production to generate heat, thus combating obesity [60]. It is well known that COX-IV supports oxidative phosphorylation. AMPKα and SIRT-1 enhance PGC-1α activity. PGC-1α is involved in the regulation of thermogenic genes, activation of PPARα, and induction of UCP-1 expression, which in turn promotes lipolysis [12,61]. Our data showed that the WIB administration increased BAT weight and regulated the expression of thermogenesis-related proteins, including SIRT1, UCP-1, PGC-1α, PPARα, and COX-IV in BAT of HFD-induced obese mice.

Although AMPK signaling is primarily regulated within individual tissues, it is plausible that enhanced AMPK activity in subcutaneous fat could influence liver metabolism through the secretion of adipokines and metabolites that act as inter-tissue communicators. Moreover, AMPK promotes the beigeing process of WAT by regulating energy metabolism, highlighting its pivotal role in linking WAT and BAT [62]. Taken together, these findings suggest that AMPK acts as a central metabolic hub connecting the liver, WAT, and BAT, thereby coordinating systemic energy homeostasis. This coordinated AMPK activation may underlie the comprehensive metabolic improvements observed with WIB treatment, providing a mechanistic basis for its anti-obesity effects.

The gut microbiota can affect obesity management [36]. Elevated levels of *Proteobacteria* can influence host energy balance by modifying the absorption and storage of dietary energy [63]. *Firmicutes* exhibit high efficiency in energy metabolism, influencing the absorption of calories [64]. Obese individuals typically have a greater abundance of *Proteobacteria* and *Firmicutes* in their gut microbiomes than non-obese individuals. In contrast, *Bacteroidetes* are known to be easily found in nonobese individuals. The differentially abundant Firmicutes and Bacteroidetes also play a critical role in obesity [7]. Significant changes in the F/B ratio denote gut microbiota dysbiosis. F/B ratios are linked to energy uptake and storage, and they provide critical insights into strategies that can be employed to prevent obesity via modulation of the microbiome [65]. As the treatment of WIB normalized the microbiome composition and F/B ratio, WIB has the potential to modulate gut microbiome composition and prevent dysbiosis. Based on our findings, we propose that the bioactivity of WIB is mediated through AMPK activation, which modulates adipose tissue formation and liver metabolism, ultimately contributing to the inhibition of lipogenesis and anti-obesity effects [66,67]. For further investigation, we examined microbiota, which is generally known to be associated with obesity [13,68,69] and found that WIB treatment significantly restored HFD-induced dysbiosis. Recently, Zhang et al. identified that intestinal AMPKα1 stimulates thermogenesis by modulating antimicrobial peptides that, in turn, influence gut microbiota and metabolites [70]. Based on this correlation, it can be inferred that WIB exerts a comprehensive effect on obesity.

Although in vivo experiments have provided valuable insights into the anti-obesity effects of WIB, the underlying molecular mechanisms have not been directly validated through in vitro assays. In addition, definitive target validation at the protein or receptor level was not conducted, which limits mechanistic interpretation. Further studies using cell-based models and target-specific approaches are warranted to confirm the signaling pathways involved. Moreover, we recognize the necessity for further investigation to assess the applicability of WIB to human subjects.

5. Conclusions

This study visualized the anti-obesity effects of WIB in HFD-induced mice. Reductions in body weight and fat mass, with advanced blood lipid profiles and adipokines, were achieved by WIB. Furthermore, WIB induced the down-regulation of p-AMPKα expression, fat accumulation, and the expression of key lipogenic transcription factors in the liver and WAT. It affects BAT by enhancing energy expenditure and metabolism-regulated protein expression. WIB's ability to modulate the gut microbiota resulted in the effect of WIB on obesity-related gut dysbiosis. These findings support the potential use of WIB as a natural therapeutic agent for obesity management.

Supplementary Materials: The following supporting information can be downloaded at: https://www.mdpi.com/article/10.3390/nu17101643/s1, Table S1: Positive and negative ion mode ESI-TOF-MS conditions for identification of WIB components; Figure S1: The blood plasma levels of GOT, GPT, and BUN. Values with the same letter are not significantly different.

Author Contributions: Formal analysis, Y.S.Y., M.-j.K. and G.P.; investigation, C.-W.L. and Y.-S.Y.; project administration, Y.-P.J. and K.-T.L.; validation, G.P. and M.C.; writing—original draft, C.-W.L.; writing—review and editing, Y.-S.Y. and K.-S.C. All authors have read and agreed to the published version of the manuscript.

Funding: This research was funded by the DALIM BIOTECH Corporation (Grant No. KHU-DALIM BIOTECH-20212131).

Institutional Review Board Statement: All procedures were executed with the Guidelines for Animal Care and Use of Kyung Hee University, and the animal model experiment was approved by the experimentation Committee of Kyung Hee University (KHSASP-22-215, Approval date: 22 July 2022).

Informed Consent Statement: Not applicable.

Data Availability Statement: The original contributions presented in this study are included in the article/Supplementary Materials; further inquiries can be directed to the corresponding author.

Conflicts of Interest: Authors Ye Seul Yoon and Mi-ju Kim were employed by the Dalim Biotech Co., Ltd. Authors Young-Seo Yoon and Kyung-Sook Chung were employed by the BELABEL BIO. Inc. The remaining authors declare that the research was conducted in the absence of any commercial or financial relationships that could be construed as a potential conflict of interest. The authors declare that this study received funding from DALIM BIOTECH Corporation. The funder was not involved in the study design, collection, analysis, interpretation of data, the writing of this article or the decision to submit it for publication.

References

1. Prattichizzo, F.; Ceriello, A.; Shah, V.N. Obesity, NAFLD/NASH, and Diabetes. *Diabetes Technol. Ther.* **2024**, *26*, S231–S240. [CrossRef]
2. Blackstone, R.P.; Blackstone, R.P. Obesity-related diseases and syndromes: Insulin resistance, type 2 diabetes mellitus, non-alcoholic fatty liver disease, cardiovascular disease, and metabolic syndrome. *Obes. Med. Pract. Essent. Guide* **2016**, 83–108.
3. Longo, M.; Zatterale, F.; Naderi, J.; Parrillo, L.; Formisano, P.; Raciti, G.A.; Beguinot, F.; Miele, C. Adipose Tissue Dysfunction as Determinant of Obesity-Associated Metabolic Complications. *Int. J. Mol. Sci.* **2019**, *20*, 2358. [CrossRef]
4. Cheng, L.; Wang, J.; Dai, H.; Duan, Y.; An, Y.; Shi, L.; Lv, Y.; Li, H.; Wang, C.; Ma, Q.; et al. Brown and beige adipose tissue: A novel therapeutic strategy for obesity and type 2 diabetes mellitus. *Adipocyte* **2021**, *10*, 48–65. [CrossRef] [PubMed]
5. Petito, G.; Cioffi, F.; Magnacca, N.; de Lange, P.; Senese, R.; Lanni, A. Adipose Tissue Remodeling in Obesity: An Overview of the Actions of Thyroid Hormones and Their Derivatives. *Pharmaceuticals* **2023**, *16*, 572. [CrossRef] [PubMed]
6. Kawai, T.; Autieri, M.V.; Scalia, R. Adipose tissue inflammation and metabolic dysfunction in obesity. *Am. J. Physiol. Cell Physiol.* **2021**, *320*, C375–C391. [CrossRef] [PubMed]
7. Han, H.-S.; Lee, H.-H.; Gil, H.-S.; Chung, K.-S.; Kim, J.-K.; Kim, D.-H.; Yoon, J.; Chung, E.K.; Lee, J.K.; Yang, W.M. Standardized hot water extract from the leaves of Hydrangea serrata (Thunb.) Ser. alleviates obesity via the AMPK pathway and modulation of the gut microbiota composition in high fat diet-induced obese mice. *Food Funct.* **2021**, *12*, 2672–2685. [CrossRef]
8. Yoon, Y.S.; Chung, K.S.; Lee, S.Y.; Heo, S.W.; Kim, Y.R.; Lee, J.K.; Kim, H.; Park, S.; Shin, Y.K.; Lee, K.T. Anti-obesity effects of a standardized ethanol extract of Eisenia bicyclis by regulating the AMPK signaling pathway in 3T3-L1 cells and HFD-induced mice. *Food Funct.* **2024**, *15*, 6424–6437. [CrossRef]
9. Abu Shelbayeh, O.; Arroum, T.; Morris, S.; Busch, K.B. PGC-1alpha Is a Master Regulator of Mitochondrial Lifecycle and ROS Stress Response. *Antioxidants* **2023**, *12*, 1075. [CrossRef]
10. Lehman, J.J.; Barger, P.M.; Kovacs, A.; Saffitz, J.E.; Medeiros, D.M.; Kelly, D.P. Peroxisome proliferator-activated receptor gamma coactivator-1 promotes cardiac mitochondrial biogenesis. *J. Clin. Investig.* **2000**, *106*, 847–856. [CrossRef]
11. Meng, D.; Yin, G.; Chen, S.; Zhang, X.; Yu, W.; Wang, L.; Liu, H.; Jiang, W.; Sun, Y.; Zhang, F. Diosgenin attenuates nonalcoholic hepatic steatosis through the hepatic SIRT1/PGC-1alpha pathway. *Eur. J. Pharmacol.* **2024**, *977*, 176737. [CrossRef] [PubMed]
12. Cheng, C.F.; Ku, H.C.; Lin, H. PGC-1alpha as a Pivotal Factor in Lipid and Metabolic Regulation. *Int. J. Mol. Sci.* **2018**, *19*, 3447. [CrossRef] [PubMed]

13. Cuevas-Sierra, A.; Ramos-Lopez, O.; Riezu-Boj, J.I.; Milagro, F.I.; Martinez, J.A. Diet, Gut Microbiota, and Obesity: Links with Host Genetics and Epigenetics and Potential Applications. *Adv. Nutr.* **2019**, *10*, S17–S30. [CrossRef]
14. Sankararaman, S.; Noriega, K.; Velayuthan, S.; Sferra, T.; Martindale, R. Gut Microbiome and Its Impact on Obesity and Obesity-Related Disorders. *Curr. Gastroenterol. Rep.* **2023**, *25*, 31–44. [CrossRef]
15. Porras, D.; Nistal, E.; Martinez-Florez, S.; Pisonero-Vaquero, S.; Olcoz, J.L.; Jover, R.; Gonzalez-Gallego, J.; Garcia-Mediavilla, M.V.; Sanchez-Campos, S. Protective effect of quercetin on high-fat diet-induced non-alcoholic fatty liver disease in mice is mediated by modulating intestinal microbiota imbalance and related gut-liver axis activation. *Free Radic. Biol. Med.* **2017**, *102*, 188–202. [CrossRef]
16. Zsálig, D.; Berta, A.; Tóth, V.; Szabó, Z.; Simon, K.; Figler, M.; Pusztafalvi, H.; Polyák, É. A review of the relationship between gut microbiome and obesity. *Appl. Sci.* **2023**, *13*, 610. [CrossRef]
17. Walker, A.W.; Parkhill, J. Microbiology. Fighting obesity with bacteria. *Science* **2013**, *341*, 1069–1070. [CrossRef] [PubMed]
18. Yarahmadi, A.; Afkhami, H.; Javadi, A.; Kashfi, M. Understanding the complex function of gut microbiota: Its impact on the pathogenesis of obesity and beyond: A comprehensive review. *Diabetol. Metab. Syndr.* **2024**, *16*, 308. [CrossRef]
19. Kimura, I.; Inoue, D.; Hirano, K.; Tsujimoto, G. The SCFA Receptor GPR43 and Energy Metabolism. *Front. Endocrinol.* **2014**, *5*, 85. [CrossRef]
20. Tak, Y.J.; Lee, S.Y. Long-Term Efficacy and Safety of Anti-Obesity Treatment: Where Do We Stand? *Curr. Obes. Rep.* **2021**, *10*, 14–30. [CrossRef]
21. Halpern, B.; Halpern, A. Safety assessment of FDA-approved (orlistat and lorcaserin) anti-obesity medications. *Expert Opin. Drug Saf.* **2015**, *14*, 305–315. [CrossRef]
22. Kim, G.N.; Shin, M.R.; Shin, S.H.; Lee, A.R.; Lee, J.Y.; Seo, B.I.; Kim, M.Y.; Kim, T.H.; Noh, J.S.; Rhee, M.H.; et al. Study of Antiobesity Effect Through Inhibition of Pancreatic Lipase Activity of Diospyros Kaki Fruit and Citrus Unshiu Peel. *BioMed Res. Int.* **2016**, *2016*, 1723042. [CrossRef] [PubMed]
23. Kang, J.G.; Park, C.Y. Anti-Obesity Drugs: A Review About Their Effects and Safety. *Diabetes Metab. J.* **2012**, *36*, 13–25. [CrossRef] [PubMed]
24. Lee, M.S.; Kim, C.T.; Kim, Y. Green tea (-)-epigallocatechin-3-gallate reduces body weight with regulation of multiple genes expression in adipose tissue of diet-induced obese mice. *Ann. Nutr. Metab.* **2009**, *54*, 151–157. [CrossRef]
25. Barrios-Nolasco, A.; Dominguez-Lopez, A.; Miliar-Garcia, A.; Cornejo-Garrido, J.; Jaramillo-Flores, M.E. Anti-Inflammatory Effect of Ethanolic Extract from *Tabebuia rosea* (Bertol.) DC., Quercetin, and Anti-Obesity Drugs in Adipose Tissue in Wistar Rats with Diet-Induced Obesity. *Molecules* **2023**, *28*, 3801. [CrossRef] [PubMed]
26. Zhang, L.; Tu, Z.C.; Yuan, T.; Wang, H.; Xie, X.; Fu, Z.F. Antioxidants and alpha-glucosidase inhibitors from Ipomoea batatas leaves identified by bioassay-guided approach and structure-activity relationships. *Food Chem.* **2016**, *208*, 61–67. [CrossRef]
27. Luo, D.; Mu, T.; Sun, H. Sweet potato (*Ipomoea batatas* L.) leaf polyphenols ameliorate hyperglycemia in type 2 diabetes mellitus mice. *Food Funct.* **2021**, *12*, 4117–4131. [CrossRef]
28. Shih, C.K.; Chen, C.M.; Varga, V.; Shih, L.C.; Chen, P.R.; Lo, S.F.; Shyur, L.F.; Li, S.C. White sweet potato ameliorates hyperglycemia and regenerates pancreatic islets in diabetic mice. *Food Nutr. Res.* **2020**, *64*. [CrossRef]
29. Lee, S.L.; Chin, T.Y.; Tu, S.C.; Wang, Y.J.; Hsu, Y.T.; Kao, M.C.; Wu, Y.C. Purple Sweet Potato Leaf Extract Induces Apoptosis and Reduces Inflammatory Adipokine Expression in 3T3-L1 Differentiated Adipocytes. *Evid. Based Complement. Altern. Med.* **2015**, *2015*, 126302. [CrossRef]
30. Lee, C.L.; Lee, S.L.; Chen, C.J.; Chen, H.C.; Kao, M.C.; Liu, C.H.; Chen, J.Y.; Lai, Y.T.; Wu, Y.C. Characterization of Secondary Metabolites from Purple Ipomoea batatas Leaves and Their Effects on Glucose Uptake. *Molecules* **2016**, *21*, 745. [CrossRef]
31. Pestel, J.; Blangero, F.; Watson, J.; Pirola, L.; Eljaafari, A. Adipokines in obesity and metabolic-related-diseases. *Biochimie* **2023**, *212*, 48–59. [CrossRef] [PubMed]
32. Cho, C.H.; Patel, S.; Rajbhandari, P. Adipose tissue lipid metabolism: Lipolysis. *Curr. Opin. Genet. Dev.* **2023**, *83*, 102114. [CrossRef]
33. Wang, L.; Li, M.; Yu, B.; Shi, S.; Liu, J.; Zhang, R.; Ayada, I.; Verstegen, M.M.A.; van der Laan, L.J.W.; Peppelenbosch, M.P.; et al. Recapitulating lipid accumulation and related metabolic dysregulation in human liver-derived organoids. *J. Mol. Med.* **2022**, *100*, 471–484. [CrossRef] [PubMed]
34. Saito, M.; Matsushita, M.; Yoneshiro, T.; Okamatsu-Ogura, Y. Brown Adipose Tissue, Diet-Induced Thermogenesis, and Thermogenic Food Ingredients: From Mice to Men. *Front. Endocrinol.* **2020**, *11*, 222. [CrossRef] [PubMed]
35. Amabebe, E.; Robert, F.O.; Agbalalah, T.; Orubu, E.S.F. Microbial dysbiosis-induced obesity: Role of gut microbiota in homoeostasis of energy metabolism. *Br. J. Nutr.* **2020**, *123*, 1127–1137. [CrossRef]
36. Xu, Z.; Jiang, W.; Huang, W.; Lin, Y.; Chan, F.K.L.; Ng, S.C. Gut microbiota in patients with obesity and metabolic disorders—A systematic review. *Genes. Nutr.* **2022**, *17*, 2. [CrossRef]
37. Obesity: Causes, consequences, treatments, and challenges. *J. Mol. Cell Biol.* **2021**, *13*, 463–465. [CrossRef]

38. Ghosh, S.; Dhar, S.; Bhattacharjee, S.; Bhattacharjee, P. Contribution of environmental, genetic and epigenetic factors to obesity-related metabolic syndrome. *Nucleus* **2023**, *66*, 215–237. [CrossRef]
39. Smits, M.M.; Van Raalte, D.H. Safety of Semaglutide. *Front. Endocrinol.* **2021**, *12*, 645563. [CrossRef]
40. Shaik Mohamed Sayed, U.F.; Moshawih, S.; Goh, H.P.; Kifli, N.; Gupta, G.; Singh, S.K.; Chellappan, D.K.; Dua, K.; Hermansyah, A.; Ser, H.L.; et al. Natural products as novel anti-obesity agents: Insights into mechanisms of action and potential for therapeutic management. *Front. Pharmacol.* **2023**, *14*, 1182937. [CrossRef]
41. Bodjrenou, D.M.; Li, X.; Lu, X.; Lei, S.; Zheng, B.; Zeng, H. Resistant starch from sweet potatoes: Recent advancements and applications in the food sector. *Int. J. Biol. Macromol.* **2023**, *225*, 13–26. [CrossRef] [PubMed]
42. Carvalho, I.S.; Cavaco, T.; Carvalho, L.M.; Duque, P. Effect of photoperiod on flavonoid pathway activity in sweet potato (*Ipomoea batatas* (L.) Lam.) leaves. *Food Chem.* **2010**, *118*, 384–390. [CrossRef]
43. Pochapski, M.T.; Fosquiera, E.C.; Esmerino, L.A.; Dos Santos, E.B.; Farago, P.V.; Santos, F.A.; Groppo, F.C. Phytochemical screening, antioxidant, and antimicrobial activities of the crude leaves' extract from *Ipomoea batatas* (L.) Lam. *Pharmacogn. Mag.* **2011**, *7*, 165–170. [CrossRef]
44. Chagas, M.; Behrens, M.D.; Moragas-Tellis, C.J.; Penedo, G.X.M.; Silva, A.R.; Goncalves-de-Albuquerque, C.F. Flavonols and Flavones as Potential anti-Inflammatory, Antioxidant, and Antibacterial Compounds. *Oxid. Med. Cell. Longev.* **2022**, *2022*, 9966750. [CrossRef] [PubMed]
45. Farhan, M. Green Tea Catechins: Nature's Way of Preventing and Treating Cancer. *Int. J. Mol. Sci.* **2022**, *23*, 10713. [CrossRef]
46. Sato, S.; Mukai, Y. Modulation of Chronic Inflammation by Quercetin: The Beneficial Effects on Obesity. *J. Inflamm. Res.* **2020**, *13*, 421–431. [CrossRef]
47. White, U. Adipose tissue expansion in obesity, health, and disease. *Front. Cell Dev. Biol.* **2023**, *11*, 1188844. [CrossRef] [PubMed]
48. Vekic, J.; Stefanovic, A.; Zeljkovic, A. Obesity and Dyslipidemia: A Review of Current Evidence. *Curr. Obes. Rep.* **2023**, *12*, 207–222. [CrossRef]
49. Huang, J.K.; Lee, H.C. Emerging Evidence of Pathological Roles of Very-Low-Density Lipoprotein (VLDL). *Int. J. Mol. Sci.* **2022**, *23*, 4300. [CrossRef]
50. Carpentier, A.C. 100(th) anniversary of the discovery of insulin perspective: Insulin and adipose tissue fatty acid metabolism. *Am. J. Physiol. Endocrinol. Metab.* **2021**, *320*, E653–E670. [CrossRef]
51. Kumar, A.; Sundaram, K.; Mu, J.; Dryden, G.W.; Sriwastva, M.K.; Lei, C.; Zhang, L.; Qiu, X.; Xu, F.; Yan, J.; et al. High-fat diet-induced upregulation of exosomal phosphatidylcholine contributes to insulin resistance. *Nat. Commun.* **2021**, *12*, 213. [CrossRef] [PubMed]
52. Yadav, A.; Kataria, M.A.; Saini, V.; Yadav, A. Role of leptin and adiponectin in insulin resistance. *Clin. Chim. Acta* **2013**, *417*, 80–84. [CrossRef]
53. Guerre-Millo, M. Adipose tissue hormones. *J. Endocrinol. Investig.* **2002**, *25*, 855–861. [CrossRef]
54. Angin, Y.; Beauloye, C.; Horman, S.; Bertrand, L. Regulation of Carbohydrate Metabolism, Lipid Metabolism, and Protein Metabolism by AMPK. *Exp. Suppl.* **2016**, *107*, 23–43. [CrossRef]
55. Zhang, S.; Yan, L.; Kim, S.M. Vanadium-protein complex inhibits human adipocyte differentiation through the activation of beta-catenin and LKB1/AMPK signaling pathway. *PLoS ONE* **2020**, *15*, e0239547. [CrossRef]
56. Ambele, M.A.; Dhanraj, P.; Giles, R.; Pepper, M.S. Adipogenesis: A Complex Interplay of Multiple Molecular Determinants and Pathways. *Int. J. Mol. Sci.* **2020**, *21*, 4283. [CrossRef]
57. Guru, A.; Issac, P.K.; Velayutham, M.; Saraswathi, N.T.; Arshad, A.; Arockiaraj, J. Molecular mechanism of down-regulating adipogenic transcription factors in 3T3-L1 adipocyte cells by bioactive anti-adipogenic compounds. *Mol. Biol. Rep.* **2021**, *48*, 743–761. [CrossRef] [PubMed]
58. Reverte-Salisa, L.; Siddig, S.; Hildebrand, S.; Yao, X.; Zurkovic, J.; Jaeckstein, M.Y.; Heeren, J.; Lezoualc'h, F.; Krahmer, N.; Pfeifer, A. EPAC1 enhances brown fat growth and beige adipogenesis. *Nat. Cell Biol.* **2024**, *26*, 113–123. [CrossRef]
59. Gaspar, R.C.; Pauli, J.R.; Shulman, G.I.; Munoz, V.R. An update on brown adipose tissue biology: A discussion of recent findings. *Am. J. Physiol. Endocrinol. Metab.* **2021**, *320*, E488–E495. [CrossRef]
60. Machado, S.A.; Pasquarelli-do-Nascimento, G.; da Silva, D.S.; Farias, G.R.; de Oliveira Santos, I.; Baptista, L.B.; Magalhaes, K.G. Browning of the white adipose tissue regulation: New insights into nutritional and metabolic relevance in health and diseases. *Nutr. Metab.* **2022**, *19*, 61. [CrossRef]
61. Carpentier, A.C.; Blondin, D.P.; Haman, F.; Richard, D. Brown Adipose Tissue—A Translational Perspective. *Endocr. Rev.* **2023**, *44*, 143–192. [CrossRef] [PubMed]
62. Wu, L.; Zhang, L.; Li, B.; Jiang, H.; Duan, Y.; Xie, Z.; Shuai, L.; Li, J.; Li, J. AMP-Activated Protein Kinase (AMPK) Regulates Energy Metabolism Through Modulating Thermogenesis in Adipose Tissue. *Front. Physiol.* **2018**, *9*, 122. [CrossRef] [PubMed]
63. Blaut, M. Gut microbiota and energy balance: Role in obesity. *Proc. Nutr. Soc.* **2015**, *74*, 227–234. [CrossRef]
64. Wu, X.; Zhang, G.; Zhang, W.; Zhou, J.; Cong, H.; Yang, G.; Liu, G. Rumen microbiota helps Tibetan sheep obtain energy more efficiently to survive in the extreme environment of the Qinghai-Tibet Plateau. *Front. Microbiol.* **2024**, *15*, 1431063. [CrossRef]

65. Stojanov, S.; Berlec, A.; Strukelj, B. The Influence of Probiotics on the Firmicutes/Bacteroidetes Ratio in the Treatment of Obesity and Inflammatory Bowel Disease. *Microorganisms* **2020**, *8*, 1715. [CrossRef] [PubMed]
66. Wang, D.; Yang, L.; Liu, Y. Targeting AMPK Signaling in the Liver: Implications for Obesity and Type 2 Diabetes Mellitus. *Curr. Drug Targets* **2022**, *23*, 1057–1071. [CrossRef]
67. Lee, S.Y.; Chung, K.S.; Son, S.R.; Lee, S.Y.; Jang, D.S.; Lee, J.K.; Kim, H.J.; Na, C.S.; Lee, S.H.; Lee, K.T. A Botanical Mixture Consisting of Inula japonica and Potentilla chinensis Relieves Obesity via the AMPK Signaling Pathway in 3T3-L1 Adipocytes and HFD-Fed Obese Mice. *Nutrients* **2022**, *14*, 3685. [CrossRef]
68. Liu, B.N.; Liu, X.T.; Liang, Z.H.; Wang, J.H. Gut microbiota in obesity. *World J. Gastroenterol.* **2021**, *27*, 3837–3850. [CrossRef] [PubMed]
69. Gomes, A.C.; Hoffmann, C.; Mota, J.F. The human gut microbiota: Metabolism and perspective in obesity. *Gut Microbes* **2018**, *9*, 308–325. [CrossRef]
70. Zhang, E.; Jin, L.; Wang, Y.; Tu, J.; Zheng, R.; Ding, L.; Fang, Z.; Fan, M.; Al-Abdullah, I.; Natarajan, R.; et al. Intestinal AMPK modulation of microbiota mediates crosstalk with brown fat to control thermogenesis. *Nat. Commun.* **2022**, *13*, 1135. [CrossRef]

nutrients

MDPI

Article

Beneficial Effects of Traditional Fermented Soybean Sauce (Kanjang) on Memory Function, Body Water, and Glucose Metabolism: Roles of Gut Microbiota and Neuroinflammation

Yu Yue [1,†], Hee-Jong Yang [2,†], Chen Li [1], Myeong-Seon Ryu [2], Ji-Won Seo [2], Do Youn Jeong [2,*] and Sunmin Park [1,3,*]

1 Department of Bioconvergence, Hoseo University, Asan 31499, Republic of Korea; yuyue6491@gmail.com (Y.Y.); lic77732@gmail.com (C.L.)

2 Department of R & D, Microbial Institute for Fermentation Industry, Sunchang 56048, Republic of Korea; godfiltss@naver.com (H.-J.Y.); rms6223@naver.com (M.-S.R.); wldnjs8769@naver.com (J.-W.S.)

3 Department of Food and Nutrition, Obesity/Diabetes Research Center, Hoseo University, Asan 31499, Republic of Korea

* Correspondence: jdy2534@korea.kr (D.Y.J.); smpark@hoseo.edu (S.P.); Tel.: +82-63-650-2001 (D.Y.J.); +82-41-540-5345 (S.P.); Fax: +82-63-650-9590 (D.Y.J.); +82-41-548-0670 (S.P.)

† These authors contributed equally to this work.

Abstract: Background: Traditional fermented soybean foods, acting as potential synbiotics, may help mitigate cognitive impairment associated with amnesia. This study investigated the neuroprotective effects of four kanjang (Korean fermented soy sauce) varieties and their underlying mechanisms. **Methods:** Male Sprague Dawley rats (n = 70) were divided into seven groups: normal control, scopolamine control, positive control (1 mg/kg bw/day of donepezil), and four scopolamine-treated groups receiving different kanjang varieties (0.5% in high-fat diet). Based on their *Bacillus* content, the kanjang samples were categorized as traditionally made kanjang (TMK) with high *Bacillus* (SS-HB), TMK with medium *Bacillus* (SS-MB), TMK with low *Bacillus* (SS-LB), and factory-made kanjang (SS-FM). **Results:** Scopolamine administration disrupted energy, glucose, and water metabolism and impaired memory function ($p < 0.05$). All kanjang treatments improved insulin sensitivity, reduced inflammation, enhanced glucose tolerance, and decreased visceral fat. SS-MB, SS-HB, and SS-FM increased skeletal muscle mass. They maintained body water homeostasis by suppressing the renin–angiotensin–aldosterone system. Kanjang treatments improved memory function, with SS-FM showing the least significant effects. The treatments reduced neuronal cell death in the hippocampal CA1 region, decreased acetylcholinesterase activity, and increased brain-derived neurotrophic factor mRNA expression. Gut microbiota analysis revealed that kanjang treatments increased Lactobacillaceae and decreased Lachnospiraceae, with SS-HB and SS-LB specifically elevating *Ligilactobacillus*. Metagenomic analysis demonstrated enhanced glycolysis/gluconeogenesis pathways and enhanced butanoate metabolism while reducing lipopolysaccharide biosynthesis and pro-inflammatory signaling. SS-MB and SS-LB increased intestinal goblet cell counts and the serum butyrate concentration. **Conclusions:** These findings suggest that kanjang consumption, particularly SS-HB and SS-LB varieties, can ameliorate memory impairment in this murine model through multiple mechanisms: metabolic improvements, enhanced neurotrophic signaling, gut microbiota modulation, and reduced neuroinflammation via gut–brain axis activation. Human clinical trials are warranted to determine if these promising neuroprotective effects translate to clinical applications.

Keywords: soy sauce; memory impairment; gut microbiota; neurotrophic signaling; gut microbiota

1. Introduction

Kanjang, a traditional Korean fermented soy sauce, has historically served as a primary source of sodium in Asian cuisine, particularly in Korea [1]. The fermentation process generates bioactive compounds, including peptides, amino acids, and phenolic compounds, a characteristic distinguishing its physiological effects from those of regular salt. In Asian cultures, mainly where rice is a staple food, fermented soybeans have traditionally been used not only as flavor enhancers but also as nutrient supplements [1]. The preservation process necessitates using salt in fermentation, leading to the development of various fermented soybean products, with kanjang emerging as a globally recognized seasoning.

Memory deficit disorders represent a growing global health concern, particularly with an increasing aging population and the rising prevalence of neurodegenerative diseases. Dietary factors play a crucial role in cognitive function, with salt intake emerging as a significant modulator. Despite the general association between high salt intake and adverse health outcomes [2], traditional fermented soybean products (jang) show inverse associations with components of the metabolic syndrome, including abdominal obesity, hypertension, dyslipidemia, and hyperglycemia, as demonstrated by the Korean Genome and Epidemiology Study (KoGES) involving a large cohort of 58,701 participants [3]. Fermented soybean consumption has been shown to reduce the sodium/potassium ratio and serum aldosterone concentrations, thereby decreasing water retention and inflammation in estrogen-deficient animal models [4]. Furthermore, these products modify the gut microbiota composition and improve intestinal permeability, establishing a potential mechanism through the gut–brain axis for improving cognitive function [5]. The composition and metabolites of the gut microbiota significantly influence cognitive performance through the production of various neuroactive metabolites acting on the gut–brain axis and affecting brain function directly or indirectly through immune and endocrine pathways [6]. Herbal extracts and probiotics have been shown to modulate gut microbiota and metagenome function, thereby enhancing cognitive function [7,8].

The present study employed male Sprague Dawley rats with scopolamine-induced memory impairment as an established model to investigate the effects and mechanisms of kanjang (traditional Korean soy sauce) on cognitive function. The scopolamine-induced amnesia model was selected for its reproducibility and translational value in studying memory impairment, as it mirrors the aspects of cholinergic dysfunction observed in human cognitive disorders [9]. This model enables the systematic examination of how different soy sauce varieties affect memory function, providing insights relevant to age-related cognitive decline in humans. The objectives of this study were as follows: (1) evaluate the effects of four different kanjang varieties on memory function in scopolamine-induced amnesic rats; (2) analyze changes in the gut microbiota composition and metagenomic functional profiles in response to different kanjang treatments; (3) investigate the relationship between gut microbiota changes, water metabolism, and cognitive performance; and (4) elucidate the underlying mechanisms by which kanjang-induced alterations in the gut microbiota influence memory function. This approach leverages the similarities between rat and human gut microbiota compositions and the conserved gut–brain axis pathways, enhancing the potential applicability of our findings to human cognitive health. Understanding these mechanisms could provide valuable insights into developing more beneficial sodium sources for improving cognitive health based on their impact on the gut microbiota and overall body physiology.

2. Materials and Methods

2.1. Kanjang Production and Sample Collection

In Korea, soy sauce is traditionally produced using two main fermentation methods: traditional fermentation (TMK) and microorganism-inoculated fermentation. TMK was produced through three sequential fermentation steps: (1) the preparation of meju (fermentation of crushed, boiled soybeans with rice straw at 20–25 °C for 40–50 days); (2) fermentation in brine (meju was soaked in 16–18% salt solution outdoors for 40–60 days); and (3) secondary fermentation (separation of liquid TMK and solid doenjang fermented for >6 months). TMK samples were collected from multiple Korean provinces to capture regional differences in bacterial communities and metabolite profiles. Initial analyses focused on measuring sodium content, identifying bacterial composition, and quantifying biogenic amine levels. For comparison, factory-made kanjang (FMK), produced through a shortened fermentation process involving inoculation with *Aspergillus* spp. and *Bacillus* spp., was also analyzed. The soy sauce (TMK) samples were classified into three categories based on *Bacillus* abundance: (1) high *Bacillus* (SS-HB), (2) medium *Bacillus* (SS-MB), and (3) low *Bacillus* (SS-LB). An additional sample type, factory-made kanjang from Sunchang (Jeollabuk-do, Republic of Korea), was labeled SS-FM.

2.2. Sodium, Aflatoxin, and Biogenic Amine Analyses of Kanjang Samples

The sodium content in the kanjang samples was measured using inductively coupled plasma atomic emission spectroscopy (ICP-AES, Thermo IRIS Intrepid II XDL, Santa Clara, CA, USA) after nitric acid digestion, with argon flow at 10.00 L/min and detection at 589.0 nm. For aflatoxin analysis, TMK was extracted with 70% methanol (1% NaCl), filtered, passed through an Afla test column, and analyzed by high-performance liquid chromatography (HPLC, Agilent 1200, Agilent Technology, Santa Clara, CA, USA) with an Ultra Grade 120 column (Shiseido Co., Osaka, Japan) using a acetonitrile/water (25:75) mobile phase at 1.0 mL/min, detected using a fluorescence detector (FLD) (ex: 360 nm; em: 450 nm).

The biogenic amine contents in the kanjang samples were derivatized with 1,7-diaminoheptane (internal standard), saturated Na_2CO_3, and 1% dansyl chloride. Histamine and tyramine standards (0.1–100 mg/L) were prepared in 0.01 N HCl. After ethyl ether extraction and evaporation, the residues were dissolved in acetonitrile for the HPLC analysis (Agilent 1200) using a Capcell Pak C18 column (Agilent 1200).

2.3. Animal Care

Seventy male 8-week-old Sprague Dawley (SD) rats (192 ± 7.4 g) were obtained from Daehan Bio Inc. (Eum-Sung, Republic of Korea) and acclimated for one week at the animal facility at Hoseo University. Each rat was housed individually in a polycarbonate cage under controlled conditions (23 °C, 12 h light/dark cycle) with ad libitum access to food and water. This study complied with the instructions provided in the Guide for the Care and Use of Laboratory Animals (8th edition, National Institutes of Health [NIH], US) and was approved by the Hoseo University Institutional Animal Care and Use Committee (HSUIACUC-23-034, May 23, 2023).

2.4. Induction of Memory Deficit in an Animal Model

Memory impairment was induced by daily intraperitoneal (IP) injections of scopolamine (2 mg/kg body weight) for 8 weeks. Scopolamine administration suppresses the parasympathetic nervous system (PNS), leading to cognitive deficits that model memory impairment. In the positive control group, donepezil (1 mg/kg body weight) was administered daily via oral gavage immediately after the scopolamine injection. The normal control group received daily IP injections of physiological saline (0.9% NaCl) of a volume equivalent to scopolamine.

2.5. Experimental Design and Diet Preparation

Sample size calculations were conducted using the G*Power 3.1 software (https://www.psychologie.hhu.de/arbeitsgruppen/allgemeine-psychologie-und-arbeitspsychologie/gpower) with power = 0.85 and effect size = 0.50, resulting in 10 rats per group to assess the main effects. No specific inclusion or exclusion criteria for animals or data points were established a priori. All animals initially enrolled in this study completed the experimental procedures without complications. Consequently, no animals or data points were excluded at any stage of the experiment or analysis. Each experimental group consisted of 10 rats (n = 10), and all animals were included in the final statistical analysis.

Male Sprague Dawley rats were randomly assigned to seven groups (n = 10 per group): normal control (high-fat diet [HFD] + saline), control (HFD + scopolamine), positive control (HFD + scopolamine + donepezil), SS-HB, SS-MB, and SS-LB (HFD + 0.5% of the respective TMK extract [HB, MB, or LB] + scopolamine), and SS-FM (HFD + 0.5% SS-FM + scopolamine) (Figure S1). Randomization was conducted using a computer-generated random sequence to ensure unbiased group allocation. To minimize potential confounding factors, animals were housed individually, and cage positions were rotated weekly. Behavioral testing and sample collection were carried out in a randomized order. Blinding was applied during outcome assessment and data analysis, with assessors unaware of group assignments. Each diet formulation was labeled with a coded number, and the animal care staff were blinded to the contents and treatment allocation of each diet.

All the diets were based on a modified polyphenol-free AIN-93 HFD containing 37% of carbohydrates, 20% of protein, 43% of lard, and essential micronutrients. This polyphenol-free diet was specifically chosen to establish a controlled baseline without dietary polyphenol interference, as TMK's potential cognitive benefits are potentially attributed to its polyphenol content. The treatment diets were supplemented with a 0.5% freeze-dried kanjang sample of a specific variety with cornstarch, casein, corn oil, and salts (NaCl) adjusted to maintain the equivalent nutrient composition (43% energy from fat, 4.65 kcal/g). The diets were stored at 4 °C until use, and rats had ad libitum access to food and water throughout the study. Food efficiency was calculated by dividing weekly food intake by weight gain in the last week of the intervention.

2.6. Oral Glucose Tolerance Test (OGTT) and Intraperitoneal Insulin Tolerance Test (IPITT)

During the 5th week of the dietary intervention, rats were fasted for 16 h overnight, followed by the oral administration of glucose at a dose of 2 g/kg body weight for OGTT. Blood samples were collected from the tail vein at 0, 15, 30, 60, and 120 min after glucose administration to measure serum glucose concentrations. In addition, serum insulin concentrations were assessed at 0, 20, 40, and 90 min to evaluate the insulin response. After completion of the OGTT, animals were returned to their normal feeding. On the following day, after a 6 h fasting period, the IPITT was conducted. Rats received an intraperitoneal insulin injection at a dose of 1 U/kg body weight, and blood samples were collected from the tail vein at 0, 15, 30, 60, and 120 min post-injection to assess serum glucose concentrations and determine insulin sensitivity.

2.7. Assessments of Memory Deficit

Memory assessments were conducted using passive avoidance, Y-maze, novel object recognition, and the Morris water maze tests at the 5–6-week intervention (Figure S1). In the passive avoidance test, the rats were placed in a light–dark shuttle box 50 min post-scopolamine injection on the day of the memory function assessment. During the acquisition trials, the rats received an electric stimulus (75 V, 0.2 mA, 50 Hz) upon entering the dark chamber. After 16 h, the latency to enter the dark chamber was recorded (cutoff: 600 s).

The Y-maze test measured spontaneous alternation behavior. The rats were placed in a Y-shaped maze (50.5 cm × 20 cm × 20 cm) for 8 min. Correct alternation was defined as sequential entry into all three arms, and the alternation percentage was calculated as correct alternations divided by total arm entries.

In the novel object recognition test, after three days of acclimation, the rats explored two identical objects for 10 min (training phase). One hour later, one object was replaced with a novel object, and exploration was recorded for 5 min. The recognition index was calculated as the time spent exploring new versus familiar objects.

Finally, the Morris water maze test evaluated hippocampal-dependent spatial memory. The rats were placed in zone 1 of a water-filled pool and trained to find a platform placed in zone 5. Training occurred over days 1, 2, and 3, and on Day 5, the rats were tested to find zone 5 without a platform. The latency time, frequency of visits, and duration spent in zone 5 were recorded with a 600 s cutoff.

2.8. Sample Collection and Biochemical Assays

After the Morris water maze test, the rats underwent 16 h of fasting before sample collection. Blood was obtained from the portal vein and inferior vena cava following ketamine–xylazine anesthesia. The epididymal and retroperitoneal fat masses were measured. The hippocampi from six randomly selected rats per group were dissected, divided, and frozen at −70 °C. The remaining four rats had their brains preserved in a 20% sucrose solution at 4 °C overnight, then frozen at −20 °C. The large intestine tissues were washed with phosphate-buffered saline (PBS) and fixed in 4% paraformaldehyde (pH 7.2). The serum was separated from the portal vein blood, and the fecal samples from the cecum were stored at −70 °C. The serum tumor necrosis factor-alpha (TNF-α) and interleukin-1 beta (IL-1β) were quantified using ELISA kits (eBioscience, Santa Clara, CA, USA).

One portion of the hippocampus was lysed in a radioimmunoprecipitation assay (RIPA) buffer, and the supernatants were used to measure triglycerides, cholesterol, and lipid peroxide levels via spectrophotometric kits (DoGenBio, Seoul, Republic of Korea). These supernatants were digested with α-amyloglucosidase (Sigma) to assess the glycogen levels using a glucose spectrophotometric kit (DoGenBio). Acetylcholinesterase (AChE) activity was measured using a rodent AChE ELISA kit (Elabscience, Houston, TX, USA). The remaining hippocampal portion was processed with a Trizol reagent (Invitrogen, Carlsbad, CA, USA) for total RNA extraction.

Serum aldosterone, renin, and angiotensin II concentrations and angiotensin-converting enzyme activity were measured using ELISA kits (eBioscience) for water metabolism.

2.9. Quantitative Real-Time PCR to Evaluate mRNA Expression in the Hippocampal Tissue

cDNA synthesis was performed by combining isolated total RNA with Superscript III reverse transcriptase and high-fidelity Taq DNA polymerase (1:1:1, *v*:*v*:*v*). The synthesized cDNA was mixed with target gene primers and SYBR Green mix for real-time quantitative PCR analysis (BioRad, Hercules, CA, USA). Target genes included a ciliary neurotrophic factor (*CNTF*), brain-derived neurotrophic factor (*BDNF*), *TNF-α*, *IL-1β*, and β-actin. Gene expression levels were analyzed using the comparative cycle threshold (CT) method [10].

2.10. Histological Analysis of the Brain and Large Intestinal Tissues

The brain was further equilibrated in a 20% sucrose solution in PBS at 4 °C for 48 h and then frozen at −20 °C. Using a cryostat microtome, the frozen brain was sectioned into 10 μm thick coronal slices, which were stained with a crystal violet solution to assess damaged cells in the hippocampal region under a microscope.

For the large intestinal tissue analysis, two serial 5 μm paraffin-embedded sections were taken from the seventh or eighth sections to avoid duplicate site analysis. The sections were stained with hematoxylin–eosin (H-E) and Alcian blue–perchloric acid–Schiff (AB-PAS) staining. Impaired cells in the H-E-stained sections were counted using a Zeiss Axiovert 5 microscope (Zeiss, Oberkochen, Germany) with the Dilation X-ray Imager (DIXI) imaging solution and scored from 0 to 5, based on the relative area of damaged cells. The percentage of goblet cells producing mucin was determined from the AB-PAS-stained sections, and their proportion within the intestinal area was calculated.

2.11. Assessment of Serum Short-Chain Fatty Acid (SCFA) Concentrations

Serum samples were treated with ethanol (Duksan, Republic of Korea), followed by 1N hydrochloric acid (HCl) (100:1 ratio). After vortexing, the mixture was centrifuged at 15,000 rpm for 15 min at 4 °C. The SCFA concentrations were determined using a gas chromatograph (GC, Clarus 680 GAS, PerkinElmer, Waltham, MA, USA) equipped with an Elite-free fatty acid phase (FFAP) capillary column (30 m × 0.25 mm × 0.25 μm) [11]. External standards for acetate, propionate, and butyrate (Sigma Co., St. Louis, MO, USA) were used for quantification.

2.12. Gut Microbiome Composition and Metagenome Analysis

The bacterial DNA from the fecal samples was extracted using the Power Water DNA Isolation Kit (Qiagen, Hilden, Germany). DNA was amplified using 16S amplicon primers, and libraries were prepared following the GS FLX plus protocol. Sequencing was performed on the Illumina MiSeq system (Genome Sequencer FLX plus; Roche Co., Basel, Switzerland) at Macrogen, Seoul. The 16S amplicon sequences were processed using Mothur v.1.36 and aligned with the Silva reference alignment v.12350 for determining bacterial taxonomy.

Taxonomic assignments and bacterial counts were analyzed using principal coordinates analysis (PCoA) in the R package. Linear discriminant analysis effect size (LEfSe) analysis identified primary bacteria in each group at the species level. Functional metabolic predictions were performed using the Phylogenetic Investigation of Communities by Reconstruction of Unobserved States (PICRUSt)2, with predicted functions mapped against the Kyoto Encyclopedia of Genes and Genomes (KEGG) Orthology database. The Sparse Correlations for Compositional Data (SparCC) algorithm was used to examine microbial species relationships, excluding taxa showing no significant differences between groups or having correlation coefficients below 0.1. The species co-occurrence network was visualized using Cytoscape version 3.4.0.

2.13. Statistical Analyses

Statistical analyses were performed using SAS version 7 (SAS Institute, Cary, NC, USA). Data were presented as means ± standard deviations (SDs). Normally distributed variables were analyzed using univariate analysis, and group comparisons were performed using one-way analysis of variance (ANOVA). When significant intergroup differences were observed in ANOVA, post hoc Tukey tests were conducted for multiple comparisons. A p-value < 0.05 was considered statistically significant.

3. Results

3.1. Characteristics of the Kanjang Samples

Four kanjang samples with varying microbial compositions, sodium content, and biogenic amine levels were selected for analysis. The samples showed distinct profiles: SS-HB predominantly contained *Bacillaceae* (82%), had high sodium content (8.59%), and moderate levels of viable bacteria (1.3 × 10^5 colony-forming units [CFU]) (Table S1, Figure S2). SS-MB was characterized by high levels of *Enterobacteriaceae* (88%), moderate levels of *Bacillaceae* (17%), lower sodium content (5.56%), and high concentrations of viable bacteria (1.0 × 10^7 CFU). SS-LB featured *Enterobacteriaceae* (20%), low *Bacillaceae* (4%), and Enterococcaceae (25%) (Table S1, Figure S2). This sample had the highest biogenic amine content (histamine and tyramine), high sodium levels (9.39%), and viable bacteria of 4.3 × 10^5. SS-FM exhibited high levels of *Enterobacteriaceae* (88%), moderate *Bacillaceae* (17%), and *Halomonadaceae* (25%), with medium sodium content (6.08%) and low viable bacterial counts (1.0 × 10^3 CFU) (Table S1, Figure S2). These varying microbial and chemical compositions influenced the metabolite profiles of each kanjang sample, potentially affecting their impact on memory impairment.

3.2. Effects of Kanjang Treatments on Weight Gain

The administration of the scopolamine injection to the control group disrupted energy metabolism compared to the normal control group without the scopolamine injection. The control group exhibited a higher final body weight and weight gain during the experimental period than the normal control group, though no significant differences were observed between the control and positive control groups (Table 1). All treatments with the kanjang samples resulted in lower weight gain than the normal control group. Interestingly, the visceral fat mass (combined retroperitoneal and epididymal fat) showed no significant differences between the control and the normal control groups. However, leg skeletal muscle mass was reduced in the control group compared to the normal control (Table 1). Among the kanjang treatments, SS-HB was the most effective at reducing body weight gain. Visceral fat contents were lower in the order of positive control = control > SS-MB = SS-FM > SS-HB> SS-LB. All the kanjang treatments, except SS-LB, restored skeletal muscle mass to levels comparable with the normal control group (Table 1). Food efficiency was not significantly different between the control and normal control groups, while all kanjang treatments showed decreased food efficiency relative to the control group. Overall, SS-HB demonstrated the maximum beneficial effects on energy metabolism by simultaneously increasing skeletal muscle mass and reducing visceral fat accumulation (Table 1).

Table 1. Visceral fat weight and energy metabolism.

	Control	Positive-C	SS-HB	SS-MB	SS-LB	SS-FM	Normal-C
Final weight (g)	356 ± 5.44 ^{a}	362 ± 6.2 ^{a}	280 ± 13.3 ^{d}	287 ± 7.22 ^{cd}	281 ± 13.9 ^{d}	299 ± 8.41 ^{c}	347 ± 5.61 ^{b}
Body weight gain (g)	182 ± 5.44 ^{a}	189 ± 6.2 ^{a}	96.6 ± 13.3 ^{d}	116 ± 7.22 ^{c}	110 ± 13.9 ^{c}	116 ± 8.41 ^{c}	175 ± 5.61 ^{b}
Retroperitoneal mass (g)	6.45 ± 0.63 ^{a}	6.99 ± 0.64 ^{a}	3.08 ± 0.45 ^{c}	4.01 ± 0.42 ^{b}	2.84 ± 0.32 ^{c}	3.9 ± 0.19 ^{b}	6.5 ± 0.39 ^{a}
Epididymal fat mass	5.14 ± 0.73 ^{a}	5.89 ± 0.41 ^{a}	1.91 ± 0.43 ^{d}	3.22 ± 0.5 ^{c}	1.36 ± 0.3 ^{e}	2.91 ± 0.33 ^{c}	5.43 ± 0.58 ^{a}
Visceral fat (% of bw)	3.18 ± 0.32 ^{a}	3.53 ± 0.18 ^{a}	1.7 ± 0.24 ^{c}	2.5 ± 0.19 ^{b}	1.47 ± 0.19 ^{d}	2.28 ± 0.1 ^{b}	2.93 ± 0.24 ^{a}
Skeletal muscle (% of bw)	4.39 ± 0.2 ^{b}	4.46 ± 0.07 ^{b}	4.79 ± 0.1 ^{a}	4.73 ± 0.2 ^{a}	4.55 ± 0.3 ^{b}	4.91 ± 0.15 ^{a}	4.76 ± 0.14 ^{a}
Food efficiency (%)	0.66 ± 0.03 ^{b}	0.74 ± 0.04 ^{a}	0.34 ± 0.05 ^{d}	0.46 ± 0.03 ^{c}	0.38 ± 0.05 ^{d}	0.45 ± 0.04 ^{c}	0.68 ± 0.04 ^{b}
Water intake (mL/day)	17.2 ± 1.27 ^{c}	18.6 ± 2 ^{c}	27.2 ± 2.27 ^{a}	29.7 ± 1.34 ^{a}	21.3 ± 1.91 ^{b}	29.4 ± 1.34 ^{a}	28.3 ± 1.88 ^{a}
Serum aldosterone level (ng/mL)	1.24 ± 0.18 ^{a}	1.18 ± 0.17 ^{a}	0.88 ± 0.11 ^{c}	0.73 ± 0.09 ^{d}	1.01 ± 0.15 ^{b}	0.76 ± 0.09 ^{cd}	0.79 ± 0.10 ^{d}
Serum renin (pg/mL)	29.4 ± 3.24 ^{a}	28.9 ± 3.05 ^{a}	22.9 ± 2.23 ^{c}	19.4 ± 2.27 ^{d}	25.3 ± 2.31 ^{b}	19.8 ± 2.32 ^{d}	19.1 ± 2.43 ^{d}
Serum Angiotensin II (ng/mL)	3.14 ± 0.32 ^{a}	3.05 ± 0.21 ^{a}	2.49 ± 0.23 ^{bc}	2.42 ± 0.32 ^{c}	2.75 ± 0.23 ^{b}	2.35 ± 0.21 ^{c}	2.32 ± 0.21 ^{c}
Angiotensin-converting-enzyme activity (U/mL)	2.07 ± 0.27 ^{a}	1.98 ± 0.24 ^{a}	1.46 ± 0.18 ^{c}	1.21 ± 0.17 ^{d}	1.67 ± 0.16 ^{b}	1.25 ± 0.16 ^{d}	1.18 ± 0.17 ^{d}

Food efficiency = food intake/body weight × 100. bw, body weight. Values represented means ± standard deviation (n = 10). ^{a,b,c,d,e} Different letters in each variable indicate significant differences in one-way ANOVA at $p < 0.05$.

3.3. *Effects of Kanjang Treatments on Water Homeostasis*

Water metabolism was significantly impaired in the scopolamine-injected control group, as indicated by elevated serum levels of renin (54%), angiotensin II (35%), and aldosterone (57%), along with a 75% increase in angiotensin-converting enzyme activity, compared to the normal control group (Table 1). Water intake in the scopolamine-injected control group decreased by approximately 39% compared to the normal control. Water metabolism did not significantly improve in the positive control group. However, all the kanjang treatments prevented increasing the serum levels of renin, angiotensin II, aldosterone concentration, and angiotensin-converting-enzyme activity, thereby improving body water homeostasis (Table 1). Among the kanjang samples, SS-MB and SS-FM showed the most improvement, restoring parameters to levels comparable to the normal control (Table 1).

3.4. *Effects of Kanjang Treatments on Glucose Metabolism*

Fasting serum glucose levels did not differ significantly between the control and normal control groups, while insulin levels were elevated in the control group. All the kanjang treatments except SS-FM reduced serum glucose levels compared to the control. Similarly, serum insulin was lower in all the kanjang groups except SS-MB and SS-FM (Table 2). The homeostatic model assessment for insulin resistance (HOMA-IR) was higher in the control (52%) and positive control (48%) groups versus the normal control. The kanjang treatments reduced HOMA-IR, with the SS-HB group achieving values comparable to normal control (Table 2).

Table 2. Glucose metabolism and lipid profiles.

	Control	Positive-C	SS-HB	SS-MB	SS-LB	SS-FM	Normal-C
Serum glucose (mg/dL)	120 ± 6.53 [ab]	125 ± 8.42 [a]	117 ± 1.69 [b]	94 ± 4.78 [c]	116 ± 4.85 [b]	120 ± 3.4 [ab]	120 ± 3.86 [ab]
Serum insulin (mg/dL)	0.25 ± 0.03 [a]	0.22 ± 0.01 [b]	0.15 ± 0.02 [b]	0.23 ± 0.02 [a]	0.18 ± 0.01 [b]	0.2 ± 0.02 [ab]	0.16 ± 0.02 [b]
HOMA-IR	6.61 ± 0.63 [a]	6.43 ± 0.52 [a]	3.95 ± 0.34 [c]	4.95 ± 0.33 [b]	4.59 ± 0.28 [b]	5.3 ± 0.31 [b]	4.35 ± 0.3 [c]
Serum TNF-α (pg/mL)	0.79 ± 0.08 [a]	0.73 ± 0.08 [a]	0.68 ± 0.09 [b]	0.65 ± 0.08 [b]	0.68 ± 0.08 [b]	0.73 ± 0.06 [a]	0.46 ± 0.05 [c]
Serum IL-1β (pg/mL)	19.5 ± 1.87 [a]	18.6 ± 1.63 [a]	15.3 ± 1.71 [b]	14.7 ± 1.54 [b]	17.5 ± 1.58 [a]	17.2 ± 1.62 [a]	11.2 ± 1.43 [c]
Hippocampus							
Glycogen (mg/g)	29.7 ± 1.4 [b]	30.8 ± 2.1 [b]	33.4 ± 2.7 [a]	34.2 ± 2.4 [a]	33.5 ± 2.5 [a]	34.8 ± 2.1 [a]	33.7 ± 2.8 [a]
Cholesterol (mg/g)	85.8 ± 8.3 [a]	62.6 ± 8.66 [c]	69.1 ± 10.1 [bc]	76.7 ± 9.26 [b]	71.6 ± 6.16 [b]	74.9 ± 2.63 [b]	76.1 ± 8.12 [b]
Triglyceride (mg/g)	68.1 ± 3.85 [a]	71.3 ± 3.5 [a]	61.7 ± 2.62 [b]	72.5 ± 3.62 [a]	63.5 ± 4.51 [b]	69.1 ± 1.93 [a]	61.1 ± 2.87 [b]
AChE activity (U/mg protein)	0.85 ± 0.10 [a]	0.36 ± 0.05 [d]	0.59 ± 0.07 [b]	0.43 ± 0.06 [c]	0.48 ± 0.23 [c]	0.67 ± 0.08 [b]	0.22 ± 0.04 [e]
Relative mRNA of TNF-α (AU)	1 [a]	0.94 ± 0.08 [a]	0.95 ± 0.09 [a]	0.62 ± 0.09 [c]	0.75 ± 0.08 [b]	0.88 ± 0.10 [b]	0.68 ± 0.09 [c]
Relative mRNA of IL-1β (AU)	1 [a]	0.78 ± 0.13 [b]	0.53 ± 0.15 [c]	0.31 ± 0.09 [e]	0.64 ± 0.12 [c]	0.51 ± 0.09 [d]	0.48 ± 0.04 [d]
Relative mRNA of BDNF (AU)	1 [e]	1.53 ± 0.38 [c]	1.90 ± 0.39 [bc]	1.47 ± 0.27 [c]	2.36 ± 0.24 [b]	1.78 ± 0.33 [c]	2.94 ± 0.16 [a]

Values represent means ± standard deviation (n = 10). HOMA-IR, homeostatic model assessment for insulin resistance; HDL, high-density lipoprotein; TG, triglyceride; LDL, low-density lipoprotein; TNF-α, tumor-necrosis factor-α; IL-1β, interleukin-1β; AChE, acetylcholinesterase; BDNF, brain-derived neurotrophic factor; MDA, malondialdehyde; AU, arbitrary unit. [a,b,c,d,e] different letters in each variable indicate significant differences in one-way ANOVA at $p < 0.05$.

Glucose intolerance was evident in the control group in the oral glucose tolerance test (OGTT). Peak glucose levels at 30 min were lower in the SS-HB, SS-MB, SS-LB, and positive control groups compared to the control (Figure 1A). The SS-HB, SS-MB, and SS-LB groups exhibited the lowest serum glucose concentrations, similar to the normal control (Figure 1A). The area under the curve for glucose (AUCG) during both phases of the OGTT was higher in the control group than in the normal control group. All the kanjang treatments except SS-FM reduced the AUC values in the first phase, while all the treatments decreased the AUC in the second phase (Figure S3A).

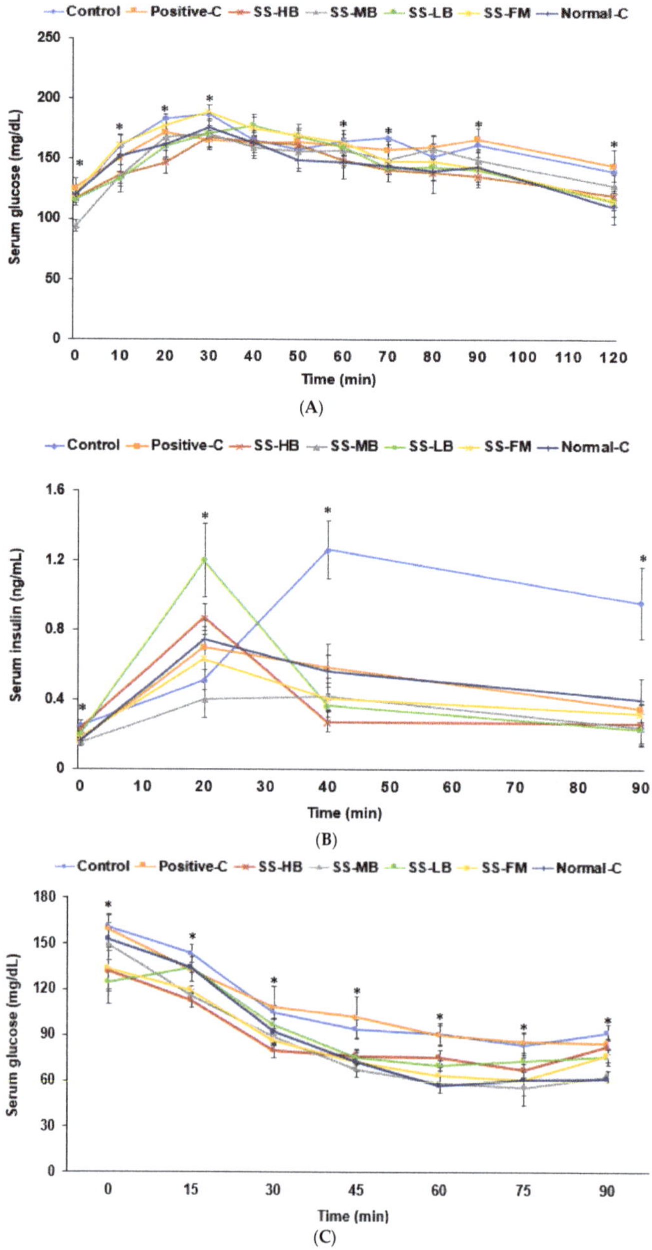

Figure 1. Serum glucose concentrations during the oral glucose tolerance test (OGTT) and intraperitoneal insulin tolerance test (IPITT). (**A**) Changes in serum glucose concentrations after oral intake of 2 g of glucose per kg of body weight (OGTT). (**B**) Changes in serum insulin concentrations during OGTT. (**C**) Changes in serum glucose concentrations after intraperitoneal injection of 1 U of insulin per kg of body weight. Dots and error bars represent the means ± standard deviations (n = 10). * indicates significant differences among the groups at each time point in one-way ANOVA at $p < 0.05$.

For the insulin response, the control group showed increased levels until 40 min, followed by a decline, while the kanjang and positive control groups peaked at 20 min. At 20 min, the SS-LB group showed higher insulin than the normal control, while at 40 min, the control group showed higher levels than all groups (Figure 1B). At 90 min, the control group displayed higher insulin levels than the other groups (Figure 1B). The first-phase insulin AUC was highest in the control and SS-LB, with the SS-MB group showing the lowest values. The second-phase AUC was the highest in the control, and it was lower in all kanjang groups than in the control group (Figure S3B). The SS-HB and SS-LB groups showed lower values than those in the normal control group (Figure S3B).

In the IPITT, fasting glucose at 6 h was higher in the control and positive control groups versus the normal control (Figure 1C). Following the insulin injection, glucose levels markedly decreased until 30 min (first phase) and fluctuated between 45 and 90 min (second phase) across all groups. The kanjang treatments decreased serum glucose concentration at 30, 45, and 90 min, with SS-MB reducing glucose to levels similar to the normal control group (Figure 1C). Notably, kanjang intake, but not donepezil (positive control), improved glucose metabolism (Figures 1C and S3C).

3.5. *Effects of Kanjang Treatments on Serum Markers of Inflammation*

Kanjang treatments affected the levels of inflammatory markers. Serum TNF-α and IL-1β concentrations, indicators of inflammation, were elevated in the control group compared to the normal control group. The levels of these markers were not significantly different in the positive control group compared to the control group. Kanjang consumption, except SS-FM, decreased serum TNF-α compared to the control group, though not to the levels observed in the normal control group (Table 2). SS-HB and SS-MB had lower serum IL-1β concentrations than the control group (Table 2).

3.6. *Effects of Kanjang Treatments on Memory Impairment*

In the passive avoidance test, the rats in the control group entered the dark room quickly, while the rats in the normal control group showed a longer latency. Treatment with kanjang and donepezil (positive control) increased latency time, indicating an improvement in short-term memory (Figure 2A). In the Y-maze test, the control group exhibited fewer correct rotations than the normal control, but SS-HB and SS-LB increased correct rotations to levels comparable with the positive control (Figure 2B). Novel object recognition analysis showed no significant difference between the control and normal control groups in the recognition index, and SS-MB increased this parameter compared to the control (Figure 2B). Locomotive activity was much lower in the control group than in the normal control group. SS-HB increased the activity levels similar to the positive control group, and SS-MB had a similar activity level to the normal control (Figure 2B).

In the Morris water maze test, the duration in zone 5 was lower in the control group than in the normal control and was similar in the SS-MB, SS-LB, and normal control groups (Figure 2C). The frequency of visits to zone 5 was higher in SS-LB than in the control group. The latency to first visit zone 5 was 3-fold higher in the control group than in the normal control. It was lower in the positive control, SS-HB, SS-MB, and SS-LB groups than in the control group, though higher than in the normal control group (Figure 2C). Thus, spatial memory improved in all the kanjang groups, except SS-FM, to levels comparable to or better than the positive control group.

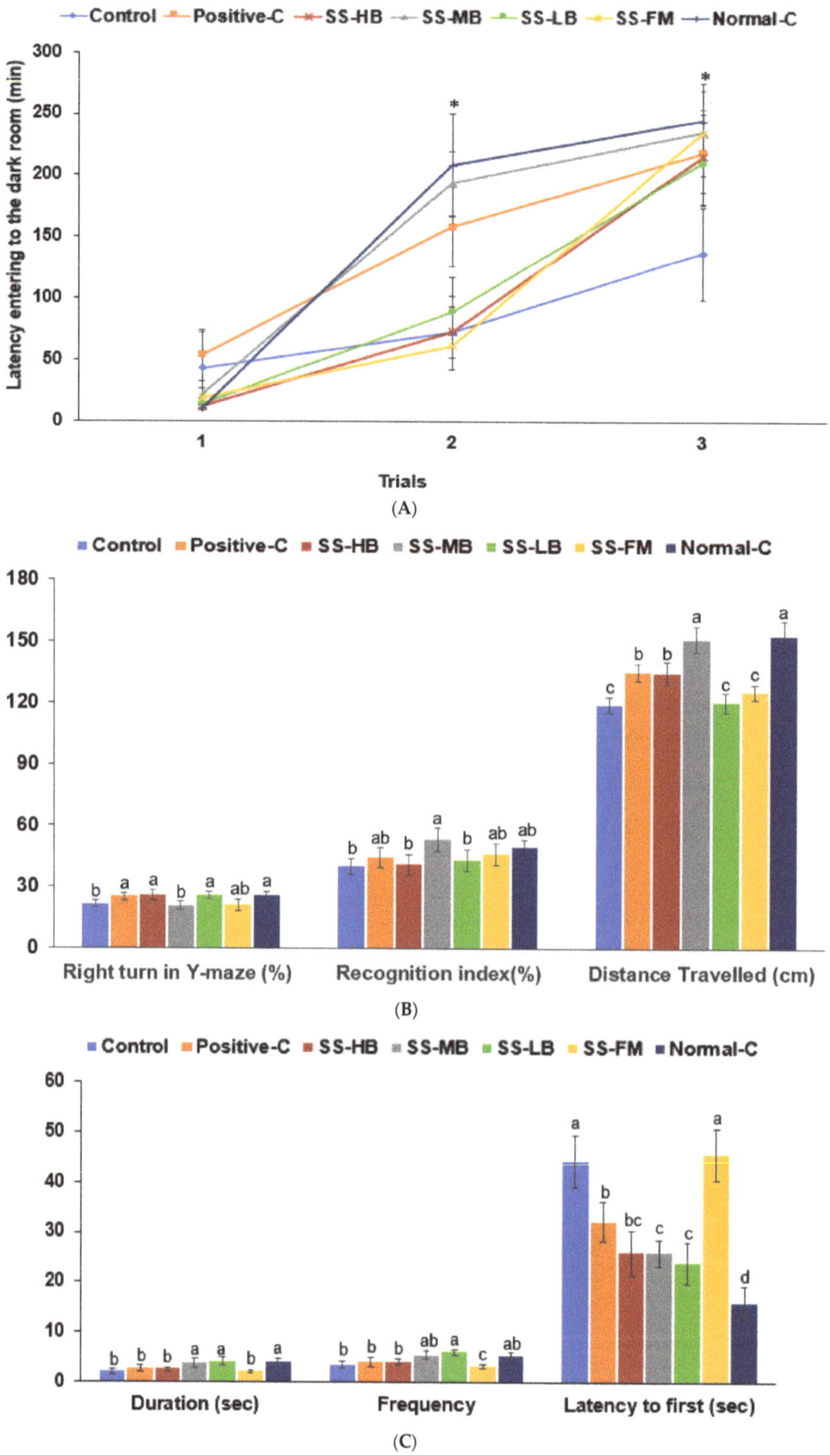

Figure 2. *Cont.*

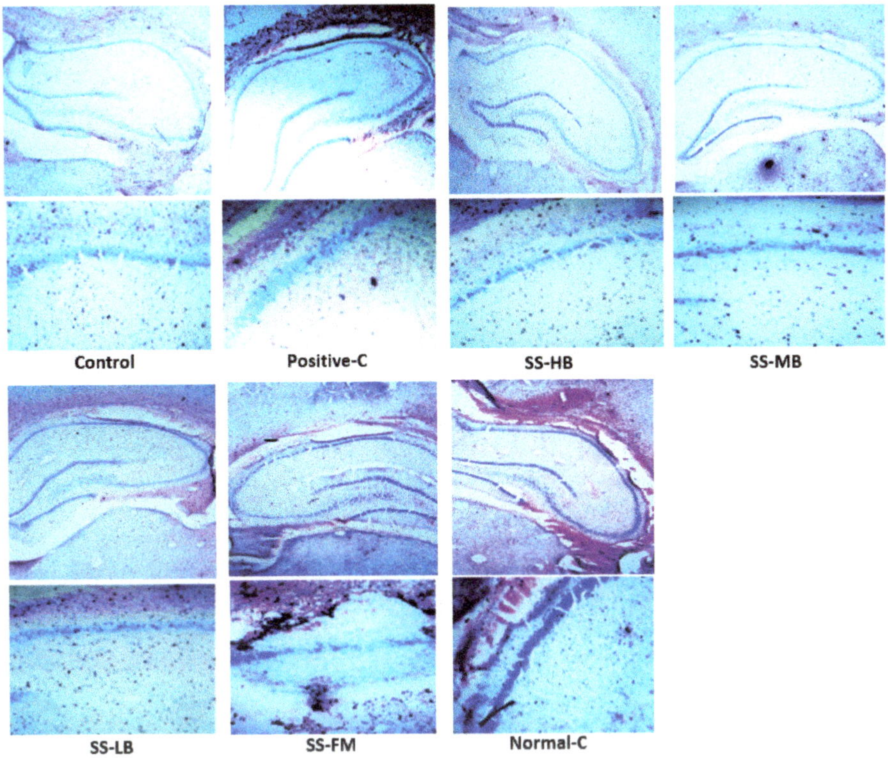

(D)

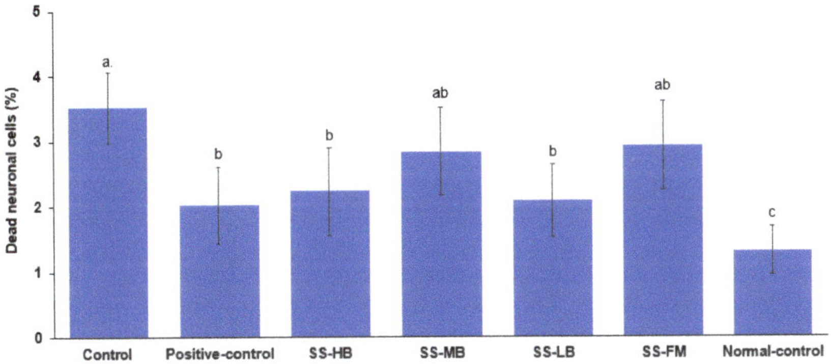

(E)

Figure 2. Memory deficits and hippocampal cornu Ammonis (CA1) neuronal cell death in rats after a scopolamine injection. At 50 min after the scopolamine injection, the passive avoidance test, Y-maze, novel object recognition, and Morris water maze test were performed, and hippocampal neuronal cell death was assessed. (**A**) Latency time (s) to enter the dark box at the first, second, and third trials. (**B**) The number of right turns among the total turns in the Y-maze test, novel object recognition index during the novel object recognition test, and distance traveled in locomotor activity measurement. (**C**) Latency time to the first visit, frequency of visiting zone 5, and duration in zone 5 in the water maze test. (**D**) The image of the hippocampal area stained with cresyl violet. Magnification was ×50 in the upper panels and ×100 in the lower panels. (**E**) Neuronal cell death (%) in the hippocampal cornu Ammonis (CA1) stained with cresyl violet. Dots or bars and error bars represent the means ± standard deviations (n = 10). * significantly different among the groups at $p < 0.05$. ^{a,b,c} different superscript letters on the bars indicated a significant difference among the groups by Tukey's test at $p < 0.05$.

3.7. Effects of Kanjang Treatments on Brain Neuronal Cell Death

Neuronal cell death in the hippocampal CA1 region was approximately 2-fold higher in the control group than the normal control. SS-HB and SS-LB significantly reduced neuronal cell death compared to the control group, with effects comparable to the positive control group, although the values were not fully restored to normal control levels (Figure 2D).

The hippocampal glycogen content was significantly lower in the control than in the normal control group, with no significant difference observed between the positive control and control groups (Table 2). All the kanjang treatments increased glycogen content to levels similar to the normal control group. Hippocampal cholesterol was elevated in the control group compared to the normal control, with the kanjang treatments further decreasing these levels. The positive control group showed lower hippocampal cholesterol than the normal control group (Table 2). The hippocampal triglyceride content was higher in the control group than in the normal control group. SS-HB and SS-LB reduced triglyceride content compared to the control, while no significant difference was observed between the positive control and the control groups.

Acetylcholinesterase activity was approximately 3.8-fold higher in the control than in the normal control group (Table 2). All the kanjang treatments reduced this activity, though not to the same extent as observed in the positive control. SS-MB and SS-LB were more effective in reducing acetylcholinesterase activity than SS-HB and SS-FM.

The mRNA expression of *TNF-α* in brain tissue was elevated in the control group relative to the normal control (Table 2). While the positive control did not show significantly reduced *TNF-α* expression, the SS-FM, SS-MB, and SS-LB treatments decreased *TNF-α* levels, and treatment with SS-MB reduced the expression to levels comparable to that of the normal control. Hippocampal *IL-1β* mRNA expression decreased in all treatment groups compared to the control group, with SS-MB showing the biggest reduction (Table 2).

BDNF mRNA expression was approximately 3-fold lower in the control group than the normal control group. All the kanjang treatments and positive control increased *BDNF* mRNA expression compared to the control, with SS-LB and SS-HB showing the most substantial effects, increasing *BDNF* mRNA expression by approximately 2-fold (Table 2).

3.8. Effects of Kanjang Treatments on Goblet Cells and Serum SCFA Concentrations

The goblet cell count was significantly reduced in the control group (1.5-fold lower) compared to the normal control. Goblet cell count increased by approximately 1.5-fold in the positive control and in all the kanjang treatment groups except for the SS-HB group, compared to the control, though it was not fully restored to normal control levels (Figure 3A,B). Mucosal length and crypt depth were lower in the control than in the normal-C group, and kanjang intake increased them (Figure S4A,B).

The serum acetate levels were elevated in the control group compared to the normal control. Both positive control and all kanjang treatments reduced serum acetate levels, with SS-LB and SS-FM decreasing acetate to levels below the normal control (Figure 3C). Serum propionate concentrations showed no significant differences among all the groups. Serum butyrate concentration was higher in the normal control group than in the control group. The serum butyrate levels were significantly higher in the positive control and SS-MB and SS-LB-treated groups compared to the control (Figure 3C). These alterations in goblet cell density and serum SCFA concentrations indicated a disruption of the gut environment, which plays a crucial role in maintaining gut–brain axis integrity.

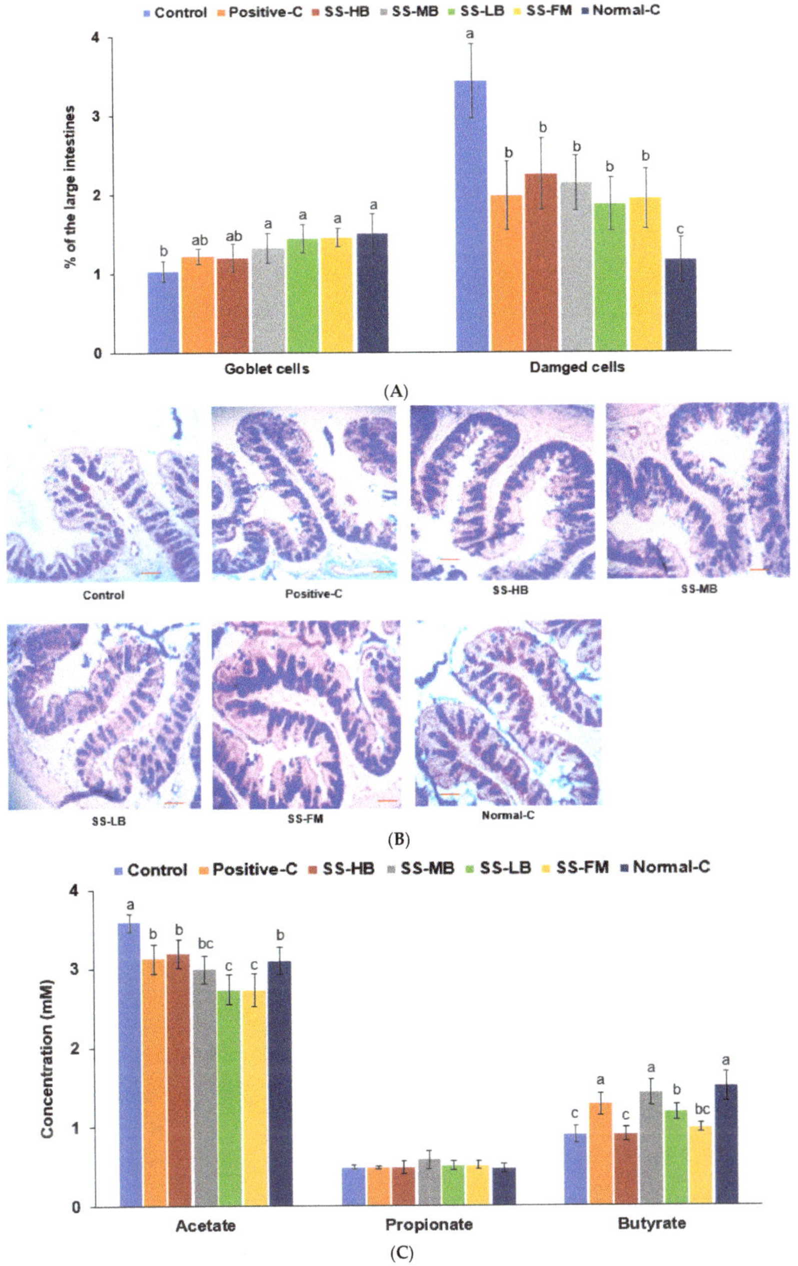

Figure 3. Large intestinal morphology and serum SCFA concentrations after the intervention. (**A**) Damaged cells and goblet cell count. (**B**) Alcian blue–perchloric acid–Schiff (AB-PAS) stain of the intestinal tissues. The violet color indicates mucin. (**C**) Serum short-chain fatty acid (SCFA) levels. The scale bar indicated 100 μm, and the magnification was ×200. Bars and error bars represent the means ± standard deviations (n = 10). [a,b,c] different letters on the bars indicate a significant difference among the groups by Tukey's test at $p < 0.05$.

3.9. *Effects of Kanjang Treatments on Gut Microbiota and Metagenome Function*

The relative abundance of Lactobacillaceae increased while Lachnospiraceae decreased in all the kanjang-treated groups, with the most pronounced effects in the SS-HB and SS-LB groups (Figure 4A). The Enterobacteriaceae levels were elevated in the control and positive control groups compared to all the kanjang treatment groups (Figure 4A). SS-MB treatment increased the abundance of Lactobacillus more than *Ligilactobacillus*. SS-HB and SS-LB treatments elevated the abundance of *Ligilactobacillus* substantially more than *Lactobacillus* (Figure 4B). *Pseudescherichia* levels were significantly higher in the control and positive control groups compared to the kanjang treatment and normal control groups. *Mediterraneibacter* was less abundant in the SS-HB and SS-LB groups compared to other groups (Figure 4B). *Akkermansia* abundance was higher in the normal control than in the control group, with only SS-HB partially restoring these levels (Figure 4B).

The LEfSE analysis revealed that the SS-MB treatment increased Bacillus-related bacteria, including *Limosilactobacillus urinaemulieris*, *Limosilactobacillus agrestis*, *Ihubacter massiliensis*, and *Bacillus velezensis* (Figure 4C). The SS-LB treatment increased *Eubacterium callanderi*, while SS-FM was associated with higher levels of *Oliverpabstia intestinalis*, *Mediterraneibacter glycyrrhizinilyticus*, and *Pagmaiobacter massiliensis* (Figure 4C). The β-diversity analysis revealed the distinct clustering of fecal bacterial communities in the kanjang-treated group, separating it from both the control and positive control groups. However, no clear separation was observed between the control and positive control groups, indicating their similar microbial compositions (Figure 4D).

Metagenomic functional analysis showed enhanced glycolysis/gluconeogenesis pathways in the normal control group compared to the control (Table 3). All the kanjang treatments except SS-MB enhanced glycolysis/gluconeogenesis and carbohydrate digestion/absorption pathways, suggesting that kanjang intake altered microbial energy metabolism toward fermentative metabolism and increased SCFA production (Table 3). These pathways were most strongly enhanced in the SS-HB and SS-LB groups, exhibiting the highest butanoate metabolism (Table 3).

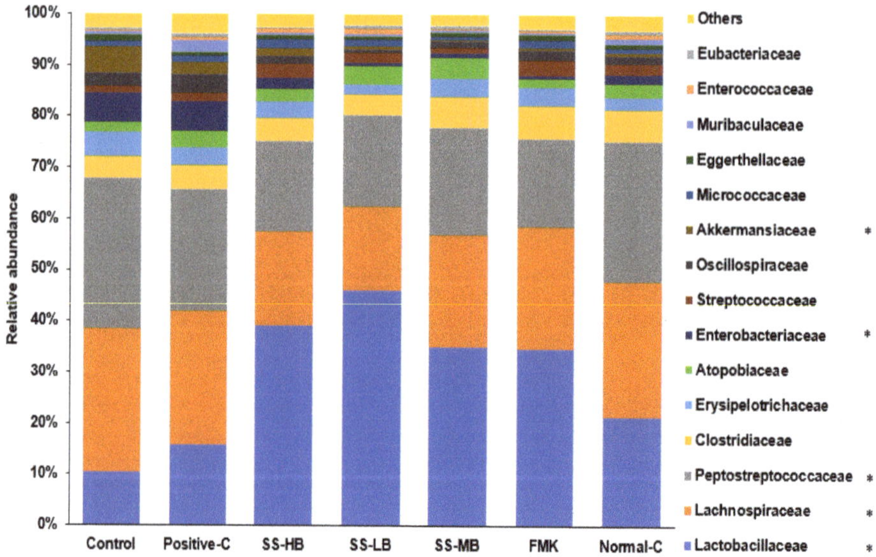

(A)

Figure 4. *Cont.*

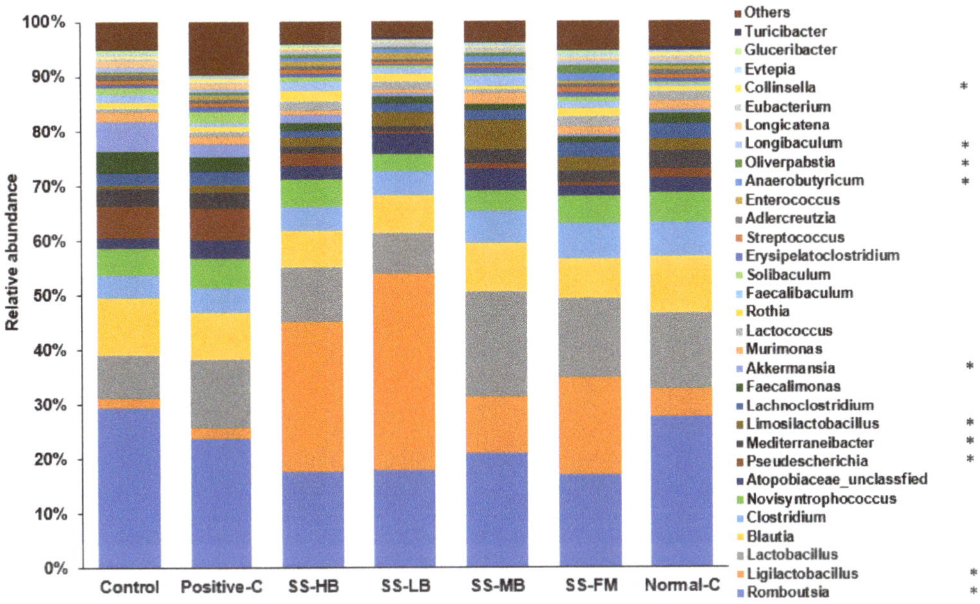

(**B**)

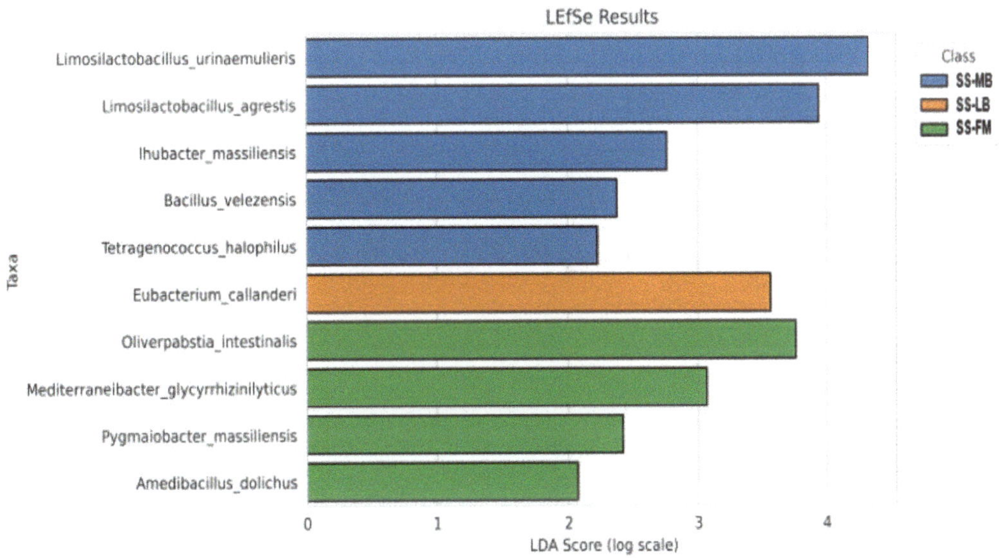

(**C**)

Figure 4. *Cont.*

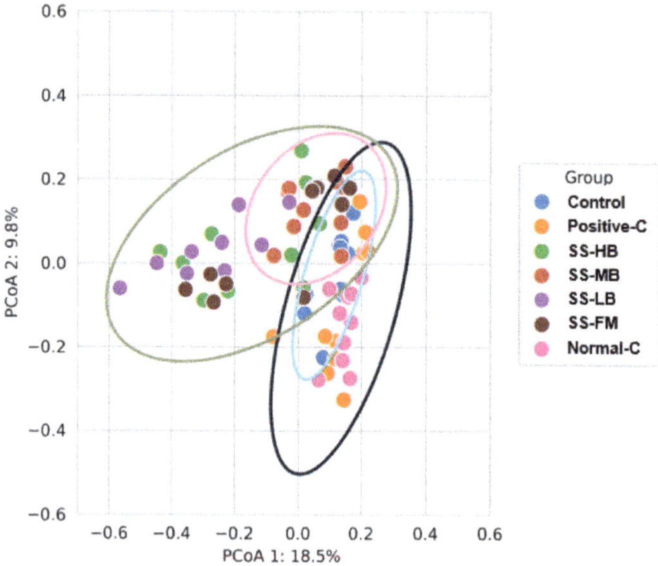

(**D**)

Figure 4. Fecal bacteria composition (**A**). Relative abundance of fecal bacteria from the cecum at the family level (**B**). Relative abundance of fecal bacteria from the cecum at the genus level (**C**). The linear discriminant analysis effect size (LEfSe) analysis (**D**). β-diversity Bars and error bars represent the means ± standard deviations (n = 10). * significantly different among the groups at $p < 0.05$. ^{a,b,c} different letters on the bars indicate a significant difference among the groups by Tukey's test at $p < 0.05$.

Table 3. Metagenome function of the fecal bacteria from the cecum.

	Control	Positive-C	SS-HB	SS-MB	SS-LB	SS-FM	Normal-C
map00010 glycolysis/gluconeogenesis (86)	2.28 ± 0.03 ^{c}	2.31 ± 0.03 ^{bc}	2.86 ± 0.09 ^{a}	2.66 ± 0.03 ^{ab}	3 ± 0.05 ^{a}	2.75 ± 0.07 ^{a}	2.44 ± 0.02 ^{b}
map04973 carbohydrate digestion and absorption (6)	0.02 ± 0.002 ^{c}	0.021 ± 0.002 ^{c}	0.044 ± 0.005 ^{a}	0.025 ± 0.002 ^{c}	0.047 ± 0.005 ^{a}	0.033 ± 0.005 ^{b}	0.022 ± 0.001 ^{c}
map03320 PPAR signaling pathway (25)	0.143 ± 0.003 ^{c}	0.148 ± 0.006 ^{bc}	0.177 ± 0.004 ^{a}	0.168 ± 0.006 ^{ab}	0.182 ± 0.004 ^{a}	0.172 ± 0.003 ^{a}	0.151 ± 0.002 ^{b}
map04066 HIF-1 signaling pathway (17)	0.528 ± 0.007 ^{c}	0.533 ± 0.013 ^{bc}	0.616 ± 0.013 ^{a}	0.616 ± 0.005 ^{a}	0.635 ± 0.006 ^{a}	0.612 ± 0.007 ^{a}	0.577 ± 0.007 ^{b}
map00480 glutathione metabolism (30)	0.327 ± 0.004 ^{c}	0.345 ± 0.003 ^{c}	0.471 ± 0.007 ^{a}	0.395 ± 0.006 ^{b}	0.497 ± 0.004 ^{a}	0.417 ± 0.008 ^{ab}	0.346 ± 0.004 ^{c}
map00540 lipopolysaccharide biosynthesis (53)	0.191 ± 0.026 ^{a}	0.204 ± 0.025 ^{a}	0.115 ± 0.017 ^{b}	0.083 ± 0.004 ^{c}	0.088 ± 0.006 ^{c}	0.089 ± 0.007 ^{c}	0.109 ± 0.011 ^{b}
map04657 IL-17 signaling pathway (11)	0.057 ± 0.002 ^{a}	0.055 ± 0.002 ^{a}	0.032 ± 0.003 ^{c}	0.041 ± 0.002 ^{c}	0.027 ± 0.002 ^{d}	0.038 ± 0.003 ^{c}	0.052 ± 0.001 ^{b}
map04137 mitophagy–animal (15)	0.009 ± 0.001 ^{a}	0.009 ± 0.001 ^{a}	0.004 ± 0.001 ^{c}	0.004 ± 0 ^{c}	0.003 ± 0 ^{c}	0.003 ± 0.001 ^{c}	0.006 ± 0 ^{b}
map00650 butanoate metabolism (96)	1.01 ± 0.01 ^{c}	1.03 ± 0.01 ^{bc}	1.1 ± 0.02 ^{a}	1.08 ± 0.01 ^{b}	1.13 ± 0.02 ^{a}	1.07 ± 0.02 ^{b}	1.03 ± 0.01 ^{bc}
map00640 propanoate metabolism (84)	1.07 ± 0.02 ^{a}	1.11 ± 0.01 ^{a}	1.01 ± 0.02 ^{b}	1.04 ± 0.01 ^{ab}	0.97 ± 0.01 ^{b}	1.03 ± 0.02 ^{ab}	1.06 ± 0.01 ^{b}

Values represent the means ± standard deviations (n = 10). (numbers) indicate the number of reactions involved in the pathways. PPAR, peroxisome proliferator-activated receptor; HIF-1, hypoxia-inducible factor-1; IL-17, interleukin-17. ^{a,b,c,d} different letters on the bars indicate a significant difference among the groups by the Tukey test at $p < 0.05$.

The peroxisome proliferator-activated receptor (PPAR) and hypoxia-inducible factor (HIF) signaling pathways were more active in the normal control group than in the control and positive control groups (Table 3). All the kanjang treatments increased the activity of these pathways compared to the control. Glutathione metabolism showed no significant differences among the control, positive control, and normal control groups but was enhanced by SS-HB, SS-LB, and SS-FM treatments.

Lipopolysaccharide biosynthesis was more pronounced in the control and positive control groups than in the normal control group, and all the kanjang treatments reduced this pathway. Pro-inflammatory IL-17 signaling was lower in all the kanjang treatment groups, particularly SS-LB, than in the control group (Table 3). Mitophagy was elevated in the control group compared to the normal control group, with all kanjang treatments reducing it. Butanoate metabolism was enhanced in all the kanjang treatment groups compared to the control, while propionate metabolism was reduced in the SS-HB and SS-LB groups (Table 3).

4. Discussion

This study examined the effects of four different kanjang varieties on memory function in rats with scopolamine-induced amnesia, revealing significant improvements in cognitive performance alongside beneficial changes in metabolism and gut microbiota composition. While all the kanjang varieties demonstrated protective effects against scopolamine-induced memory impairment, the magnitude and mechanisms of these effects somewhat varied among them.

Among the kanjang varieties evaluated, SS-HB and SS-LB consistently improved cognitive performance across multiple behavioral paradigms, including the Y-maze and Morris water maze tests. In contrast, SS-MB demonstrated selective cognitive enhancement, as evidenced by prolonged latency in the passive avoidance test, a higher novel object recognition index in the novel object recognition test, and an increased traveled distance in locomotor activity. These results suggest that SS-MB exerts targeted effects on recognition memory and exploratory behavior. At the molecular level, the cognitive benefits of SS-MB were supported by the marked suppression of hippocampal pro-inflammatory cytokines (TNF-α and IL-1β), the upregulation of BDNF expression, and reduced AChE activity. Together, these changes imply enhancements in synaptic plasticity, neurotrophic signaling, and cholinergic neurotransmission. While SS-HB and SS-LB also produced favorable outcomes in memory-related behaviors and neuroinflammatory markers, SS-FM showed only modest cognitive effects.

These behavioral outcomes were further corroborated by reduced neuronal cell death in the hippocampal CA1 region and elevated *BDNF* mRNA expression, indicating improved neuronal survival and neuroplasticity. Notably, each kanjang variety exhibited distinct cognitive effects, suggesting that differences in fermentation-derived microbial compositions—such as bacterial species and metabolite profiles—may differentially modulate specific memory domains. These findings are consistent with previous studies, demonstrating that isoflavonoids and *Bacillus*-fermented soybean products improve cognitive function through mechanisms involving *BDNF* upregulation and oxidative stress attenuation in aged or cognitively impaired rodent models [12–14]. The high efficacy of SS-HB, which contains a notable abundance of Bacillaceae, aligns with earlier reports showing improvements in memory function and menopausal symptoms in estrogen-deficient rats administered *Bacillus*-fermented soybean products [4]. Similarly, other studies have reported that *Bacillus*-containing fermented foods enhance hippocampal neurogenesis and spatial learning in mouse models of Alzheimer's disease [15], further reinforcing the neuroprotective role of specific bacterial strains found in SS-HB.

In all kanjang-treated groups, acetylcholinesterase (AChE) activity in the hippocampus was reduced, though not to the extent observed with donepezil in the positive control group. This aligns with previous findings that isoflavone-rich fermented soybeans can inhibit AChE activity in vivo [16–18], although less potent than pharmaceutical cholinesterase inhibitors. These results support the potential of kanjang as a dietary strategy for cholinergic modulation, offering complementary cognitive support through nutritional intervention.

Collectively, these findings underscore the critical role of microbial ecology and fermentation processes in shaping the neurofunctional potential of traditional fermented soybean products. A comparative overview of the behavioral and molecular outcomes is presented in Table 4, illustrating the differential cognitive efficacy and underlying mechanisms associated with each kanjang variety.

Table 4. Integrated summary of neurocognitive and neurochemical effects of different kanjang varieties.

Kanjang Variety	Improved Memory Function	Neuroinflammation by the Hippocampal mRNA Expression	Neuroplasticity (BDNF)	Cholinergic Function (AChE)	Overall Brain Health Effects
SS-HB	Y-maze, locomotive activity, and passive avoidance	↓ TNF-α, ↓↓ IL-1β	↑ BDNF	↓ AChE	Strong multi-dimensional effect
SS-MB	Locomotive activity, novel object recognition, water maze, and passive avoidance	↓↓ TNF-α, ↓↓↓ IL-1β	↑ BDNF	↓↓ AChE	Best behavioral outcome; good mechanistic support
SS-LB	Y-maze, water maze, and passive avoidance	↓↓ TNF-α, ↓↓ IL-1β	↑↑ BDNF	↓↓ AChE	Strong anti-inflammatory and plasticity-related effects
SS-FM	Passive avoidance	Mild anti-inflammatory	↑ BDNF	↓ AChE	Weaker behavioral and molecular effects

Improvements are categorized by hippocampal biochemical markers, inflammation, neuroplasticity, and behavioral cognitive performance. Symbols indicate the direction and relative strength of observed effects compared to the control group. ↑, ↑↑, ↓, ↓↓: Direction/magnitude of improvement. TNF-α, tumor-necrosis factor-α; IL-1β, interleukine-1β; AChE, acetylcholinesterase; BDNF, brain-derived neurotrophic factor.

The metabolic improvements observed following kanjang supplementation—particularly enhanced insulin sensitivity, improved glucose tolerance, and reduced fat accumulation—align with previous studies, demonstrating that fermented soybean products ameliorate insulin resistance and metabolic dysfunction in high-fat-diet-induced models [14]. In our study, these effects were most pronounced in the SS-MB group, which showed the greatest reductions in fasting glucose, HOMA-IR, and glucose levels during IPITT, indicating a significant enhancement of systemic insulin sensitivity.

A particularly novel aspect of our findings is the consistent modulation of water metabolism observed in all kanjang-treated groups. Kanjang intake led to increased water consumption and decreased circulating levels of aldosterone, renin, and angiotensin II, suggesting the effective inhibition of the renin–angiotensin–aldosterone system (RAAS). This response was especially marked in SS-MB and SS-FM, both of which exhibited the highest water intake and lowest RAAS activity. As RAAS suppression is associated with reductions in blood pressure, fluid retention, and improved insulin signaling, these findings provide a compelling link between fluid balance regulation and metabolic enhancement. These results are consistent with earlier reports showing that fermented soy consumption attenuates RAAS activity and hypertension [10,19].

In addition to glycemic improvements, several kanjang varieties showed favorable effects on body composition, as shown in a previous study [11]. The SS-HB group demonstrated the most significant reductions in final body weight, visceral fat mass, and food efficiency, suggesting anti-obesity potential. Meanwhile, SS-LB was characterized by elevated insulin levels during OGTT, indicating a possible insulinotropic mechanism that supports glycemic control via increased insulin secretion. These distinct metabolic profiles highlight the role of microbial composition and fermentation characteristics in shaping the functional properties of each kanjang variety. A detailed comparative summary of the metabolic effects—including glucose regulation, insulin sensitivity, RAAS suppression, and body weight control—is presented in Table S2.

Importantly, these metabolic improvements may also contribute to the cognitive enhancements observed in kanjang-treated groups. The interconnection between metabolic health, neuroinflammation, and cognitive function is well established [20,21]. In our study, kanjang intake led to a reduced hippocampal expression of pro-inflammatory cytokines, consistent with previous research demonstrating that fermented soybean extracts inhibit microglial activation and neuroinflammation in LPS-challenged models [22,23]. Notably, SS-MB showed the most robust suppression of hippocampal TNF-α expression, supporting its dual role in improving both metabolic and cognitive function.

Emerging evidence suggests that specific microbial metabolites derived from fermented foods exert anti-inflammatory effects through the inhibition of the NF-κB signaling pathway, a critical mediator of both metabolic and neuroimmune inflammation. Together, our findings support the potential of kanjang varieties—particularly SS-MB, SS-HB, and SS-LB—as multifunctional dietary agents capable of enhancing glucose metabolism, regulating water homeostasis, and attenuating neuroinflammation, with downstream cognitive benefits. The comparative profiles of metabolic outcomes across kanjang types are summarized in Table S2, highlighting their differential efficacy and therapeutic potential.

The alterations in gut microbiota composition induced by the kanjang treatments represent a novel finding extending beyond previous research. Several studies have demonstrated that fermented soy products can modify gut microbiota in different animal models and humans [24–28]. Our study sought to comprehensively analyze the relationship between specific bacterial compositions in kanjang and their effects on host gut microbiota in modifying cognitive function in an amnesic animal model. The increased abundance of *Lactobacillaceae* and *Ligilactobacillus* in the SS-HB and SS-LB groups parallels findings [29–31], which reported similar shifts in microbiota following the consumption of fermented soybean foods. Furthermore, our metagenomic functional analysis provides deeper insights into the metabolic consequences of these changes in the microbiota, revealing enhanced glycolysis/gluconeogenesis pathways and butanoate metabolism. Consistent with the metagenome function, the serum butyrate concentration was higher in the SS-MB and SS-LB groups, and a recent study also revealed that soy sauce (kanjang) increased *Agathobacter rectalis* to elevate butyrate production [32]. Elevating serum butyrate levels in the SS-MB and SS-LB groups supports the study that butyrate supplementation improved memory in a mouse model of vascular dementia [33]. Similarly, other studies have shown that butyrate administration enhanced memory formation through increased histone acetylation in the hippocampus, providing a potential mechanism for the cognitive improvements observed in our study [34,35].

The increases in goblet cell count observed in the kanjang-treated groups suggest enhanced gut barrier integrity, consistent with studies which have demonstrated that fermented soybean products strengthen intestinal barrier function and reduce intestinal inflammation in colitis models [36,37]. Our findings extend this work by linking improved gut barrier function to cognitive benefits, supporting the emerging concept that gut permeability plays a crucial role in neurological disorders. Furthermore, kanjang consumption improves memory function through bidirectional gut–brain axis communication. This model aligns with the growing body of evidence linking gut microbiota to cognitive function, potentially through the vagus nervous system [38–40]. However, our study is among the first to demonstrate that different varieties of the same traditional fermented food can exert varying effects on this axis, depending on their microbial composition. The superior performance of SS-HB and SS-LB may be attributed to their unique bacterial compositions, which more effectively modulated these pathways. This finding is consistent with recent work, which demonstrated the strain-specific effects of fermented food-derived bacteria on cognitive function and neuroinflammation [18,41].

The estimated sodium intake from the kanjang-supplemented diet was approximately 5.95 mg/day per rat, which, after adjusting for the actual sodium content in fresh kanjang (7%), corresponds to ~19.8 mg/day. Using standard body surface area-based conversion, this equates to approximately 773 mg/day of sodium in a 60 kg adult human, or ~39% of the WHO's recommended upper intake limit of 2000 mg/day. This sodium level is well within the recognized safety thresholds, supporting the tolerability and translational relevance of the dosage used in this study.

Importantly, no signs of toxicity or adverse effects were observed in the animal model, including no significant differences in food intake among groups. Although the kanjang-treated animals exhibited a lower weight gain, this was attributed to reduced food efficiency rather than reduced appetite or metabolic distress, suggesting a potential metabolic shift rather than harmful effects. These findings, combined with the realistic human-equivalent sodium intake, indicate that dietary supplementation with kanjang is safe and tolerable within the typical sodium range found in traditional diets, particularly when used as a functional substitute for table salt.

Clinical Implications and Future Directions

These findings have significant implications for developing dietary interventions aimed at preventing cognitive decline. Unlike previous studies that typically examined a single fermented product [42–44], our comparative approach across kanjang varieties—each with distinct microbial compositions—underscores the importance of standardizing fermentation processes when developing evidence-based functional foods. The varying cognitive efficacy among different kanjangs also suggests that traditional food processing method, including salt concentrations (typically 8–10%), may provide the empirical knowledge of optimal microbial ecosystems for health benefits. This aligns with a growing interest in traditional fermented foods as sources of next-generation probiotics [45,46]. As the current findings are based on a murine model, future clinical trials will be essential to determine whether the observed improvements in memory, the modulation of neuroinflammation, and gut–brain interaction translate to human cognitive health outcomes.

5. Conclusions

This study demonstrates that kanjang consumption, particularly of the SS-HB and SS-LB varieties containing approximately 8–10% sodium, effectively ameliorates scopolamine-induced cognitive dysfunction through a multifaceted mechanistic approach in a murine model. By revealing the interconnected effects on metabolic regulation, neurotrophic signaling, gut microbiota composition, and neuroinflammation, our findings elucidate the complex physiological pathways underlying the cognitive-enhancing properties of kanjang (Figure 5). While high sodium content in fermented foods is typically viewed as unfavorable for health, our results suggest that excessively reducing sodium levels in kanjang may compromise its functional benefits. Traditional fermentation processes require adequate salt concentrations to support the growth of specific microbial communities and the production of bioactive compounds essential for neuroprotection. Our investigation was distinguished by (1) a comparative analysis of kanjang varieties with distinct bacterial compositions, (2) an exploration of microbial metabolites and their role in cognitive function, (3) comprehensive metagenomic functional profiling, and (4) the systems-level integration of metabolic, microbial, and neurological pathways into a unified mechanistic model. The bioactive compounds and microbial signatures identified in kanjang represent a promising foundation for developing targeted nutraceuticals, bridging traditional fermented food knowledge with modern functional food research. Overall, our findings provide not only novel insights into diet-based cognitive interventions but also establish a robust scientific framework for future clinical investigations into the neuroprotective potential of fermented soybean products.

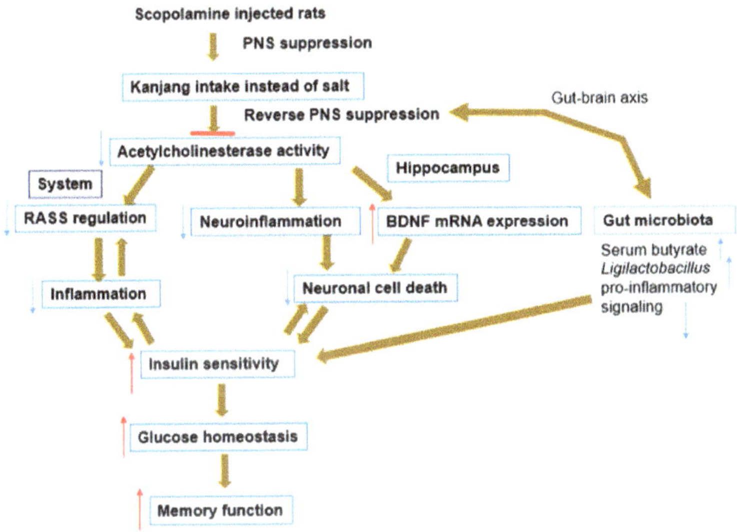

Figure 5. Mechanisms of kanjang intake in reversing scopolamine-induced memory impairment and neuronal cell death. Schematic illustrates the comprehensive mechanisms by which kanjang intake mitigates scopolamine-induced memory impairment and neuronal cell death by parasympathetic nervous system (PSN) suppression with scopolamine injection: (1) reverses PNS suppression, partially by gut microbiota modulation, (2) inhibits acetylcholinesterase activity, (3) increases BDNF mRNA expression and prevents neuronal cell death, (4) modulates the renin–angiotensin–aldosterone system (RASS) and neuroinflammation, and (5) enhances insulin sensitivity. Brown arrows depict interconnected pathways that result in improved memory function and neuronal survival. Small red and blue arrows indicated increase and decrease, respectively. Horizontal red line indicated block of the acetylcholinesterase activity.

Supplementary Materials: The following supporting information can be downloaded at: https://www.mdpi.com/article/10.3390/nu17101617/s1, Figure S1. Experimental design; Figure S2. Microbiome composition of kanjang samples; Figure S3. Area under the curve (AUC) of serum glucose and insulin concentrations during the oral glucose tolerance (OGTT) and AUC of serum glucose during the intraperitoneal insulin tolerance test (IPITT); Figure S4. Large intestinal morphology after the intervention. (A) Hematoxylin-eosin staining of the intestinal tissues. (B) Mucosal length, crypt width, and crypt depth; Table S1. General characteristics of kanjang samples. Table S2. Integrated summary of the metabolic effects of different kanjang varieties across key domains: energy balance, water regulation, glucose metabolism, and inflammatory status.

Author Contributions: S.P.: Conceptualization, Methodology, Supervision, Writing—Original Draft, and Funding Acquisition; Y.Y. and H.-J.Y.: Conceptualization, Formal Analysis, Visualization, and Visualization. C.L., M.-S.R., and J.-W.S.: Formal Analysis and Methodology. D.Y.J.: Conceptualization, Supervision, Visualization, and Writing—Review and Editing. All authors have read and agreed to the published version of the manuscript.

Funding: This work was supported by "functional research of fermented soybean food (safety monitoring)" under the Ministry of Agriculture, Food and Rural Affairs in 2025.

Institutional Review Board Statement: This study complied with the instructions provided in the Guide for the Care and Use of Laboratory Animals (8th edition, National Institutes of Health [NIH], US) and was approved by the Hoseo University Institutional Animal Care and Use Committee (HSUIACUC-23-034, 23 May 2023).

Informed Consent Statement: Not applicable.

Data Availability Statement: The original contributions presented in this study are included in the article/Supplementary Material. Further inquiries can be directed to the corresponding author(s).

Conflicts of Interest: The authors do not have any financial or personal interest in the work incorporated in this manuscript.

References

1. Kim, S.-H.; Ko, J.; Kwon, D.Y. Jang, Korean fermented soybean product, the result of endeavors of ancients for the best taste of Korean diet. *J. Ethn. Foods* **2023**, *10*, 33. [CrossRef]
2. Faraco, G.; Brea, D.; Garcia-Bonilla, L.; Wang, G.; Racchumi, G.; Chang, H.; Buendia, I.; Santisteban, M.M.; Segarra, S.G.; Koizumi, K.; et al. Dietary salt promotes neurovascular and cognitive dysfunction through a gut-initiated TH17 response. *Nat. Neurosci.* **2018**, *21*, 240–249. [CrossRef] [PubMed]
3. Jeong, S.J.; Yang, H.J.; Yang, H.G.; Ryu, M.S.; Ha, G.; Jeong, D.Y.; Park, S. Inverse association of daily fermented soybean paste ("Jang") intake with metabolic syndrome risk, especially body fat and hypertension, in men of a large hospital-based cohort. *Front. Nutr.* **2023**, *10*, 1122945. [CrossRef] [PubMed]
4. Park, S.; Zhang, T.; Yue, Y.; Jeong, S.J.; Ryu, M.S.; Wu, X.; Yang, H.J.; Jeong, D.Y. Alleviation of metabolic disturbance by substituting kanjang high in Bacillus for salt through modulation of gut microbiota in estrogen-deficient Rats. *Foods* **2022**, *11*, 1951. [CrossRef]
5. Zheng, Y.; Bonfili, L.; Wei, T.; Eleuteri, A.M. Understanding the gut-brain axis and Its therapeutic implications for neurodegenerative disorders. *Nutrients* **2023**, *15*, 4631. [CrossRef]
6. Lu, S.; Zhao, Q.; Guan, Y.; Sun, Z.; Li, W.; Guo, S.; Zhang, A. The communication mechanism of the gut-brain axis and its effect on central nervous system diseases: A systematic review. *Biomed. Pharmacother.* **2024**, *178*, 117207. [CrossRef]
7. Skalny, A.V.; Aschner, M.; Gritsenko, V.A.; Martins, A.C.; Tizabi, Y.; Korobeinikova, T.V.; Paoliello, M.M.B.; Tinkov, A.A. Modulation of gut microbiota with probiotics as a strategy to counteract endogenous and exogenous neurotoxicity. *Adv. Neurotoxicol.* **2024**, *11*, 133–176. [CrossRef]
8. Martin, M.; Boulaire, M.; Lucas, C.; Peltier, A.; Pourtau, L.; Gaudout, D.; Layé, S.; Pallet, V.; Joffre, C.; Dinel, A.-L. Plant extracts and ω-3 improve short-term memory and modulate the microbiota–gut–brain axis in D-galactose model mice. *J. Nutr.* **2024**, *154*, 3704–3717. [CrossRef]
9. Poceviciute, I.; Brazaityte, A.; Buisas, R.; Vengeliene, V. Scopolamine animal model of memory impairment. *Behav. Brain Res.* **2025**, *479*, 115344. [CrossRef]
10. Mun, E.G.; Sohn, H.S.; Kim, M.S.; Cha, Y.S. Antihypertensive effect of Ganjang (traditional Korean soy sauce) on Sprague-Dawley rats. *Nutr. Res. Pract.* **2017**, *11*, 388–395. [CrossRef]
11. Lee, E.J.; Song, J.; Park, C.H.; Mun, E.G.; Wang, J.; Han, A.; Park, J.E.; Cha, Y.S. Soy sauce lowers body weight and fat mass in high-fat diet-induced obese rats. *J. Med. Food* **2023**, *26*, 858–867. [CrossRef] [PubMed]
12. Graham, S.E.; Clarke, S.L.; Wu, K.-H.H.; Kanoni, S.; Zajac, G.J.M.; Ramdas, S.; Surakka, I.; Ntalla, I.; Vedantam, S.; Winkler, T.W.; et al. The power of genetic diversity in genome-wide association studies of lipids. *Nature* **2021**, *600*, 675–679. [CrossRef] [PubMed]
13. Ke, B.; Zhang, T.; An, T.; Lu, R. Soy isoflavones ameliorate the cognitive dysfunction of Goto-Kakizaki rats by activating the Nrf2-HO-1 signaling pathway. *Aging* **2020**, *12*, 21344–21354. [CrossRef] [PubMed]
14. Gopikrishna, T.; Suresh Kumar, H.K.; Perumal, K.; Elangovan, E. Impact of Bacillus in fermented soybean foods on human health. *Ann. Microbiol.* **2021**, *71*, 30. [CrossRef]
15. Kim, B.V.; Yoon, S.; Kim, J.E. A review of fermented foods with beneficial effects on brain and cognitive function. *Prev. Nutr. Food Sci.* **2016**, *21*, 297–305. [CrossRef]
16. do Prado, F.G.; Pagnoncelli, M.G.B.; de Melo Pereira, G.V.; Karp, S.G.; Soccol, C.R. Fermented soy products and their potential health benefits: A review. *Microorganisms* **2022**, *10*, 1606. [CrossRef]
17. Qiao, Y.; Zhang, K.; Zhang, Z.; Zhang, C.; Sun, Y.; Feng, Z. Fermented soybean foods: A review of their functional components, mechanism of action and factors influencing their health benefits. *Food Res. Int.* **2022**, *158*, 111575. [CrossRef]

18. Ryu, M.S.; Yue, Y.; Li, C.; Yang, H.-J.; Zhang, T.; Wu, X.; Jeong, D.Y.; Park, S. Moderate capsaicin-containing kochujang alleviates memory impairment through the gut-brain axis in rats with scopolamine-induced amnesia. *Biomed. Pharmacother.* **2024**, *178*, 117091. [CrossRef]
19. Zhong, B.; Mun, E.-G.; Wang, J.-X.; Cha, Y.-S. Chinese traditional fermented soy sauce exerts protective effects against high-fat and high-salt diet-induced hypertension in Sprague-Dawley rats by improving adipogenesis and renin-angiotensin-aldosterone system activity. *Fermentation* **2021**, *7*, 52. [CrossRef]
20. Zaprovalna, O.E.; Kolesnikova, O.V.; Potapenko, A.V.; Radchenko, A.O. Association between metabolic parameters and cognitive dysfunction in different age groups. *Atherosclerosis* **2022**, *355*, 156–157. [CrossRef]
21. Yulug, B.; Altay, O.; Li, X.; Hanoglu, L.; Cankaya, S.; Lam, S.; Velioglu, H.A.; Yang, H.; Coskun, E.; Idil, E.; et al. Combined metabolic activators improve cognitive functions in Alzheimer's disease patients: A randomized, double-blinded, placebo-controlled phase-II trial. *Transl. Neurodegener.* **2023**, *12*, 4. [CrossRef] [PubMed]
22. Shalal, O.S. Anti-inflammatory activity of fermented soybean (Glycine max) extract on macrophages by inhibiting cytokines expression. *Gene Rep.* **2023**, *30*, 101729. [CrossRef]
23. Das, D.; Sarkar, S.; Borsingh Wann, S.; Kalita, J.; Manna, P. Current perspectives on the anti-inflammatory potential of fermented soy foods. *Food Res. Int.* **2022**, *152*, 110922. [CrossRef] [PubMed]
24. Arcusa, R.; Villaño, D.; Marhuenda, J.; Cano, M.; Cerdà, B.; Zafrilla, P. Potential role of ginger (Zingiber officinale Roscoe) in the prevention of neurodegenerative diseases. *Front. Nutr.* **2022**, *9*, 809621. [CrossRef]
25. Muniyappan, M.; Shanmugam, S.; Park, J.H.; Han, K.; Kim, I.H. Effects of fermented soybean meal supplementation on the growth performance and apparent total tract digestibility by modulating the gut microbiome of weaned piglets. *Sci. Rep.* **2023**, *13*, 3691. [CrossRef]
26. Zhang, L.; Su, H.; Wang, S.; Fu, Y.; Wang, M. Gut microbiota and neurotransmitter regulation: Functional effects of four traditional Chinese fermented soybeans (Sojae Semen praeparatum). *Foods* **2025**, *14*, 671. [CrossRef]
27. Song, E.-J.; Kim, M.J.; Jung, C.H.; Chung, W.-H.; Nam, Y.-D.; Lim, M.Y. Early response of the gut microbiome and serum metabolites to Cheonggukjang intake in healthy Korean subjects. *J. Funct. Foods* **2023**, *101*, 105420. [CrossRef]
28. Karbownik, M.S.; Mokros, Ł.; Dobielska, M.; Kowalczyk, M.; Kowalczyk, E. Association between consumption of fermented food and food-derived prebiotics with cognitive performance, depressive, and anxiety symptoms in psychiatrically healthy medical students under psychological stress: A prospective cohort study. *Front. Nutr.* **2022**, *9*, 850249. [CrossRef]
29. Zhu, J.-j.; Gao, M.-x.; Song, X.-j.; Zhao, L.; Li, Y.-w.; Hao, Z.-h. Changes in bacterial diversity and composition in the feces and colon of weaned piglets after feeding fermented soybean meal. *J. Med. Microbiol.* **2018**, *67*, 1181–1190. [CrossRef]
30. Jang, S.-E.; Kim, K.-A.; Han, M.J.; Kim, D.-H. Doenjang, a fermented Korean soybean paste, inhibits lipopolysaccharide production of gut microbiota in mice. *J. Med. Food* **2014**, *17*, 67–75. [CrossRef]
31. Lim, H.J.; Park, I.S.; Seo, J.W.; Ha, G.; Yang, H.J.; Jeong, D.Y.; Kim, S.Y.; Jung, C.H. Anti-inflammatory effect of Korean soybean sauce (Ganjang) on mice with induced colitis. *J. Microbiol. Biotechnol.* **2024**, *34*, 1501–1510. [CrossRef] [PubMed]
32. Hayashi, K.; Uchida, R.; Horiba, T.; Kawaguchi, T.; Gomi, K.; Goto, Y. Soy sauce-like seasoning enhances the growth of Agathobacter rectalis and the production of butyrate, propionate, and lactate. *Biosci. Microbiota Food Health* **2024**, *43*, 275–281. [CrossRef] [PubMed]
33. Fernando, W.M.A.D.B.; Martins, I.J.; Morici, M.; Bharadwaj, P.; Rainey-Smith, S.R.; Lim, W.L.F.; Martins, R.N. Sodium butyrate reduces brain amyloid-β levels and improves cognitive memory performance in an Alzheimer's disease transgenic mouse model at an early disease stage. *J. Alzheimers Dis.* **2020**, *74*, 91–99. [CrossRef] [PubMed]
34. Ziemka-Nalecz, M.; Jaworska, J.; Sypecka, J.; Polowy, R.; Filipkowski, R.K.; Zalewska, T. Sodium butyrate, a histone deacetylase inhibitor, exhibits neuroprotective/neurogenic effects in a rat model of neonatal hypoxia-ischemia. *Mol. Neurobiol.* **2017**, *54*, 5300–5318. [CrossRef]
35. Ge, X.; Zheng, M.; Hu, M.; Fang, X.; Geng, D.; Liu, S.; Wang, L.; Zhang, J.; Guan, L.; Zheng, P.; et al. Butyrate ameliorates quinolinic acid-induced cognitive decline in obesity models. *J. Clin. Investig.* **2023**, *133*, e154612. [CrossRef]
36. Basson, A.R.; Ahmed, S.; Almutairi, R.; Seo, B.; Cominelli, F. Regulation of intestinal inflammation by soybean and soy-derived compounds. *Foods* **2021**, *10*, 774. [CrossRef]
37. Wu, X.; Zhang, T.; Zhang, T.; Park, S. The impact of gut microbiome enterotypes on ulcerative colitis: Identifying key bacterial species and revealing species co-occurrence networks using machine learning. *Gut Microbes* **2024**, *16*, 2292254. [CrossRef]
38. Tooley, K.L. Effects of the Human gut microbiota on cognitive performance, brain structure, and function: A narrative review. *Nutrients* **2020**, *12*, 3009. [CrossRef]
39. Park, S.; Wu, X. Modulation of the gut microbiota in memory impairment and Alzheimer's disease via the inhibition of the parasympathetic nervous system. *Int. J. Mol. Sci.* **2022**, *23*, 13574. [CrossRef]
40. Han, Y.; Wang, B.; Gao, H.; He, C.; Hua, R.; Liang, C.; Zhang, S.; Wang, Y.; Xin, S.; Xu, J. Vagus nerve and underlying impact on the gut microbiota-brain axis in behavior and neurodegenerative diseases. *J. Inflamm. Res.* **2022**, *15*, 6213–6230. [CrossRef]

41. Balasubramanian, R.; Schneider, E.; Gunnigle, E.; Cotter, P.D.; Cryan, J.F. Fermented foods: Harnessing their potential to modulate the microbiota-gut-brain axis for mental health. *Neurosci. Biobehav. Rev.* **2024**, *158*, 105562. [CrossRef] [PubMed]
42. Bhatt, P.C.; Pathak, S.; Kumar, V.; Panda, B.P. Attenuation of neurobehavioral and neurochemical abnormalities in an animal model of cognitive deficits of Alzheimer's disease by fermented soybean nano nutraceutical. *Inflammopharmacology* **2018**, *26*, 105–118. [CrossRef] [PubMed]
43. Lee, H.J.; Hwang, Y.H.; Kim, D.H. Lactobacillus plantarum C29-fermented soybean (DW2009) alleviates memory impairment in 5XFAD transgenic mice by regulating microglia activation and gut microbiota composition. *Mol. Nutr. Food Res.* **2018**, *62*, e1800359. [CrossRef] [PubMed]
44. Jeong, D.Y.; Ryu, M.S.; Yang, H.J.; Park, S. γ-PGA-rich chungkookjang, short-term fermented soybeans: Prevents memory impairment by modulating brain insulin sensitivity, neuro-inflammation, and the gut-microbiome-brain axis. *Foods* **2021**, *10*, 221. [CrossRef]
45. Nithya, A.; Misra, S.; Panigrahi, C.; Dalbhagat, C.G.; Mishra, H.N. Probiotic potential of fermented foods and their role in non-communicable diseases management: An understanding through recent clinical evidence. *Food Chem. Adv.* **2023**, *3*, 100381. [CrossRef]
46. Valentino, V.; Magliulo, R.; Farsi, D.; Cotter, P.D.; O'Sullivan, O.; Ercolini, D.; De Filippis, F. Fermented foods, their microbiome and its potential in boosting human health. *Microb. Biotechnol.* **2024**, *17*, e14428. [CrossRef]

nutrients

MDPI

Article

Gene–Lifestyle Interactions in Renal Dysfunction: Polygenic Risk Modulation via Plant-Based Diets, Coffee Intake, and Bioactive Compound Interactions

Meiling Liu [1,†], Da-Sol Kim [2,†] and Sunmin Park [2,*]

1 Department of Chemical Engineering, Shanxi Institute of Science and Technology, Jincheng 048011, China; liumeiling@sxist.edu.cn

2 Department of Food and Nutrition, Obesity/Diabetes Research Center, Hoseo University, 20 Hoseoro97bun-gil, BaeBang-Yup, Asan 41399, ChungNam-Do, Republic of Korea; tpfptm14@daum.net

* Correspondence: smpark@hoseo.edu; Tel.: +82-41-540-5345; Fax: +82-41-548-0670

† These authors contributed equally to this work.

Abstract: Background: This study aimed to investigate genetic variants associated with the estimated glomerular filtration rate (eGFR) and their interactions with lifestyle factors and bioactive compounds in large hospital-based cohorts, assessing their impact on renal dysfunction risk. **Methods:** Participants were categorized into two groups based on eGFR: High-GFR (control; n = 51,084) and Low-GFR (renal dysfunction; n = 7617), using an eGFR threshold of 60 mL/min/1.73 m^2. Genetic variants were identified through a genome-wide association analysis, and their interactions with lifestyle factors were assessed a using generalized multifactor dimensionality reduction (GMDR) analysis. Additionally, interactions between polygenic risk scores (PRS) and nutrient intake were examined. **Results:** Low eGFR was associated with higher urinary protein levels (4.67-fold) and correlated with a Western-style diet and with saturated fat, arginine, and isoleucine intakes but not sodium intake. The genetic model for low eGFR included variants linked to energy production and amino acid metabolism, such as rs1047891_*CPS1*, rs3770636_*LRP2*, rs5020545_*SHROOM3*, rs3812036_*SLC34A1*, and rs4715517_*HCRTR2*. A high PRS was associated with a 1.78-fold increased risk of low eGFR after adjusting for sociodemographic and lifestyle factors. The PRS from the 6-SNP model interacted with plant-based diets (PBDs) and coffee intake, where individuals with higher PBD and coffee consumption had a lower risk of renal dysfunction. Additionally, *CPS1* rs1047891 interacted with vitamin D intake (p = 0.0436), where the risk allele was linked to lower eGFR with low vitamin D intake but not with high intake. Molecular docking showed that vitamin D3 had a lower binding energy to the CPS1 mutant type (−9.9 kcal/mol) than the wild type (−7.5 kcal/mol), supporting a potential gene–nutrient interaction influencing renal function. **Conclusions:** Middle-aged and elderly individuals with a high genetic risk for renal dysfunction may benefit from a plant-based diet, moderate coffee consumption, and sufficient vitamin D intake.

Keywords: polygenic-risk score; glomerular filtration rates; plant-based diet; coffee; renal dysfunction

1. Introduction

Chronic kidney disease (CKD) affects approximately 10% of the global adult population, with the prevalence increasing steadily over the past two decades [1]. Among adults aged 35 years or older, CKD prevalence reaches approximately 14%, with higher rates observed in elderly populations due to demographic aging trends [1]. People of Asian descent appear to have a higher prevalence of CKD compared to other ethnicities, though this remains a subject of ongoing investigation [2]. CKD is strongly associated with metabolic syndrome (MetS), cardiovascular disease (CVD), cognitive dysfunction, and premature mortality. Importantly, CKD can be prevented through lifestyle modifications [3].

Renal function is measured as the filtration rate of fluid through the kidneys [4]. The gold standard measurement involves collecting a urinary volume over a 24 h period, which presents practical challenges in clinical settings [4]. Alternatively, creatinine—a breakdown product of creatine and creatine phosphate that freely passes through the glomerulus—is a useful biomarker. The creatinine clearance rate represents the glomerular filtration rate (GFR), a key indicator of kidney function. GFR correlates inversely with serum creatinine concentration and directly with urinary creatinine concentration and urine flow [4]. Significant nephron loss results in elevated serum creatinine levels [4]. Estimated GFR (eGFR) is calculated using serum creatinine levels, age, and sex to determine the blood filtration capacity per minute relative to the body surface area [5]. An eGFR ≤ 60 mL/min/1.73 m^2 indicates reduced kidney function and potential CKD [6].

Multiple risk factors influence eGFR and CKD development, including aging, obesity, hypertension, impaired glucose tolerance, dyslipidemia, cognitive dysfunction, MetS, and CVD [7,8]. Various lifestyle factors also affect eGFR, though research on these factors remains limited. Smoking is a well-established lifestyle risk factor for reduced eGFR [7,8]. Other factors including sodium and potassium intake, alcohol and coffee consumption, and physical activity have been examined in cohort studies and meta-analyses, with inconsistent results [9]. High sodium intake (>4.6 g/day) has been associated with lower eGFR in some systematic reviews [7–10]. These inconsistencies may be attributable to genetic differences among populations.

Reduced kidney function reflects interactions between genetic and environmental factors [9,10]. Genes affecting eGFR may influence not only kidney function but also liver function, muscle mass, inflammation, and other physiological processes [11,12]. Ethnicity-related genetic differences are known to impact eGFR, with dietary factors—particularly high salt intake among Asians—interacting with genetic predispositions [13,14]. However, eGFR-related genetic variants remain understudied in certain Asian populations, and gene–lifestyle interactions require further investigation.

Exploring the direct metabolic effects of genetic variants in large cohort studies presents significant challenges. Consequently, molecular docking has emerged as a valuable approach for investigating gene–lifestyle interactions, especially for missense mutations affecting protein–ligand interactions. Previous research on obesity-related genetic variants such as brain-derived neurotrophic factor (*BDNF*) rs6265 has employed molecular docking to identify bioactive compounds influencing genetic risk [10]. Missense genetic variants influence renal function differently by interacting with bioactive compounds and lowering the binding energy. This study aims to identify the genetic variants associated with eGFR, analyze their interactions with lifestyle factors and bioactive compounds, and assess their impact on renal dysfunction risk in large hospital-based Asian cohorts.

2. Methods

2.1. Participants

This cohort study recruited individuals aged over 40 who visited multi-center hospitals in major Korean cities between 2010 and 2014. The study protocol received approval from the Institutional Review Board (IRB) of the Korea National Institute of Health and Hoseo University (approval numbers: KBP-2019-055 and 1041231-150811-HR-034-01). All participants provided written informed consent before enrollment.

2.2. Demographic, Anthropometric, and Biochemical Measurements

At baseline, participants completed comprehensive demographic questionnaires covering age, gender, education, income, and residential information. Trained research assistants performed anthropometric measurements, with the participants wearing light clothing and no footwear, following standardized protocols previously described.

Blood pressure was measured by a physician with participants in a seated position. Three consecutive readings were taken using a standard sphygmomanometer, and the mean values of systolic blood pressure (SBP) and diastolic blood pressure (DBP) were recorded for analysis [9].

Blood samples were collected after a minimum 12 h fasting period in tubes with and without heparin and ethylenediaminetetraacetic acid (EDTA) [9]. Fasting plasma glucose was analyzed using a Hitachi 7600 Automatic Analyzer (Hitachi, Tokyo, Japan), while hemoglobin A1c (HbA1c) concentrations were measured with an automatic analyzer (ZEUS 9.9; Takeda, Tokyo, Japan). Serum parameters, including total cholesterol, high-density lipoprotein cholesterol (HDL), triglycerides (TG), alanine aminotransferase (ALT), aspartate aminotransferase (AST), blood urea nitrogen (BUN), total bilirubin, and creatinine, were measured using an Hitachi 7600 Automatic Analyzer. High-sensitivity C-reactive protein (hs-CRP) concentrations were determined using a high-sensitivity ELISA kit (ThermoFisher, Waltham, MA, USA). Insulin resistance was calculated using the homeostatic model assessment of insulin resistance (HOMA-IR) [15,16].

Daily alcohol consumption (g/day) was calculated by assessing intake patterns of different beverage types (beer, wine, and spirits). For each beverage type, consumption frequency was multiplied by the average amount per intake, and these values were summed to determine total alcohol consumption [17]. Daily coffee intake was similarly calculated by multiplying consumption frequency by the amount per intake. Smoking status was categorized as follows: current smokers ($\geq$20 cigarettes in the past six months), past smokers (>20 cigarettes in lifetime but none in the past six months), and never smokers [17]. Regular exercise was defined as engaging in moderate physical activity for more than 30 min on three or more days per week.

2.3. Assessment of Kidney Function

Kidney function was evaluated using the Modification of Diet in Renal Disease (MDRD) equation, as follows: 186 $\times$ serum creatinine concentration$^{-1.154}$ $\times$ age$^{-0.203}$ $\times$ 0.742 for women and 1 for men [18]. The MDRD equation was selected because the study population had a mean age of 53.7 years (SD = 8.0). This selection was supported by comparative studies of the MDRD and Chronic Kidney Disease Epidemiology Collaboration (CKD-EPI) equations across different age groups in a Chinese population, which found that the MDRD and CKD-EPI exhibited similar trends in eGFR, with the MDRD showing a reasonable decline in eGFR with age compared to the CKD-EPI [19]. The eGFR was standardized to a body surface area of 1.73 m^2. Renal dysfunction was defined as an eGFR $\leq$ 60 mL/min/1.73 m^2 or current use of kidney disease medication. Based on these criteria, participants were categorized into the following two groups: the Low-GFR group (n = 7617) and the High-GFR group (eGFR > 60 mL/min/1.73 m^2, with no kidney disease medication; n = 51,084). The mean eGFR was significantly lower in the Low-GFR group (55.3 $\pm$ 0.34 mL/min/1.73 m^2) than in the High-GFR group (87.1 $\pm$ 0.06 mL/min/1.73 m^2), confirming an appropriate stratification of renal function between groups.

2.4. Usual Food Intake Assessment Using a Semi-Quantitative Food Frequency Questionnaire (SQFFQ)

The participants' habitual food intake was evaluated using an SQFFQ specifically designed for the study population's typical dietary patterns, covering the preceding 12 months [20]. The questionnaire comprised 106 commonly consumed food items, with participants documenting both consumption frequencies and portion sizes. Consumption frequencies were categorized as follows: never or seldom, once per month, two to three times per month, once or twice weekly, three or four times weekly, five or six times weekly, daily, twice daily, and three or more times daily. Portion sizes were recorded as 0.5, 1, or 2 times the standard portion size, which was visually represented through 106 food photographs. The SQFFQ's reproducibility and validity were confirmed by comparison against three-day food records collected across all four seasons [21]. Daily food intake (g/day) was calculated by multiplying the median frequency of daily consumption by the reported portion size. Daily intake of energy, macronutrients (carbohydrates, proteins, amino acids, and fats), vitamins, and minerals were determined using Can-Pro 2.0 nutrient assessment software (Korean Nutrition Society, Seoul, Republic of Korea). Nutrient intake levels were categorized as low or high based on either established Dietary Reference Intake (DRI) cutoffs or study-specific percentiles, depending on the nutrient. For nutrients with well-defined DRI thresholds, these values were used to distinguish between low and high intakes. When no specific DRI cutoff was available or intake levels were highly variable, the 33rd and 66th percentiles of the study population's intake distribution were used for classification according to the nutrients' characteristics. For example, low vitamin D intake was defined as <2.53 μg/day, corresponding to the 33rd percentile in our study, rather than the DRI of 10 μg/day. The specific cutoff values for each nutrient are detailed in the corresponding tables and figure legends.

2.5. Dietary Pattern Classification and Inflammatory Index

Dietary patterns were classified using principal component analysis (PCA) based on 30 predefined food groups derived from the 106 individual food items. Using eigenvalues > 1.5 and orthogonal rotation (varimax), we identified the following four distinct dietary patterns: Asian-style balanced diet (ABD), plant-based diet (PBD), Western-style diet (WSD), and rice-based diet (RBD) [21,22]. Food groups with factor-loading values ≥ 0.40 were considered primary contributors to each pattern, as detailed in Supplemental Table S1.

The Dietary Inflammatory Index (DII) was calculated using a prediction equation incorporating food and nutrient intakes with corresponding dietary inflammatory weights [23]. This equation included energy, 32 nutrients, four food products, four spices, and caffeine [24]. Four components (garlic, ginger, saffron, and turmeric) were excluded from the DII calculation as they were not included in the SQFFQ. The final DII was computed as the sum of scores for the 38 included foods and nutrients, divided by 100.

2.6. Genotyping and Quality Control

Genomic DNA was extracted from participants' whole blood samples and genotyped using a K-Chip (Affymetrix, Santa Clara, CA, USA) specifically designed to detect disease-related single-nucleotide polymorphisms (SNPs) in regional, rural, and urban hospital-based cohorts. Genotypes were imputed using 1000-genome sequence data or Asian HapMap data [25] and evaluated for accuracy using a Bayesian learning algorithm for robust general linear models [9,26]. Genotyping quality control was performed based on the following criteria: (1) genotyping accuracy $\geq$ 98%, (2) missing genotype call rate < 4%, (3) heterozygosity < 30%, and (4) absence of gender bias. Genetic variants were excluded from analysis if they failed to meet the threshold of $p \leq 0.05$ for the Hardy–Weinberg equilibrium (HWE) or had a minor allele frequency (MAF) $\leq$1% [26].

2.7. Selection and Characterization of the Genetic Variants Associated with Renal Dysfunction Risk

The process of genetic variant selection and interaction analysis is illustrated in Figure S1. A genome-wide association study (GWAS) was conducted using the urban hospital-based cohort to identify genetic variants associated with renal function risk between the Low-GFR and High-GFR groups (significance threshold: $p < 1 \times 10^{-6}$). Genetic bias was assessed using a Manhattan plot and the genetic inflation factor (lambda) of the quantile-quantile (Q–Q) plot. The Manhattan plot displayed the negative logarithms of association p-values for renal function. The Q–Q plot evaluated GWAS genotype quality by comparing the quantile distribution of observed p-values (y-axis) against expected p-values (x-axis). Genotypes were considered ideal when the lambda value approached 1.

From an initial pool of 3787 genetic variants, 364 were excluded for failing to meet minor allele frequency (MAF < 1%) and Hardy–Weinberg equilibrium ($p < 0.05$) criteria, as determined using g:Profiler (https://biit.cs.ut.ee/gprofiler/snpense, accessed on 5 March 2024). Additionally, 3245 SNPs with high linkage disequilibrium (D′ $\geq$ 0.2) were excluded as they provided redundant genetic information. The remaining 178 genetic variants met the linkage disequilibrium criteria (D′ < 0.2), as assessed using Haploview 4.2 in PLINK. Another 103 variants were removed because of unidentifiable gene names, leaving 75 genetic variants. From these, we selected 22 genetic variants involved in a common genetic pathway identified using Genemania (https://genemania.org/, accessed on 29 March 2024). This pathway was linked to renal-function-associated genetic variants (p for Bonferroni correction <0.05) and was selected using MAGMA gene-set analysis in SNP2GENE of the Functional Mapping and Annotation of Genetic Associations (FUMA) web application, available through the git repository (https://github.com/Kyoko-wtnb/FUMA-webapp/, accessed on 10 April 2024).

An expression quantitative trait locus (eQTL) analysis was employed to directly assess how genetic variants at risk loci influence candidate gene expression. This approach helped determine the gene expressions associated with genetic variants linked to hypo-HDL risk using the Genotype-Tissue Expression (GTEx) × eQTL calculator (https://gtexportal.org/home/testyourown, accessed on 30 April 2024).

2.8. PRS Development and Gene–Lifestyle Interactions

From the 22 SNPs identified through the generalized multifactor dimensionality reduction (GMDR), we selected 10 for the best model of SNP–SNP interactions related to renal dysfunction risk. Selection criteria for the optimal model included $p < 0.001$ for the sign test of testing-balanced accuracy (TEBA) and 10-fold cross-validation consistency (CVC) in the exhaustive search type after covariate adjustment. The following two adjustment models were considered: model 1 (covariates: age, gender, residence area, education, and income) and model 2 (model 1 covariates plus energy, sodium, and alcohol intake; regular exercise; and smoking status). Ten-fold cross-validation was employed because of the large sample size (>1000) [27].

We calculated the polygenic risk score (PRS) by summing the number of risk alleles from each selected SNP in the best gene–gene interaction model. Risk allele values were assigned as follows: homozygous risk genotype (for example, "TT") = 2; heterozygous genotype (for example, "TC") = 1; and homozygous non-risk genotype (for example, "CC") = 0. The PRS values were categorized into Low-PRS (0–4 for the 6-SNP model; 0–5 for the 7-SNP model), Medium-PRS (5–6 for the 6-SNP model; 6–7 for the 7-SNP model), and

High-PRS (>6 for the 6-SNP model and >7 for the 7-SNP model). We selected the model with the fewest SNPs for the lifestyle interaction analyses.

2.9. Molecular Docking Analysis of Missense Mutation with Food Compounds

Both wild-type and mutated protein structures were obtained in the Protein Data Bank (PDB) format via the Iterative Threading Assembly Refinement (I-TASSER) website (https://zhanggroup.org/I-TASSER/, accessed on 14 May 2024). These protein structures were converted to PDB, partial charge (Q), and atom type (T) (PDBQT) files using AutoDock Tools 1.5.6, provided by the Molecular Graphics Laboratory at the Scripps Research Institute (La Jolla, CA, USA) [28]. Active sites within the proteins were identified using ProteinsPlus (https://proteins.plus/, accessed on 29 May 2024), with both active functional pockets and mutated sites included in the active site for molecular docking. Concurrently, approximately 20,000 food compounds were transformed into the PDBQT file format, with any water molecules attached to the ligands removed [28]. Food components were selected based on binding energy thresholds of less than −10 kcal/mol [29]. Lower binding free energy values indicate a lower binding energy between the protein and ligand, suggesting a more stable interaction.

2.10. Statistical Analysis

Statistical analyses were conducted using SAS (version 9.3; SAS Institute, Cary, NC, USA). The study included 58,701 participants, providing sufficient statistical power to detect significance at $\alpha = 0.05$ and $\beta = 0.99$, as well as an odds ratio (OR) of 1.05 in the logistic regression analysis, as determined by the G-power calculation.

For the categorical variables, frequency distributions were calculated, and chi-square tests assessed statistical differences in low eGFR (eGFR $\leq$ 60 mL/min/1.73 m^2). For continuous variables, adjusted means with standard errors were calculated after controlling for covariates, including age, gender, residence area, education, income, daily energy intake, sodium intake, alcohol consumption, smoking status, and physical activity. Differences between the Low-GFR and High-GFR groups were evaluated using one-way analysis of covariance (ANCOVA) with covariate adjustment [30]. When ANCOVA revealed significant differences, Tukey's test was applied for post hoc multiple comparisons.

The association between low eGFR and metabolic parameters was examined through logistic regression with covariate adjustment. The results are presented as an adjusted OR with the 95% confidence interval (CI) for each metabolic parameter. The following two adjustment models were implemented: Model 1, including age, residence area, survey year, education, and income as covariates; Model 2, incorporating all Model 1 covariates plus energy intake, alcohol consumption, sodium intake, physical activity, and smoking status.

Interactions between PRS or carbamoyl-phosphate synthase-1 (*CPS1*) rs1047891 (Thr1406Asn in protein) and lifestyle-related parameters were analyzed using two-way ANCOVA. Participants were categorized into high or low groups based on dietary reference intake values or the 66th percentiles of each lifestyle variable. Within these high and low lifestyle parameter groups, the OR and 95% CI for the low eGFR were determined using logistic regression analysis. Additionally, chi-square tests assessed statistical differences in low eGFR prevalence across PRS groups within the stratified lifestyle parameter categories.

3. Results

3.1. Demographic and Lifestyle Characteristics

Table 1 presents the general characteristics of participants stratified by renal function. Participants in the Low-GFR group were significantly older than those in the High-GFR group, with older individuals having a 2.16 times higher risk of renal dysfunction. Interestingly, the female gender showed an inverse association with renal dysfunction compared to males. Educational attainment did not significantly differ between the groups, indicating no association between education level and eGFR (Table 1). While the Low-GFR group contained more former and current smokers than the High-GFR group, smoking status showed no significant association with eGFR after covariate adjustment (Table 1).

Table 1. Parameters related to metabolic diseases according to the estimated glomerular filtration rates (eGFR) [1].

	High-GFR (n = 51,084)	Low-GFR (n = 7617)	Adjusted OR and 95% CI
Age (years) [2]	53.3 ± 0.03	56.5 ± 0.08 ***	2.156 (1.975–2.354)
Gender (male, N %)	16,105 (33.6)	3332 (43.7) +++	0.701 (0.649–0.756)
Education			
<High school	7268 (19.6)	1223 (21.2)	1
High school	27,133 (73.2)	4172 (72.2)	1.130 (0.978–1.306)
>High school	2687 (7.24)	412 (7.09)	1.194 (0.912–1.562)
MetS (N, %) [3]	6998 (13.7)	2148 (28.2) +++	1.991 (1.781–2.225)
CVD (N, %) [4]	1890 (3.72)	799 (10.5) +++	1.920 (1.625–2.268)
BMI (kg/m^2) [5]	23.9 ± 0.03	24.3 ± 0.05 ***	1.374 (1.244–1.518)
Waist Cir. (cm) [6]	80.6 ± 0.03	81.7 ± 0.18 ***	1.304 (1.168–1.456)
Serum glucose (mg/dL) [7]	95.1 ± 0.09	97.6 ± 0.48 **	1.853 (1.632–2.105)
Blood HbA1c (%) [8]	5.71 ± 0.004	5.96 ± 0.026 ***	1.598 (1.339–1.908)
Serum HDL (mg/dL) [9]	53.9 ± 0.06	51.1 ± 0.31 ***	0.662 (0.598–0.733)
Serum LDL (mg/dL) [10]	118 ± 0.15	120 ± 0.39 ***	1.277 (1.143–1.427)
Serum TG (mg/dL) [11]	124 ± 0.39	130 ± 1.00 ***	1.340 (1.210–1.483)
SBP (mmHg) [12]	122 ± 0.07	122 ± 0.17	1.142 (1.032–1.263)
DBP (mmHg) [13]	75.7 ± 0.04	75.8 ± 0.11	1.103 (0.943–1.289)
Hypertension (N, %)	2814 (5.51)	1150 (15.1) +++	2.089 (1.887–2.312)
Insulin resistance (N, %)	3918 (7.67)	975 (12.8)***	1.473 (1.271–1.707)
Serum CRP (mg/dL) [14]	0.137 ± 0.002	0.154 ± 0.005 **	1.714 (1.254–2.344)
Serum creatinine (mg/dL)	0.79 ± 0.001	1.24 ± 0.003	
Serum uric acid (mg/dL) [15]	4.60 ± 0.005	5.24 ± 0.01 ***	4.531 (4.036–5.087)
Blood urinary nitrogen (mg/dL) [16]	14.4 ± 0.02	18.2 ± 0.05	3.247 (2.935–3.591)
Albumin (mg/dL) [17]	4.62 ± 0.001	4.59 ± 0.006 ***	0.753 (0.683–0.831)
AST (U/L) [18]	23.6 ± 0.11	24.7 ± 0.30 ***	1.189 (0.957–1.477)
ALT (U/L) [19]	22.3 ± 0.11	23.0 ± 0.29 *	1.170 (1.010–1.355)
Total bilirubin [20]	0.73 ± 0.002	0.74 ± 0.005 *	2.432 (2.306–2.565)
Urinary protein [21]	1.09 ± 0.002	1.33 ± 0.01 ***	4.653 (3.919–5.524)

[1] The MDRD Study's equation using serum creatinine concentrations and the High-GFR and Low-GFR groups were defined as > and ≤60 mL/min/1.73 m^2 of eGFR. OR, odds ratio; CI, confidence intervals. The cutoff points for moderate exercise in the logistic regression were as follows: [2] <55 years old. [3] Metabolic syndrome (MetS) criteria. [4] Cardiovascular diseases (CVDs). [5] <25 kg/m^2 for body mass index (BMI). [6] <90 cm for men and 85 cm for women waist circumferences (Cir.). [7] <126 mL/dL fasting serum glucose plus diabetic drug intake. [8] <6.5% hbA1c plus diabetic drug intake. [9] >40 mg/dL for men and 50 mg/dL for women serum HDL cholesterol. [10] <160 mg/dL serum LDL cholesterol. [11] <150 mg/dL serum triglyceride (TG). [12] <140 mmHg systolic blood pressure (SBP). [13] <90 mmHg diastolic blood pressure (DBP) plus hypertension medication. [14] <0.5 mg/dL serum high-sensitivity C-reactive protein (hs-CRP). [15] <7 mg/dL for men and 6 mg/dL for women serum uric acid. [16] <24 mg/dL blood urinary nitrogen (BUN). [17] <4.8 mg/dL serum albumin concentrations. [18] <40 U/L Aspartate aminotransferase (AST). [19] <35 U/L alanine aminotransferase (ALT). [20] <1.2 mg/dL serum total bilirubin concentrations. [21] Negative urinary protein. Covariates: sex, age, residence area, lean body mass, education, income, married status, lean body mass, energy and sodium intake, smoking, alcohol drinking, and exercise. * Significant differences by GFR at $p < 0.05$, ** $p < 0.01$, and *** $p < 0.001$. +++ Significantly different from the control group in the χ^2 test at $p < 0.001$.

3.2. Biochemical Parameters Related to Metabolic Syndrome

MetS prevalence was significantly higher in the Low-GFR group compared to the High-GFR group (Table 1). Serum creatinine concentration demonstrated strong positive correlations with both blood urea nitrogen (r^2 = 0.3595, $p < 0.0001$) and uric acid (r^2 = 0.475,

$p < 0.0001$). Individuals with MetS had a 1.991-fold higher risk of renal dysfunction (Table 1). The association between CVD and renal dysfunction followed a similar pattern to that observed with MetS. Anthropometric measures including body mass index (BMI) and waist circumference were significantly elevated in the Low-GFR group compared to the High-GFR group, with adjusted odds ratios positively associated with low eGFR (1.37 for BMI and 1.30 for waist circumference; Table 1). Metabolic parameters including fasting serum glucose, HbA1c, LDL cholesterol, and triglycerides were all significantly higher in the Low-GFR group and demonstrated positive associations with low eGFR, with odds ratios ranging from 1.277 to 1.853 (Table 1). Conversely, serum HDL cholesterol showed an inverse association with low eGFR (OR = 0.66; Table 1).

Although systolic blood pressure (SBP) and diastolic blood pressure (DBP) did not differ significantly between the Low-GFR and High-GFR groups, SBP showed a positive association with eGFR (Table 1). Hypertension prevalence was significantly higher in the Low-GFR group, with hypertensive individuals having a 2.09 times higher risk of developing renal dysfunction (Table 1). Insulin resistance, as determined by HOMA-IR, was also positively associated with low eGFR (OR = 1.47; Table 1). The inflammatory marker high-sensitivity C-reactive protein (hs-CRP) was significantly lower in the High-GFR group, and individuals with elevated hs-CRP (>0.5 mg/dL) had a 1.71-fold higher risk of renal dysfunction (Table 1).

Beyond the MetS parameters, eGFR was also associated with markers of liver function. Serum uric acid, BUN, and total bilirubin concentrations were substantially higher in the Low-GFR group compared to the High-GFR group, with strong positive associations with low eGFR (OR = 2.43–4.53; Table 1). Serum albumin concentrations were lower in the Low-GFR group and inversely associated with low eGFR (Table 1). Among liver enzymes, only serum alanine aminotransferase (ALT) activity showed a positive association with eGFR (Table 1).

3.3. *Lifestyles and Nutrient Intake*

Participants in the Low-GFR group demonstrated significantly lower energy intake than those in the High-GFR group. Carbohydrate and protein intakes did not differ significantly between the Low-GFR and High-GFR groups, and neither was associated with low eGFR (Table S1). Despite similar total protein intake between groups, both essential amino acid and animal protein consumption were significantly higher in the Low-GFR group, showing positive associations with low-GFR. However, the amino acid analysis revealed that participants in the Low-GFR group consumed higher amounts of arginine and isoleucine than the High-GFR group, with these amino acids positively linked to low-GFR. Conversely, cysteine intake demonstrated an inverse association with low eGFR (Table S1). Fat intake was significantly higher among participants in the Low-GFR group than the High-GFR group and showed an inverse relationship with low eGFR. However, no significant differences were observed between groups regarding saturated, monounsaturated, and polyunsaturated fatty acid consumption. Sodium intake was similar between the Low-GFR and High-GFR groups and showed no association with low eGFR (Table S1). Several micronutrients and dietary quality indicators including calcium, vitamin D, vitamin C, flavonoid intake, and DII showed no significant differences between groups and were not associated with low eGFR (Table S1). Among the four dietary patterns analyzed, WSD consumption was significantly higher in the Low-GFR group compared to the High-GFR group, with WSD intake positively associated with low eGFR. The other dietary patterns—ABD, PBD, and RMD—showed no association with low eGFR (Table S1).

Alcohol consumption was significantly lower in the Low-GFR group compared to the High-GFR group and demonstrated an inverse association with renal dysfunction

(Table S1). Similarly, coffee intake was lower among participants in the Low-GFR group and showed an inverse association with low eGFR. In contrast, tea consumption did not differ between groups and showed no association with eGFR. While the proportion of individuals engaging in regular exercise was higher in the Low-GFR group than in the High-GFR group, no significant association was observed between regular exercise and eGFR after covariate adjustment (Table S1).

3.4. Polygenic Variants and Their Interaction Related to Renal Dysfunction Risk

The GWAS revealed multiple genetic variants associated with renal dysfunction as measured by eGFR. The Manhattan plot (Figure S2A) illustrates the statistical associations of the genetic variants across all chromosomes. The Q–Q plot demonstrated good consistency between observed and expected *p*-values, with a genome inflation factor (λ) of 1.054, confirming no significant inflation in the GWAS results (Figure S2B).

Following our selection criteria ($p < 1 \times 10^{-6}$ for GWAS, D′ < 0.2 for linkage disequilibrium, $p \geq 0.05$ for Hardy–Weinberg equilibrium, and minor allele frequency ≥0.01), we identified 22 SNPs associated with renal dysfunction. Among these, the following 10 genetic variants were selected based on genetic variant–genetic variant interaction analysis: rs1047891_*CPS1*, rs3770636_LDL receptor-related protein-2 (*LRP2*), rs5020545_Shroom family member-3 (*SHROOM3*), rs3812036_solute carrier family 34 member-1 (*SLC34A1*), rs4715517_hypocretin receptor-2 (*HCRTR2*), rs140652052_BRI1-associated kinase 1 (*BAK1*), rs139132767_suppression of tumorigenicity 7 (*ST7*), rs141574969_coiled-coil domain containing 63 (*CCDC63*), rs1031755_WD repeat domain 72 (*WDR72*), and rs6001939_myocardin-related transcription factor A (*MRTFA*) (Table 2). All variants demonstrated significant associations with renal dysfunction risk in the city hospital-based cohort ($p < 5 \times 10^{-7}$). Three variants—rs3770636 (*LRP2*), rs1031755 (*WDR72*), and rs6001939 (*MRTFA*)—showed inverse associations with low eGFR, while the remaining seven variants were positively associated with increased risk (Table 2). Most identified variants were located in intronic regions. Notably, rs4715517 (*HCRTR2*) was found in the 5′-untranslated region (UTR) and rs140652052 (*BAK1*) in the nonsense-mediated decay (NMD) transcripts, with rs1047891 (*CPS1*) representing a missense variant (Table 2).

Table 2. Characteristics of the ten genetic variants selected for estimated glomerular filtration rates.

CHR [1]	SNP [2]	Position	Mi [3]	Ma [4]	OR [5]	SE [6]	Adjusted *p*-Value [7]	Adjusted *p*-Value [8]	MAF [9]	*p*-Value for HWE [10]	Gene Names	Location
2	rs1047891 (Thr1406Asn)	211540507	A	C	1.172	0.0241	4.61×10^{-11}	2.98×10^{-5}	0.179	0.1156	*CPS1*	Missense
2	rs3770636	170202833	G	T	0.881	0.0245	2.3×10^{-7}	0.00692	0.200	0.0692	*LRP2*	Intron
4	rs5020545	77414988	T	C	1.149	0.0247	1.83×10^{-8}	0.00724	0.171	0.6204	*SHROOM3*	Intron
5	rs3812036	176813404	T	C	1.122	0.0227	3.97×10^{-7}	0.0003224	0.219	0.7723	*SLC34A1*	Intron
6	rs4715517	54973761	A	C	1.283	0.0396	2.88×10^{-10}	0.0002845	0.054	0.3498	*HCRTR2*	5′-UTR
6	rs140652052	33547810	C	A	1.259	0.0464	6.95×10^{-7}	0.009824	0.038	0.8193	*BAK1*	Intron
7	rs139132767	116726021	G	A	1.579	0.0616	1.22×10^{-13}	0.008934	0.018	0.2941	*ST7*	Intron
12	rs141574969	111319366	G	A	1.142	0.0257	2.15×10^{-7}	0.007747	0.159	0.1384	*CCDC63*	Intron
15	rs1031755	53951435	C	A	0.8967	0.0198	3.49×10^{-8}	0.00043	0.403	0.4817	*WDR72*	Intron
22	rs6001939	40892794	T	C	0.9098	0.0213	9.21×10^{-7}	0.001771	0.293	0.2773	*MRTFA*	Intron

[1] Chromosome. [2] Single-nucleotide polymorphism. [3] Minor allele. [4] Major allele. [5] Adjusted odds ratio for renal dysfunction in a hospital-based cohort. [6] Standard error. [7] p-Value for the OR in the urban hospital-based cohort (case: n = 1361, control: n = 12,237). [8] *p*-Value for OR in the Ansan/Ansung + Nong-chon cohort (case: n = 7617, control: n = 51,084). [9] Minor allele frequency. [10] Hardy–Weinberg equilibrium. Covariates: sex, age, residence area, lean body mass, education, income, married status, lean body mass, energy and sodium intake, smoking, alcohol drinking, and exercise.

The eQTL analysis revealed that the risk allele (T) of *SHROOM3*_rs5020545 was associated with significantly reduced gene expression compared to the non-risk allele (C) in liver tissue (coefficient: −0.2, p = 0.00015). Conversely, the risk allele (A) of *CPS1*_rs1047891 exhibited a markedly increased expression relative to the non-risk allele (C) specifically in the hypothalamus.

GMDR analysis identified models with 6–10 SNPs that met the sign test criteria for TEBA ($p < 0.05$) and CVC (10/10), indicating significant interactions among genetic variants influencing low eGFR (Table S2). The six-SNP model included *LRP2*_rs3770636, *CPS1*_rs1047891, *SHROOM3*_rs5020545, *CCDC63*_rs141574969, *SLC34A1*_rs3812036, and *MRTFA*_rs6001939. The seven-SNP model incorporated these six variants plus *WDR72*_rs491567 (Table S2).

PRS was calculated to assess the predictive value of selected models. The six-SNP model showed significant association with low eGFR, with odds ratios of 1.761 (95% CI: 1.526–1.984) and 1.772 (95% CI: 1.509–2.020) in models 1 and 2, respectively, after adjusting for different covariates (Figure 1). Similarly, the seven-SNP model yielded odds ratios of 1.737 (95% CI: 1.480–1.996) and 1.782 (95% CI: 1.492–2.061) in models 1 and 2, respectively (Figure 1). These results suggest that the six-SNP model represents the optimal model for predicting renal dysfunction risk.

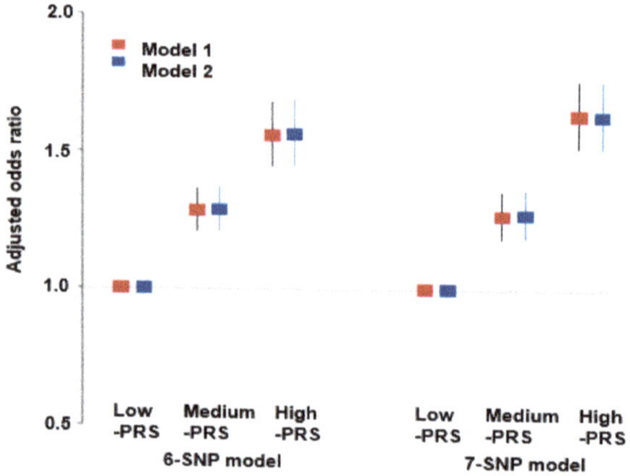

Figure 1. Adjusted odds ratio (OR) and 95% confidence intervals (CI) of 6-SNP PRS and 7-SNP PRS for renal dysfunction risk measured by estimated glomerular filtration rates. PRS was generated with the sum of the number of risk alleles in each genetic variant and classified into Low-PRS, Middle-PRS, and High-PRS, respectively, in the 6- and 7-SNP models. Low-PRS (0–4; 0–5), Medium-PRS (5–6; 6–7), and High-PRS (>6; >7) in 6-SNP and 7-SNP models, respectively. SNP: Single-nucleotide polymorphism; PRS: Polygenic risk score.

3.5. Metabolic Functions Related to Genes Involved in the Hypo-eGFR

Functional analysis revealed that genes associated with low eGFR were linked to multiple biological processes and pathways, including energy production through ATP synthase activity; protein autoprocessing; regulation of receptor recycling; liver functions, such as liver cancer, thiazolidinedione regulation, LDL pathways, estrogen receptor 1 (*ESR1*) targets, and insulin signaling; and skeletal muscle function through myosin activity, neuromuscular process, and oligodendrocyte differentiation (Table 3). Notably, the identified genes were not directly associated with renal filtering processes but rather with ATP-producing pathways and the production of nitrogen-composed waste from the liver and skeletal muscles (Table 3).

Table 3. Pathways related to genetic variants influencing renal function determined by estimated glomerular filtration rates.

Gene Set	No. Genes	Beta	Beta SD	SE	p-Value
GO BP: Protein autoprocessing	28	0.59988	0.02312	0.15852	7.73×10^{-5}
GO BP: Regulation of receptor recycling	22	0.66108	0.02259	0.17705	9.46×10^{-5}
Acevedo liver cancer dn	516	0.1403	0.02291	0.03774	0.0001007
GO BERT: Core oligodendrocyte differentiation	40	0.48444	0.02231	0.14096	0.0002951
GO CC: Neuronal ribonucleoprotein granule	3	1.6359	0.02065	0.48121	0.0003383
Biocarta LDL pathway	6	1.2646	0.02257	0.37738	0.0004037
Bhat esr1 targets via akt1 up	273	0.17603	0.02104	0.05297	0.0004456
GO CC: Proton transporting atp synthase complex catalytic core f1	6	1.0336	0.01845	0.31139	0.0004519
GO BP: Negative regulation of receptor recycling	5	1.0453	0.01703	0.31814	0.0005096
GO BP: Negative regulation of myosin light chain phosphatase activity	5	1.4803	0.02412	0.4553	0.0005756

SD, standard deviation; SE, standard error; GO, gene ontology; CC, cellular compartment; BP, biological process.

3.6. Genetic Variants-Lifestyle Interaction with Hypo-eGFR

An analysis of the interactions between the PRS of the 6-SNP model and lifestyle factors revealed significant interactions with PBD ($p = 0.0415$) and coffee intake ($p = 0.0092$) in relation to low eGFR risk (Table 4). Participants with higher consumption of PBD and coffee demonstrated an attenuated association between PRS and low eGFR, suggesting potential protective effects of these dietary factors (Figure 2A,B). In contrast, no significant interactions were observed between PRS and either alcohol consumption or regular exercise concerning renal dysfunction risk (Table 4).

Table 4. Adjusted odds ratios and 95% confidence intervals for renal dysfunction risk by polygenetic risk scores (PRS) of the 6-SNP model or *CPS1* rs1047891 after covariate adjustments according to lifestyle patterns.

PRS 6	Low-PRS (n = 17,680)	Medium-PRS (n = 26,672)	High-PRS (n = 9476)	PRS Interaction p-Value
Low-ABD [1]	1	1.247 (1.151–1.351)	1.534 (1.390–1.693)	0.2522
High-ABD	1	1.396 (1.250–1.558)	1.665 (1.452–1.910)	
Low-PBD [1]	1	1.371 (1.266–1.484)	1.628 (1.475–1.797)	0.0215
High-PBD	1	1.162 (1.039–1.299)	1.457 (1.275–1.686)	
Low-WSD [1]	1	1.305 (1.199–1.420)	1.555 (1.400–1.728)	0.9430
High-WSD	1	1.285 (1.162–1.421)	1.611 (1.424–1.822)	
Low-RMD [1]	1	1.331 (1.230–1.440)	1.592 (1.444–1.755)	0.0756
High-RMD	1	1.232 (1.100–1.379)	1.558 (1.354–1.792)	
Low-Sodium [2]	1	1.301 (1.179–1.435)	1.501 (1.328–1.697)	0.8257
High-Sodium	1	1.298 (1.191–1.414)	1.649 (1.484–1.833)	
Low-Alcohol [3]	1	1.226 (1.124–1.336)	1.526 (1.376–1.694)	0.2312
High-Alcohol	1	1.391 (1.261–1.534)	1.639 (1.445–1.859)	

Table 4. *Cont.*

PRS 6	Low-PRS (n = 17,680)	Medium-PRS (n = 26,672)	High-PRS (n = 9476)	PRS Interaction p-Value
Non-smoker	1	1.284 (1.187–1.388)	1.620 (1.472–1.784)	0.4421
Former + Current smokers	1	1.338 (1.192–1.502)	1.522 (1.318–1.757)	
Low Exercise	1	1.140 (1.033–1.259)	1.431 (1.267–1.615)	0.0596
Regular Exercise [4]	1	1.419 (1.304–1.545)	1.709 (1.538–1.898)	
Low-Coffee [5]	1	1.311 (1.220–1.409)	1.655 (1.513–1.809)	0.0092
High-Coffee	1	1.248 (1.078–1.445)	1.344 (1.121–1.611)	
Low-Tea [6]	1	1.307 (1.212–1.409)	1.609 (1.466–1.765)	0.2290
High-Tea	1	1.272 (1.119–1.446)	1.496 (1.275–1.754)	
Low-Vitamin D [7]	1	1.327 (1.169–1.505)	1.574 (1.440–1.721)	0.2066
High-Vitamin D	1	1.280 (1.191–1.376)	1.521 (1.300–1.780)	
CPS1 rs1047891	Major	Heterozygote	Minor	
Low-Vitamin D [7]	1	1.235 (1.099–1.388)	1.393 (1.190–1.632)	0.0436
High-Vitamin D	1	1.176 (1.099–1.257)	1.124 (0.833–1.517)	

The cutoffs of the logistic regression analysis were as follows: [1] <66th percentiles; [2] 2 g/day sodium intake; [3] 140 g/week alcohol intake; [4] moderate activity for 150 min/week; [5] 3 g/day coffee intake; [6] <45 g/day tea intake; and [7] <2.53 μg/day vitamin D intake (33rd percentile). The High-GFR and Low-GFR groups were defined as ≥ and <60 mL/min/1.73 m^2 of eGFR. Low-PRS (0–4), Medium-PRS (5–6), and High-PRS (>6) in the 6-SNP model. Covariates: sex, age, residence area, lean body mass, education, income, married status, lean body mass, energy and sodium intake, smoking, alcohol drinking, and exercise. ABD, Asian balanced diet; PBD, plant-based diet; WSD, Western-style diet; RMD, rice—main diet.

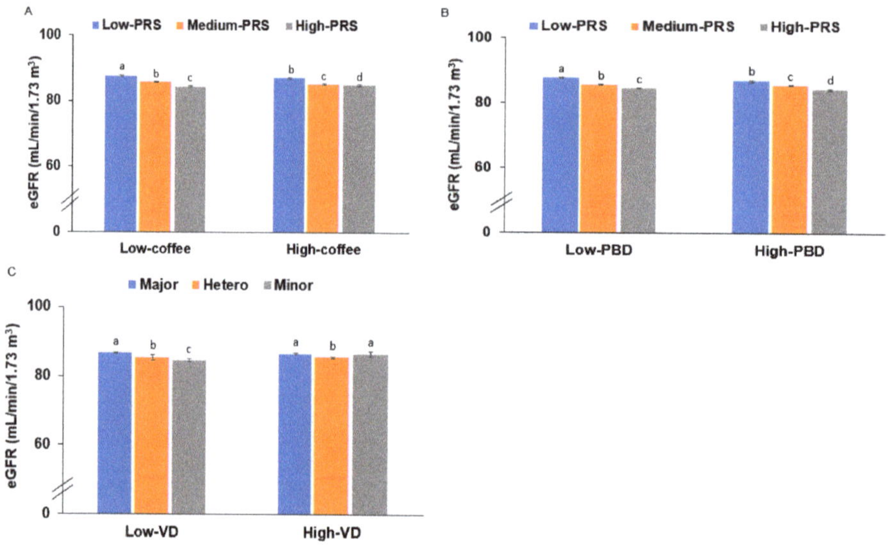

Figure 2. Estimated glomerular filtration rates (eGFRs) according to the polygenic risk scores (PRS) of the 6-SNP model or CPS1 alleles and different lifestyles: (**A**) plant-based diet and PRS (cutoff: 66th percentile); (**B**) coffee intake and PRS (cutoff: 3 g/day); (**C**) vitamin D3 intake and CPS1 WT and MT (cutoff: 2.53 μg/day; 33rd percentile). Low-PRS (0–4), Medium-PRS (5–6), and High-PRS (>6) in the 6-SNP model. [a,b,c] Different letters on the bars indicate significant differences among the PRS groups in Tukey's test at $p < 0.05$.

Further analysis identified a significant interaction between *CPS1* rs1047891 and vitamin D intake ($p = 0.0477$; Table 4). Specifically, individuals carrying the risk allele of *CPS1* rs1047891 exhibited lower eGFR when vitamin D intake was low, whereas this adverse effect was substantially mitigated among those with high vitamin D intake (Figure 2C).

3.7. Bioactive Compound Interaction with CPS1 rs1047891 Missense Mutation (Thr1406) and Molecular Docking

To investigate the potential molecular mechanisms underlying the observed gene–diet interactions, we conducted molecular docking analyses of approximately 1100 polyphenol compounds from vegetables and fruits, including anthocyanidins, flavonoids, carotenoids, and saponins, with the CPS1 protein. Our analysis identified 19 bioactive compounds that exhibited lower binding energy with the wild-type (WT) CPS1 protein (Thr1406) compared to the mutant-type (MT) protein (1406Asn) (Table 5). This differential binding suggests these compounds may preferentially interact with the WT protein.

Table 5. Bioactive compounds lower intermolecular binding energy with CPS1 (Thr1406Asn) wild type (WT) than the mutated type (MT).

Food Components	Foods	WT	MT
		Docking Energy, ΔG (kcal mol^{-1})	
Cichoriin	Chicory	−10.1	−8.6
Malvidin 3-alpha-L-galactoside	Blue berry	−10.1	−8.6
Glyceollin II	Soybeans	−10.6	−8.7
Stigmasteryl glucoside	Soybean oil	−10.2	−8.5
alpha-Carotene	Carrot	−10.9	−8.6
(5R,5′R,6S,8′R)-Luteochrome	Sweet potato	−10.2	−7.3
Tuberoside B	Allium tuberosum	−10.6	−8.7
Cycloartanyl ferulate	Rice bran oil	−10.3	−8.6
delta-Carotene	Carrot tomatoes	−10.5	−7.7
19′-Hexanoyloxymytiloxanthin	Mussel	−10.2	−8
(R)-Hispaglabridin A	Licorice	−10.2	−8.6
5,6,7,8-Tetrahydroxy-3′,4′-dimethoxyflavone	Seville orange	−10.6	−8.7
(3S,3′S,all-E)-Zeaxanthin	Shrimp	−10.9	−8.3
(E)-4-(3,7-Dimethyl-2,6-octadienyl)-1,3,5-trihydroxyxanthone	Garcinia livingstonei	−10.1	−8.5
28-Hydroxymangiferonic acid	Mango	−10.5	−8.5
Soyasaponin ag	Soybeans, pulses	−11.3	−8.2
(S)-Nerolidol 3-O-[a-L-Rhamnopyranosyl-(1->4)-a-L-rhamnopyranosyl-(1->2)-[4-(4-hydroxy-3-methoxycinnamoyl)-(E)-a-L-rhamnopyranosyl-(1->6)]-b-D-glucopyranoside]	Eriobotrya japonica	−10.5	−8.6
3alpha-12-Ursene-3,24-diol	Boswellia serrata	−10.6	−8.5
Hovenidulcioside B2	Hovenia dulcis	−10.5	−8.6
Vitamin D3	Egg yolk, liver, tuna	−7.6	−9.9

Among these compounds, soyasaponin ag demonstrated the most pronounced difference in binding energy between WT and MT CPS1. The interaction between WT CPS1 and soyasaponin ag involved multiple binding forces, including hydrogen bonds, Van der Waals forces, alkyl interactions, π-alkyl interactions, and carbon–hydrogen bonds (Figure S3A). In contrast, the interaction between MT CPS1 and soyasaponin ag was primarily mediated by Van der Waals forces alone (Figure S3B).

Molecular docking analysis with vitamin D3 supported our cohort study findings. Vitamin D3 exhibited a lower binding energy to the mutant (MT) CPS1 protein (−9.9 kcal/mol) compared to the wild-type (WT) protein (−7.5 kcal/mol). In the WT CPS1 protein, van der Waals forces primarily mediated the interaction with vitamin D3, whereas, in the MT CPS1 protein, π-alkyl and alkyl interactions were more prominent, contributing to greater binding stability and reduced binding energy (Figure S4A,B). This aligns with our cohort study's results, in which the adverse effect of the CPS1 rs1047891 risk allele on eGFR was observed only in individuals with low vitamin D intake ($p = 0.0436$; Table 4, Figure S4A,B). These findings collectively suggest that vitamin D intake may modify the impact of the CPS1 risk allele on renal function, potentially mitigating its negative effect (Figure 2C).

Despite identifying 19 bioactive compounds from plant-based foods with differential binding affinities to CPS1 WT versus MT protein in our molecular docking analyses, our cohort study did not demonstrate significant interactions between CPS1 rs1047891 and consumption of specific fruits or vegetables. While our molecular docking suggested potential interactions between CPS1 and various bioactive compounds from plant sources, these specific molecular interactions did not translate to detectable gene–diet interactions in our cohort study, unlike the clear interaction observed with vitamin D. This suggests that the protective effect of a PBD on eGFR observed at the PRS level may involve mechanisms beyond direct interactions with CPS1 or may reflect the cumulative effects of multiple dietary components acting through various pathways.

4. Discussion

Declined eGFR represents a progressive loss of kidney function and is positively associated with urinary protein [31]. The present study confirmed this relationship, demonstrating that low eGFR was associated with urinary protein by 4.7 times. This indicates that decreased eGFR and increased urinary protein can serve as complementary indices of CKD. Importantly, reduced eGFR is linked not only to CKD but also to MetS and CVD.

A meta-analysis of GWAS data from European ancestry populations (61,286 controls and 5807 cases) identified 23 susceptible loci for reduced renal function [32]. In a follow-up study [32] with 22,982 replication samples, 13 loci were associated with renal function and CKD (*LASS2, GCKR, ALMS1, TFDP2, DAB2, SLC34A1, VEGFA, PRKAG2, PIP5K1B, ATXN2, DACH1, UBE2Q2*, and *SLC7A9*), while seven loci were involved in creatinine production and secretion (*CPS1, SLC22A2, TMEM60, WDR37, SLC6A13, WDR72*, and *BCAS3*). Our findings align with these previous studies, as the genetic variants with $p < 1 \times 10^{-6}$ related to low eGFR were primarily identified as being involved in creatinine production and secretion rather than kidney function and CKD directly. Furthermore, the genetic variants associated with low eGFR were identified as being associated with liver function, ATP production, myosin synthesis, and neuromuscular processes but not kidney function in the present study. The PRS from the selected genetic variants interacted with the PBD and coffee intake to affect low eGFR in the present study: high PBD and coffee intakes protected against low eGFR risk, especially in middle-aged and older people with a high PRS. These results can be applied to personalized nutrition.

In this study, we utilized the MDRD equation for eGFR estimation as our primary method for assessing kidney function. While the assessment of agreement between the CKD-EPI and MDRD equations was not a primary objective of our genetic association analysis, we verified the appropriateness of using MDRD in our Asian cohort. The verification showed strong concordance between the methods, with MDRD being highly predictive of CKD classification (OR = 0.115, 95% CI: 0.089–0.148). Given that the mean age of our study population was 53.7 years (SD: 8.0), we selected the MDRD equation as it has been shown to provide more stable eGFR estimates in aging adults without excessive CKD classification bias. This decision aligns with previous research in Chinese populations, which found that the MDRD exhibited a more gradual decline in eGFR with age than the CKD-EPI [19]. While the MDRD served the purposes of our genetic and lifestyle interaction analyses, we acknowledge that future studies investigating genetic determinants of kidney function in Asian populations should consider incorporating multiple eGFR estimation methods, including the CKD-EPI, to ensure robust phenotyping. This would be particularly important when evaluating gene–environment interactions across different age groups, as estimation methods may influence the detection and interpretation of genetic associations with kidney function.

Renal function is closely related to metabolic diseases [33]. As kidney function decreases, the metabolic pathways are altered to induce metabolic diseases such as MetS, CVD, gout, and cognitive dysfunction [6]. The changes could include altered blood volume and pressure, disturbed mineral metabolism, an activated renin-angiotensin system, oxidative stress, and increased inflammatory cytokines [34]. As a result, renal dysfunction contributes to increased insulin resistance to induce MetS and cardiac remodeling, which could progress to systolic and/or diastolic left ventricular failure [33]. The present study showed consistent results. Participants with a low eGFR had higher BMI and serum glucose and lipid concentrations than those with a high eGFR, indicating they were at a higher risk of MetS. Those with low eGFR had a higher prevalence of CVD and higher BUN and serum uric acid, AST, ALT, and hs-CRP concentrations. However, the serum albumin concentration was lower in participants with a low eGFR than in those with a high eGFR [33]. Therefore, renal function is closely connected with MetS, CVD, and gout and is linked to increased insulin resistance.

The relationship between eGFR and nutrient intake has been widely studied, focusing primarily on protein, sodium, and anti-inflammatory foods, but findings remain inconsistent. In this study, we found that high intakes of animal protein, essential amino acids, and fat were positively associated with low eGFR, while arginine intake, linked to the urea cycle, also showed a positive association. Previous studies have reported that high-fat intake (>35 En%) increases CKD risk (OR = 1.94, 95% CI: 1.39–2.71), while moderate protein intake (13–15 En%) may reduce risk (OR = 0.50, 95% CI: 0.35–0.72) in Mendelian randomization analyses using UK Biobank data [35]. However, longitudinal studies have suggested that high protein intake may accelerate eGFR decline in middle-aged adults [36]. While protein restriction (<10% total energy intake) may prevent renal decline, it can also lead to reduced lean body mass [37]. Given these findings, an optimal protein intake (~0.8 g/kg body weight) should be maintained to preserve renal function while preventing sarcopenia, particularly in older adults [38].

Although sodium intake has been linked to eGFR decline, findings remain inconsistent [39]. A high sodium intake was associated with eGFR decline in a longitudinal study [40], while a meta-analysis of eight randomized trials found that salt reduction lowered blood pressure and proteinuria in CKD patients [41]. In the present study, sodium and potassium intakes were lower in the Low-GFR group, but no association with low eGFR was found, possibly due to dietary sodium restriction as part of clinical recommendations. However, the potassium-to-sodium ratio was positively associated with low eGFR, consistent with prior cross-sectional findings [40]. These results suggest that sodium reduction may help maintain kidney function, though further longitudinal studies are needed to confirm this relationship.

Genetic variants influence renal function and creatinine metabolism, with multiple loci identified in European and Asian populations [42]. While many eGFR-associated variants are pleiotropic and shared across populations, some are unique to specific ancestries. Our study identified variants in *SHROOM3* and *SLC34A1*, previously associated with CKD risk, and others, including *CPS1*, *WDR37*, and *WDR72*, linked to creatinine metabolism and secretion. Given that *CPS1* plays a central role in nitrogen metabolism and ammonia detoxification via the urea cycle, genetic variation in *CPS1* could affect renal function through altered amino acid metabolism and nitrogen balance.

In this study, we found that the PRS of the 6-SNP model for low eGFR interacted with PBD and coffee intake but not with WSD, high protein, or sodium intake. The impact of high PRS was lower in participants with a high PBD intake, though a PBD itself was not associated with renal function in the overall population. This aligns with previous studies in US and Chinese populations, where higher adherence to a PBD and vegetarian diets was inversely associated with low eGFR in middle-aged adults [43,44]. These findings suggest that a PBD may provide a protective effect on eGFR, particularly in individuals with genetic susceptibility to renal dysfunction.

The protective effects of polyphenols from plant-based foods on renal function likely involve multiple mechanisms. Polyphenols are known to exert antioxidant and anti-inflammatory effects, which may protect against oxidative stress and inflammation-induced kidney damage [45]. Additionally, polyphenols may modulate signaling pathways involved in renal cell survival and function. Our molecular docking analyses suggest a potential direct interaction between certain polyphenolic compounds and CPS1, which could influence nitrogen metabolism and subsequently impact kidney function. However, the absence of specific interactions between CPS1 and the majority of plant-derived bioactive compounds in our molecular docking studies, coupled with the observed protective effect of a PBD on renal function in our cohort, suggests that the beneficial effects of polyphenols may be mediated through broader metabolic pathways rather than direct modulation of CPS1 activity alone.

Additionally, our results support a beneficial effect of coffee intake on kidney function, consistent with prior research showing that drinking more than daily one cup of coffee is associated with higher eGFR and lower albuminuria in Mendelian randomization analyses [46]. A meta-analysis of 12 studies also found that coffee consumption was linked to a lower risk of CKD (RR = 0.86, 95% CI: 0.76–0.97) and albuminuria (OR = 0.81, 95% CI: 0.68–0.97) [47]. In the present study, coffee intake was inversely associated with renal dysfunction, and the PRS-low eGFR association was weaker in those with high coffee intake, indicating a gene–diet interaction influencing renal function. These findings suggest that coffee consumption may help protect against renal dysfunction, particularly in individuals at higher genetic risk.

Our study also revealed a significant interaction between *CPS1* rs1047891 and vitamin D intake, where low vitamin D intake was associated with decreased eGFR in risk allele carriers, while high vitamin D intake mitigated this effect. Prior studies have shown that vitamin D plays a key role in kidney health by regulating calcium-phosphate homeostasis, immune function, and oxidative stress [48,49]. Additionally, CPS1 is a key enzyme in nitrogen metabolism, and mutations in CPS1 have been linked to urea cycle disorders, hyperammonemia, and impaired metabolic function [50]. To further explore this interaction, molecular docking analysis was performed using AutoDock Vina, demonstrating that vitamin D3 exhibited a lower binding energy to CPS1 mutant-type (−9.9 kcal/mol) than wild-type (−7.5 kcal/mol). This finding aligns with our cohort results showing that vitamin D intake modifies the effect of the CPS1 risk allele on renal function and provides a potential molecular mechanism for this gene–nutrient interaction.

It is worth noting that while our molecular docking analyses identified differential binding patterns between vitamin D3 and *CPS1* variants that correspond with our cohort findings, similar correlations were not observed for bioactive compounds from plant-based foods. Despite identifying 19 compounds from vegetables and fruits with different binding energies to wild-type versus mutant *CPS1*, our cohort study did not demonstrate significant interactions between specific fruits or vegetables and *CPS1* rs1047891. This suggests that the protective effect of a PBD on eGFR observed at the PRS level may involve complex mechanisms beyond direct interactions with *CPS1*, potentially including synergistic effects of multiple polyphenols acting through various pathways. This complexity highlights the limitations of in silico analyses in predicting functional outcomes and emphasizes the importance of validation through biological assays and human studies.

The major limitation of this study was that the cause-and-effect relationship could not be established because of its case–control design. Second, renal function was estimated using eGFR calculated with the MDRD equation, which, while suitable for our study population, may have limitations in assessing acute kidney injury and could differ from other eGFR estimation methods, such as CKD-EPI. Third, alcohol intake was analyzed as total daily consumption, without distinguishing the potential differential effects of beer, wine, and spirits on renal function. Finally, dietary intake was assessed with an SQFFQ for the previous six months. However, since the SQFFQ (106 food items) was validated against 3-day food records collected across four seasons, it is likely to provide a reliable estimate of the usual intake in this population.

5. Conclusions

The present study reveals a significant association between renal dysfunction and insulin resistance and dietary factors like WSD, with fast-food intake exacerbating this relationship. Genetic variants linked to renal function also showed connections to metabolic pathways in the liver and skeletal muscle. Notably, our 6-SNP polygenic risk score demonstrated a 1.782-fold increased risk for renal dysfunction and interacted with a PBD and coffee consumption. These findings suggest that dietary modifications—particularly a PBD and moderate coffee intake—may mitigate genetic risk for renal dysfunction in middle-aged and elderly individuals. These results support integrating genetic risk assessments into personalized nutritional recommendations for kidney health, potentially enhancing CKD prevention strategies in at-risk populations. Future research should validate these findings through longitudinal studies and explore the underlying mechanisms through functional studies of relevant genetic variants and bioactive compounds.

Supplementary Materials: The following supporting information can be downloaded at: https://www.mdpi.com/article/10.3390/nu17050916/s1, Table S1: Nutrient intake according to estimated glomerular filtration rates (eGFR); Table S2: Generalized multifactor dimensionality reduction (GMDR) results of multi-locus interaction with genes related to glomerular filtration rate risk; Figure S1: A flow chart to generate the polygenic risk score (PRS) linked to duodenal ulcers by SNP–SNP interaction and its interaction with lifestyle factors; Figure S2: Distribution of genetic variants associated with duodenal ulcers based on the genome-wide association study (GWAS); Figure S3: Molecular docking of CPS1 WT protein (Thr1406) (A) and MT (1406Asn) (B) with soyasaponin ag; Figure S4: Molecular docking of CPS1 WT protein (Thr1406) (A) and MT (1406Asn) (B) with vitamin D3.

Author Contributions: M.L., D.-S.K., Study coordination, data collection, data quality assurance, and data analysis; S.P., data management, data analysis, interpretation of results, and writing. All authors have read and agreed to the published version of the manuscript.

Funding: This study was supported by the Academic Research Fund of Hoseo University in 2023 (20230307).

Institutional Review Board Statement: The study protocol received approval from the Institutional Review Board (IRB) of the Korea National Institute of Health and Hoseo University (approval numbers: KBP-2019-055 and 1041231-150811-HR-034-01, 16 August 2019).

Informed Consent Statement: All participants provided written informed consent before enrollment.

Data Availability Statement: The data were deposited in Korean biobank (Osong, Korea) and provided for the research.

Conflicts of Interest: All authors declare no competing interests.

References

1. Kovesdy, C.P. Epidemiology of chronic kidney disease: An update 2022. *Kidney Int. Suppl.* **2022**, *12*, 7–11. [CrossRef] [PubMed]
2. Teo, B.W.; Chan, G.C.; Leo, C.C.H.; Tay, J.C.; Chia, Y.-C.; Siddique, S.; Turana, Y.; Chen, C.-H.; Cheng, H.-M.; Hoshide, S.; et al. Hypertension and chronic kidney disease in Asian populations. *J. Clin. Hypertens.* **2021**, *23*, 475–480. [CrossRef] [PubMed]
3. Bragadottir, G.; Redfors, B.; Ricksten, S.-E. Assessing glomerular filtration rate (GFR) in critically ill patients with acute kidney injury—True GFR versus urinary creatinine clearance and estimating equations. *Crit. Care* **2013**, *17*, R108. [CrossRef] [PubMed]
4. Shahbaz, H.; Gupta, M. *Creatinine Clearance*; StatPearls: Treasure Island, FL, USA, 2021.
5. Teo, B.W.; Zhang, L.; Guh, J.Y.; Tang, S.C.W.; Jha, V.; Kang, D.H.; Tanchanco, R.; Hooi, L.S.; Praditpornsilpa, K.; Kong, X.; et al. Glomerular Filtration Rates in Asians. *Adv. Chronic Kidney Dis.* **2018**, *25*, 41–48. [CrossRef]
6. Yanai, H.; Adachi, H.; Hakoshima, M.; Katsuyama, H. Molecular, Biological, and Clinical Understanding of the Pathophysiology and Treatments of Hyperuricemia and Its Association with Metabolic Syndrome, Cardiovascular Diseases and Chronic Kidney Disease. *Int. J. Mol. Sci.* **2021**, *22*, 9221. [CrossRef]
7. Schrauben, S.J.; Hsu, J.Y.; Amaral, S.; Anderson, A.H.; Feldman, H.I.; Dember, L.M. Effect of Kidney Function on Relationships between Lifestyle Behaviors and Mortality or Cardiovascular Outcomes: A Pooled Cohort Analysis. *J. Am. Soc. Nephrol.* **2021**, *32*, 663–675. [CrossRef]
8. Kelly, J.T.; Su, G.; Zhang, L.; Qin, X.; Marshall, S.; González-Ortiz, A.; Clase, C.M.; Campbell, K.L.; Xu, H.; Carrero, J.-J. Modifiable Lifestyle Factors for Primary Prevention of CKD: A Systematic Review and Meta-Analysis. *J. Am. Soc. Nephrol.* **2021**, *32*, 239–253. [CrossRef]
9. Kim, Y.; Han, B.G. Cohort Profile: The Korean Genome and Epidemiology Study (KoGES) Consortium. *Int. J. Epidemiol.* **2017**, *46*, e20. [CrossRef]
10. Zhang, T.; Park, S. Energy Intake-Dependent Genetic Associations with Obesity Risk: BDNF Val66Met Polymorphism and Interactions with Dietary Bioactive Compounds. *Antioxidants* **2025**, *14*, 170. [CrossRef]
11. Böger, C.A. It's not only the kidneys—Genetic determinants of glomerular filtration marker levels. *Nephrol. Dial. Transplant.* **2013**, *28*, 2397–2398. [CrossRef]
12. Ryu, J.; Lee, C. Association of glycosylated hemoglobin with the gene encoding CDKAL1 in the Korean Association Resource (KARE) study. *Hum. Mutat.* **2012**, *33*, 655–659. [CrossRef] [PubMed]
13. Montasser, M.E.; Shimmin, L.C.; Gu, D.; Chen, J.; Gu, C.; Kelly, T.N.; Jaquish, C.E.; Rice, T.K.; Rao, D.C.; Cao, J.; et al. Variations in genes that regulate blood pressure are associated with glomerular filtration rate in Chinese. *PLoS ONE* **2014**, *9*, e92468. [CrossRef] [PubMed]
14. Yoshida, T.; Kato, K.; Fujimaki, T.; Yokoi, K.; Oguri, M.; Watanabe, S.; Metoki, N.; Yoshida, H.; Satoh, K.; Aoyagi, Y.; et al. Association of genetic variants with chronic kidney disease in Japanese individuals. *Clin. J. Am. Soc. Nephrol.* **2009**, *4*, 883–890. [CrossRef]
15. Daily, J.W.; Park, S. Interaction of BDNF rs6265 variants and energy and protein intake in the risk for glucose intolerance and type 2 diabetes in middle-aged adults. *Nutrition* **2017**, *33*, 187–194. [CrossRef] [PubMed]
16. Park, S.; Daily, J.W.; Zhang, X.; Jin, H.S.; Lee, H.J.; Lee, Y.H. Interactions with the MC4R rs17782313 variant, mental stress and energy intake and the risk of obesity in Genome Epidemiology Study. *Nutr. Metab.* **2016**, *13*, 38. [CrossRef]
17. Park, S.; Ahn, J.; Lee, B.K. Self-rated Subjective Health Status Is Strongly Associated with Sociodemographic Factors, Lifestyle, Nutrient Intakes, and Biochemical Indices, but Not Smoking Status: KNHANES 2007-2012. *J. Korean Med. Sci.* **2015**, *30*, 1279–1287. [CrossRef]
18. Michels, W.M.; Grootendorst, D.C.; Verduijn, M.; Elliott, E.G.; Dekker, F.W.; Krediet, R.T. Performance of the Cockcroft-Gault, MDRD, and New CKD-EPI Formulas in Relation to GFR, Age, and Body Size. *Clin. J. Am. Soc. Nephrol.* **2010**, *5*, 1003–1009. [CrossRef]
19. Ma, Y.; Zhan, J.; Xu, G. Reference values of glomerular filtration rate for healthy adults in southern China: A cross-sectional survey. *Ther. Adv. Chronic Dis.* **2021**, *12*, 20406223211035287. [CrossRef]
20. Park, S.; Zhang, X.; Lee, N.R.; Jin, H.S. TRPV1 Gene Polymorphisms Are Associated with Type 2 Diabetes by Their Interaction with Fat Consumption in the Korean Genome Epidemiology Study. *J. Nutrigenet. Nutrigenom.* **2016**, *9*, 47–61. [CrossRef]
21. Ahn, Y.; Kwon, E.; Shim, J.E.; Park, M.K.; Joo, Y.; Kimm, K.; Park, C.; Kim, D.H. Validation and reproducibility of food frequency questionnaire for Korean genome epidemiologic study. *Eur. J. Clin. Nutr.* **2007**, *61*, 1435–1441. [CrossRef]
22. Steel, R.G.; Torrie, J.H.; Dickey, D.A. *Principles and Procedures of Statistics: A Biological Approach*; McGraw-Hill: New York, NY, USA, 1997.
23. Hébert, J.R.; Shivappa, N.; Wirth, M.D.; Hussey, J.R.; Hurley, T.G. Perspective: The Dietary Inflammatory Index (DII)-Lessons Learned, Improvements Made, and Future Directions. *Adv. Nutr.* **2019**, *10*, 185–195. [CrossRef]

24. van Woudenbergh, G.J.; Theofylaktopoulou, D.; Kuijsten, A.; Ferreira, I.; van Greevenbroek, M.M.; van der Kallen, C.J.; Schalkwijk, C.G.; Stehouwer, C.D.; Ocké, M.C.; Nijpels, G.; et al. Adapted dietary inflammatory index and its association with a summary score for low-grade inflammation and markers of glucose metabolism: The Cohort study on Diabetes and Atherosclerosis Maastricht (CODAM) and the Hoorn study. *Am. J. Clin. Nutr.* **2013**, *98*, 1533–1542. [CrossRef] [PubMed]
25. Lee, S.K.; Kim, M.K. Relationship of sodium intake with obesity among Korean children and adolescents: Korea National Health and Nutrition Examination Survey. *Br. J. Nutr.* **2016**, *115*, 834–841. [CrossRef] [PubMed]
26. Rabbee, N.; Speed, T.P. A genotype calling algorithm for Affymetrix SNP arrays. *Bioinformatics* **2006**, *22*, 7–12. [CrossRef]
27. Uma Jyothi, K.; Reddy, B.M. Gene-gene and gene-environment interactions in the etiology of type 2 diabetes mellitus in the population of Hyderabad, India. *Meta Gene* **2015**, *5*, 9–20. [CrossRef] [PubMed]
28. Yuan, H.; Liu, L.; Zhou, J.; Zhang, T.; Daily, J.W.; Park, S. Bioactive Components of Houttuynia cordata Thunb and Their Potential Mechanisms Against COVID-19 Using Network Pharmacology and Molecular Docking Approaches. *J. Med. Food* **2022**, *25*, 355–366. [CrossRef]
29. Yang, Y.; Shi, C.-Y.; Xie, J.; Dai, J.-H.; He, S.-L.; Tian, Y. Identification of potential dipeptidyl peptidase (DPP)-IV inhibitors among Moringa oleifera phytochemicals by virtual screening, molecular docking analysis, ADME/T-based prediction, and in vitro analyses. *Molecules* **2020**, *25*, 189. [CrossRef]
30. SAS Inc. *SAS/STAT® 14.2 User's Guide*; SAS Inc.: Cary, NC, USA, 2016.
31. Inaguma, D.; Kitagawa, A.; Yanagiya, R.; Koseki, A.; Iwamori, T.; Kudo, M.; Yuzawa, Y. Increasing tendency of urine protein is a risk factor for rapid eGFR decline in patients with CKD: A machine learning-based prediction model by using a big database. *PLoS ONE* **2020**, *15*, e0239262. [CrossRef]
32. Köttgen, A.; Pattaro, C.; Böger, C.A.; Fuchsberger, C.; Olden, M.; Glazer, N.L.; Parsa, A.; Gao, X.; Yang, Q.; Smith, A.V.; et al. New loci associated with kidney function and chronic kidney disease. *Nat. Genet.* **2010**, *42*, 376–384. [CrossRef]
33. Kaesler, N.; Babler, A.; Floege, J.; Kramann, R. Cardiac Remodeling in Chronic Kidney Disease. *Toxins* **2020**, *12*, 161. [CrossRef]
34. Silveira Rossi, J.L.; Barbalho, S.M.; Reverete de Araujo, R.; Bechara, M.D.; Sloan, K.P.; Sloan, L.A. Metabolic syndrome and cardiovascular diseases: Going beyond traditional risk factors. *Diabetes/Metab. Res. Rev.* **2022**, *38*, e3502. [CrossRef] [PubMed]
35. Park, S.; Lee, S.; Kim, Y.; Lee, Y.; Kang, M.W.; Kim, K.; Kim, Y.C.; Han, S.S.; Lee, H.; Lee, J.P.; et al. Causal effects of relative fat, protein, and carbohydrate intake on chronic kidney disease: A Mendelian randomization study. *Am. J. Clin. Nutr.* **2021**, *113*, 1023–1031. [CrossRef] [PubMed]
36. Cirillo, M.; Lombardi, C.; Chiricone, D.; De Santo, N.G.; Zanchetti, A.; Bilancio, G. Protein intake and kidney function in the middle-age population: The contrast between cross-sectional and longitudinal data. *Nephrol. Dial. Transplant.* **2014**, *29*, 1733–1740. [CrossRef] [PubMed]
37. Oosterwijk, M.M.; Navis, G.; Bakker, S.J.L.; Laverman, G.D. Personalized Nutrition in Patients with Type 2 Diabetes and Chronic Kidney Disease: The Two-Edged Sword of Dietary Protein Intake. *J. Pers. Med.* **2022**, *12*, 300. [CrossRef]
38. Jung, H.W.; Kim, S.W.; Kim, I.Y.; Lim, J.Y.; Park, H.S.; Song, W.; Yoo, H.J.; Jang, H.C.; Kim, K.; Park, Y.; et al. Protein Intake Recommendation for Korean Older Adults to Prevent Sarcopenia: Expert Consensus by the Korean Geriatric Society and the Korean Nutrition Society. *Ann. Geriatr. Med. Res.* **2018**, *22*, 167–175. [CrossRef]
39. He, J.; Mills, K.T.; Appel, L.J.; Yang, W.; Chen, J.; Lee, B.T.; Rosas, S.E.; Porter, A.; Makos, G.; Weir, M.R.; et al. Urinary Sodium and Potassium Excretion and CKD Progression. *J. Am. Soc. Nephrol.* **2016**, *27*, 1202–1212. [CrossRef]
40. Cirillo, M.; Bilancio, G.; Cavallo, P.; Palladino, R.; Terradura-Vagnarelli, O.; Laurenzi, M. Sodium intake and kidney function in the general population: An observational, population-based study. *Clin. Kidney J.* **2021**, *14*, 647–655. [CrossRef]
41. McMahon, E.J.; Campbell, K.L.; Bauer, J.D.; Mudge, D.W. Altered dietary salt intake for people with chronic kidney disease. *Cochrane Database Syst. Rev.* **2015**, *18*, CD010070. [CrossRef]
42. Okada, Y.; Sim, X.; Go, M.J.; Wu, J.-Y.; Gu, D.; Takeuchi, F.; Takahashi, A.; Maeda, S.; Tsunoda, T.; Chen, P.; et al. Meta-analysis identifies multiple loci associated with kidney function-related traits in East Asian populations. *Nat. Genet.* **2012**, *44*, 904–909. [CrossRef]
43. Kim, H.; Caulfield, L.E.; Garcia-Larsen, V.; Steffen, L.M.; Grams, M.E.; Coresh, J.; Rebholz, C.M. Plant-Based Diets and Incident CKD and Kidney Function. *Clin. J. Am. Soc. Nephrol.* **2019**, *14*, 682–691. [CrossRef]
44. Xu, K.; Cui, X.; Wang, B.; Tang, Q.; Cai, J.; Shen, X. Healthy adult vegetarians have better renal function than matched omnivores: A cross-sectional study in China. *BMC Nephrol.* **2020**, *21*, 268. [CrossRef] [PubMed]
45. Ashkar, F.; Bhullar, K.S.; Wu, J. The Effect of Polyphenols on Kidney Disease: Targeting Mitochondria. *Nutrients* **2022**, *14*, 3115. [CrossRef] [PubMed]
46. Kennedy, O.J.; Pirastu, N.; Poole, R.; Fallowfield, J.A.; Hayes, P.C.; Grzeszkowiak, E.J.; Taal, M.W.; Wilson, J.F.; Parkes, J.; Roderick, P.J. Coffee Consumption and Kidney Function: A Mendelian Randomization Study. *Am. J. Kidney Dis.* **2020**, *75*, 753–761. [CrossRef] [PubMed]

47. Kanbay, M.; Siriopol, D.; Copur, S.; Tapoi, L.; Benchea, L.; Kuwabara, M.; Rossignol, P.; Ortiz, A.; Covic, A.; Afsar, B. Effect of Coffee Consumption on Renal Outcome: A Systematic Review and Meta-Analysis of Clinical Studies. *J. Ren. Nutr.* **2021**, *31*, 5–20. [CrossRef]
48. Vervloet, M.G.; Hsu, S.; de Boer, I.H. Vitamin D supplementation in people with chronic kidney disease. *Kidney Int.* **2023**, *104*, 698–706. [CrossRef]
49. Yeung, W.-C.G.; Toussaint, N.D.; Badve, S.V. Vitamin D therapy in chronic kidney disease: A critical appraisal of clinical trial evidence. *Clin. Kidney J.* **2024**, *17*, sfae227. [CrossRef]
50. Nitzahn, M.; Lipshutz, G.S. CPS1: Looking at an ancient enzyme in a modern light. *Mol. Genet. Metab.* **2020**, *131*, 289–298. [CrossRef]

nutrients

MDPI

Review

Combating Sarcopenia Through Nutrition: Anti-Inflammatory and Antioxidant Properties of *Aronia melanocarpa*

Kalina Metodieva *, Iliyan Dimitrov and Anelia Bivolarska

Department of Medical Biochemistry, Faculty of Pharmacy, Medical University of Plovdiv, 4002 Plovdiv, Bulgaria; iliyan.dimitrov@mu-plovdiv.bg (I.D.); anelia.bivolarska@mu-plovdiv.bg (A.B.)
* Correspondence: kalina.metodieva@mu-plovdiv.bg; Tel.: +359-897729991

Abstract: Introduction: Sarcopenia, the progressive age-related decline in skeletal muscle mass, strength, and function, represents a major contributor to morbidity, frailty, and reduced quality of life in older adults. Oxidative stress and chronic low-grade inflammation are increasingly recognized as central mechanisms driving its onset and progression, through pathways involving mitochondrial dysfunction, impaired satellite cell activity, and dysregulated protein turnover. Objective: The purpose of the following manuscript is to summarize current research on the molecular and cellular interactions between oxidative stress and inflammation in sarcopenia, as well as to assess *Aronia melanocarpa*'s potential as a nutritional intervention. Methods: A narrative review was conducted by searching PubMed, Scopus, and Web of Science for peer-reviewed literature published between 2000 and 2024. Keywords included "sarcopenia", "oxidative stress", "inflammation", "*Aronia melanocarpa*", "polyphenols", and even "functional foods". Eligible publications provided mechanistic, preclinical, or clinical findings on skeletal muscle biology and *A. melanocarpa* bioactivity. Results: This narrative review examines the relationship between oxidative stress and inflammation in sarcopenia, focusing on NF-κB-mediated inflammatory signaling, Nrf-2-dependent antioxidant defenses, myokines like myostatin and irisin, and macrophage polarization in muscle homeostasis. *Aronia melanocarpa* (black chokeberry) is highlighted as a polyphenol-rich fruit with a distinct profile of anthocyanins and proanthocyanidins that have strong antioxidant and anti-inflammatory properties. According to preclinical, clinical, and nutritional studies, *A. melanocarpa* bioactives modulate redox balance, suppress pro-inflammatory cytokine production, increase antioxidant enzyme activity, and regulate metabolic and regenerative signaling pathways important for skeletal muscle health. Conclusions: Overall, the data suggest *A. melanocarpa*'s potential as a functional food and nutraceutical candidate for the prevention and treatment of sarcopenia. However, further translational and clinical research is needed to determine the appropriate intake, bioavailability, and long-term efficacy in human populations.

Keywords: sarcopenia; oxidative stress; chronic inflammation; *Aronia melanocarpa*; polyphenols; functional foods

1. Introduction

The aging process undergoes a dynamic and complex development, progressing over time. According to numerous studies, aging accelerates significantly after the fourth decade, ultimately leading to a terminal outcome. In essence, aging is a complex interaction of biological, physiological, and social elements, and its manifestation in every individual is different [1].

What is common among all, however, is the decline in organ function, which threatens the overall physiological state. This decline is closely linked to a reduced regenerative capacity of stem cells, which compromises tissue maintenance and repair [2]. At the cellular level, aging is associated with a permanent arrest of the cell cycle and cessation of mitosis [3]. In addition to irreversible cell cycle arrest, cellular senescence is characterized by profound alterations in chromatin structure, gene expression, organelle function, and overall cell morphology. Senescent cells change their secretory phenotype, transitioning to a senescence-associated secretory phenotype, which includes the secretion of proinflammatory cytokines [4]. This proinflammatory mediation alters the extracellular matrix, impairs stem cell function, and induces cellular transdifferentiation, which could spread the senescent phenotype to surrounding cells. In combination, these effects contribute to the development of systemic chronic low-grade inflammation, a hallmark of aging, also known as "inflammaging" [5]. In older individuals, this aseptic, chronic low-grade systemic inflammation is increasingly recognized as a common denominator of many age-related diseases [6].

Sarcopenia, as a skeletal muscle age-related disease, poses significant clinical, social, and economic challenges worldwide. The growing elderly population, particularly in both Western and rapidly developing countries, underscores the urgent need to elucidate the underlying mechanisms of sarcopenia to inform effective preventive and therapeutic strategies [7]. A molecular relationship between oxidative stress and inflammation has been hypothesized in the genesis of sarcopenia. Improved understanding of the immune mediators involved in skeletal muscle atrophy may provide valuable insights into the pathophysiological consequences of the diseases [8]. Bone marrow-derived immune cells, particularly infiltrating myeloid cells such as macrophages, neutrophils, and their progenitors, have a specific role in regulating cell proliferation, angiogenesis, and immune surveillance. A pathway of particular interest involves the generation and release of reactive oxygen species (ROS) by these myeloid cells under chronic inflammatory conditions [9]. The disrupted equilibrium between ROS production and antioxidant defense mechanisms in the elderly contributes to lipid peroxidation of cellular membranes and alterations in protein synthesis. These processes collectively result in diminished cellular proliferative capacity, increased susceptibility to mechanical injury, and a heightened inflammatory response, ultimately leading to compromised antioxidant defense and reduced regenerative potential of skeletal muscles in advancing age [10].

Robust evidence supports the critical role of nutrition in maintaining muscle mass, strength, and function among older adults, positioning nutritional interventions as key components in sarcopenia prevention and management [11]. For instance, *Aronia melanocarpa* extract promotes myogenic differentiation through protein kinase B (AKT) pathway activation, resulting in enhanced muscle mass and strength. It further upregulates both glycolytic and oxidative myofiber gene expression, regulating muscle-specific and metabolic pathways, suggesting its potential as a nutraceutical agent for mitigating muscle weakness and atrophy [12].

2. Materials and Methods

2.1. Methodology of Literature Review

This article presents a narrative review that synthesizes evidence from mechanistic, preclinical, and clinical studies examining the interplay between oxidative stress, chronic inflammation, and sarcopenia, with a particular focus on the antioxidant and anti-inflammatory potential of *Aronia melanocarpa*. A narrative review was chosen rather than a systematic or scoping review because the current body of literature is heterogeneous in study designs, outcomes, and models (ranging from cell-based assays and animal models to small clinical trials). This diversity makes it difficult to apply the strict requirements of systematic reviews, but a scoping review would be too wide and descriptive, not permitting in-depth exploration of mechanistic discoveries. The narrative format thus enables a focused integration of diverse findings and the identification of mechanistic themes and translational gaps that require further study.

2.1.1. Databases and Search Strategy

A literature search was conducted in PubMed, Scopus, and Web of Science covering the period January 2000–December 2024. Search strategies combined relevant terms using Boolean operators. An example PubMed query was "sarcopenia" OR "skeletal muscle atrophy"; "oxidative stress" OR "reactive oxygen species"; "inflammation" OR "inflammaging" AND "NF-kB"; "*Aronia melanocarpa*" OR "black chokeberry" OR "polyphenols". Equivalent adapted strings were applied to Scopus and Web of Science.

2.1.2. Inclusion Criteria

Inclusion criteria were peer-reviewed studies in English reporting experimental, mechanistic, preclinical, or clinical findings relevant to skeletal muscle biology, oxidative stress, inflammation, or the bioactivity of *Aronia melanocarpa*.

2.1.3. Exclusion Criteria

Exclusion criteria were commentaries, conference abstracts, publications not related to skeletal muscle or sarcopenia, and studies not addressing *Aronia melanocarpa* or its bioactive compounds.

2.1.4. Filters

Searches were filtered by year of publication (2000–2024), language (English), and document type (meta-analysis, reviews, corrected and republished articles, original research articles, and clinical trials). Relevant articles were screened by title and abstract, followed by full-text assessment, and those meeting the eligibility criteria were synthesized narratively. This approach enabled the integration of diverse findings and highlighted current gaps that require further research.

2.1.5. Strategies for Handling Conflicting Results

Since chronic inflammation is a key mechanism in sarcopenia, studies were included if they investigated oxidative stress or *Aronia melanocarpa* bioactivity, even when chronic inflammation was not the primary endpoint. The collected studies were organized into thematic categories, including mechanisms of sarcopenia and the roles of oxidative stress and inflammation; antioxidant and anti-inflammatory properties of *Aronia melanocarpa*, and potential interactions with muscle-specific regulatory factors such as myostatin and irisin. Within each theme, findings were qualitatively analyzed and narratively described, highlighting consistencies, discrepancies, and translational implications.

2.2. *Application of AI in Manuscript Preparation*

In the process of writing this publication, the creators utilized ChatGPT (OpenAI, version GPT-4 and GPT-5) to assist with the organization, formatting, and structural refinement of the text, as well as translation from Bulgarian into English, verification and correction of the manual translation, paraphrasing, refinement of language and academic phrasing, and reformatting the bibliography into the MDPI reference style. The writers carefully read, revised, and validated the manuscript, and they accept full responsibility for its final version. The scientific information was not created by artificial intelligence.

3. Results

3.1. Overview of Sarcopenia: Definition, Prevalence, and Clinical Relevance

Sarcopenia is an illness commonly defined by a gradual decrease in skeletal muscle mass and function, which is directly related to negative health outcomes [13]. As a consequence of an imbalance between protein synthesis and proteolysis, the ensuing muscle atrophy progressively compromises essential physical functions, including respiration, locomotion, and mobility [14]. Sarcopenia contributes significantly to the deterioration of quality of life and increases susceptibility to secondary conditions such as dyslipidemia, immunosuppression, metabolic syndrome, and cardiovascular disease [15–17]. A 2019 systematic review and meta-analysis, which included 41 studies and nearly 35,000 participants, found that sarcopenia affected about 11% of men and 9% of women. Prevalence rates were substantially higher among nursing home residents—around 51% for men and 31% for women—and among hospitalized older adults, where it reached roughly 23% for men and 24% for women [18].

The development of sarcopenia is influenced by multiple factors, including genetic predisposition, nutritional status, and comorbid clinical conditions [7]. Beyond primary sarcopenia, which is primarily age-related, secondary sarcopenia can arise due to various diseases such as diabetes mellitus and chronic obstructive pulmonary disease. Early identification and analysis of risk factors are critical for preventing the progression and complications associated with sarcopenia [19]. Factors such as physical inactivity, malnutrition, smoking, excessive sleep duration, diabetes, and other comorbidities have been implicated in increasing the incidence of sarcopenia [20,21]. Isometric muscle strength and power both decline significantly with advancing age; however, the annual loss of muscle power exceeds that of isometric strength. Consequently, muscle power has been proposed as a more sensitive indicator for the early detection of sarcopenia [22]. While sarcopenia is often associated with aging, secondary causes can induce sarcopenic changes in younger individuals. Contributory factors include metabolic syndrome, physical inactivity, poor nutrition, congenital and perinatal conditions, vitamin D deficiency, endocrine disorders, gut microbiota dysbiosis, neuromuscular diseases, organ failure, cancer, and other inflammatory states [23].

At the molecular level, several key factors are implicated in age-related sarcopenia. In elderly individuals, disruptions in mitochondrial function and biogenesis within skeletal muscle significantly contribute to declines in muscle mass and performance [24,25]. Aging increases skeletal muscle susceptibility to oxidative stress, particularly during periods of rest and disuse atrophy, underscoring oxidative stress as a central driver of muscle loss in these contexts. Chronic oxidative stress also plays a pivotal role in the pathogenesis of diseases that promote muscle wasting [26]. However, mitochondrial dysfunction and increased oxidative stress are the central driving forces for age-related skeletal muscle abnormalities. Excess oxidative stress in aged muscle leads to excitation–contraction uncoupling, disrupted calcium homeostasis, apoptosis-mediated fiber loss, atrophy of residual fibers, satellite cell dysfunction, and impaired muscle regeneration—all contributing to reduced muscle mass, strength, and function [27]. The primary enzymatic antioxidant defenses counteracting oxidative stress include superoxide dismutase (SOD), catalase (CAT), and glutathione peroxidase (GPx). The activities of these enzymes are modulated by factors such as physical exercise, nutritional status, and the aging process. Furthermore, dietary and endogenous antioxidants play a critical role in maintaining the redox homeostasis of muscle cells, thereby mitigating ROS-induced intracellular damage and preserving muscle function [28].

ROS generation occurs in multiple cellular compartments, including the cytoplasm, plasma membrane, endoplasmic reticulum, mitochondria, and peroxisomes, as well as via enzymes such as NADPH (nicotinamide adenine dinucleotide phosphate) oxidase. The effects of ROS vary depending on their origin and cellular localization, exerting both physiological and pathological functions [29]. The remarkable interplay between oxidative stress and inflammation reflects how ROS regulate the transcription of nuclear factor kappa B (NF-κB)-dependent genes, while ROS themselves modulate NF-κB activity. NF-κB transcription factors, in turn, play a pivotal role in coordinating inflammatory responses and maintaining immune function, thereby underscoring the bidirectional association of oxidative stress and inflammation [30].

Chronic inflammation in skeletal muscle impairs regenerative capacity, affecting satellite cell activation, and promotes accumulation of fibro-adipogenic progenitors and extracellular matrix deposition, impeding effective muscle repair and differentiation [31]. Satellite cell function is impaired by increased oxidative stress in aging muscle. Alongside changes in systemic factors, many of which remain largely unknown, this leads to compromised muscle regeneration and accelerates the progression of sarcopenia [32].

The antioxidant and anti-inflammatory molecules contained in *Aronia melanocarpa* may influence these pathophysiological processes by limiting oxidative stress and modulating the immune response in older individuals [33].

Mass-spectrometry-based proteomic analyses of aging human and animal skeletal muscle reveal a consistent trend: a fiber-type shift from fast-twitch (Type II) to slow-twitch (Type I) fibers during aging, most likely due to the preferential susceptibility of fast-twitch fibers to atrophy (Table 1). These changes are reflected in the differential expression of contractile proteins, including various myosin heavy and light chains, actin, troponin, and tropomyosin, which serve as biomarkers for fiber-type transitions in sarcopenic muscles [34]. Since fast type II fibers are particularly susceptible to atrophy, the polyphenols from *A. melanocarpa* may exert a protective effect by enhancing mitochondrial function and reducing inflammation-induced damage in these fibers [12].

Table 1. Features of skeletal muscle fiber types. The following table outlines the key structural and functional properties of the three major skeletal muscle fiber types: Type I, Type IIa, and Type IIx/IIb. Type I fibers, also known as slow-twitch fibers, have the slowest contraction speed, a high mitochondrial density, low glycogen content, red pigmentation, and excellent fatigue resistance, making them ideal for endurance and continuous activity. Type IIa fibers exhibit an intermediate phenotype, with moderate contraction speed, fewer mitochondria than Type I, high glycogen content, red color, and moderate fatigue resistance, allowing for a balance of power production and endurance. Type IIx/IIb, also known as fast-twitch fibers, contract the fastest, have the fewest mitochondria, a high glycogen content, white pigmentation, and low fatigue resistance, making them ideal for rapid, high-intensity, short-duration movements. Collectively, these characteristics illustrate the metabolic and functional diversity of skeletal muscle fibers, which underlies their distinct contributions to muscle performance and adaptation.

Features	Type I Fibers	Type IIa Fibers	Type IIb/IIx Fibers
Speed of contraction	Slowest	Intermediate	Fastest
Mitochondria	Many	Fewer	Least
Glycogen content	Low	High	High
Color	Red	Red	White
Fatigue resistance	High	Moderate	Low
Activity duration	Long	Moderate	Short

3.2. *Aronia melanocarpa: A Nutritional Powerhouse for Reducing Oxidative Stress and Inflammation*

Functional foods are specially designed to include bioactive compounds or beneficial microorganisms at concentrations that are both safe and effective, aiming to support health maintenance and reduce disease risk. These formulations often incorporate nutrients, dietary fibers, phytochemicals, or probiotics, which contribute to their physiological benefits beyond basic nutrition [35]. Fruits and vegetables contribute essential micronutrients to the diet, including a wide range of vitamins and minerals, and serve as rich sources of phytochemicals that exert antioxidant, estrogenic, anti-inflammatory, and other protective biological effects [36].

Aronia melanocarpa, commonly known as black chokeberry, is an underutilized fruit species increasingly recognized for its high nutritional value and potent antioxidant properties, particularly due to its rich polyphenol content [37]. Native to eastern North America, this deciduous shrub was traditionally employed by Indigenous peoples such as the Abnaki and Potawatomi tribes for therapeutic purposes, including cold treatments. In recent years, *A. melanocarpa* has gained popularity in Eastern European countries and Russia, where it is cultivated for the production of various food products, including juices, jams, teas, wines, and natural colorants [38].

Extracts from *Aronia* have been demonstrated to possess geroprotective properties, as potential mechanisms of action involve hormesis, activation of antioxidant defenses, and anti-inflammatory activity [39].

The chemical composition of black chokeberries has been extensively studied, particularly concerning the bioactive compounds that contribute to their health benefits. Phytochemical profiling has demonstrated that *A. melanocarpa* is an abundant source of phenolic compounds, including procyanidins, anthocyanins, phenolic acids, and their derivatives [40]. Among the most significant nutritional constituents are polyphenols, carbohydrates, essential minerals, and vitamins, all of which contribute to its documented physiological and health-promoting effects. A growing body of in vitro and in vivo research has confirmed the wide-ranging biological activities of these compounds, which include antioxidant [41], anti-inflammatory [42], cardioprotective [43], antiviral [44], anticancer [45], antiplatelet [46], and antidiabetic properties [47].

Polyphenols in *Aronia* can be broadly classified into two main categories: flavonoids and phenolic acids. Flavonoids exist in plants either as free aglycones or as glycosidic conjugates, including O- and C-glycosides [48]. The major flavonoid subgroups present in *Aronia* include anthocyanins, flavonoids, and flavanols, while the phenolic acid profile is dominated by chlorogenic acid and its isomers. Among these, proanthocyanidins have been identified as the principal contributors to the fruit's antioxidant capacity. The predominant anthocyanins are cyanidin derivatives, particularly cyanidin-3-O-arabinoside and cyanidin-3-O-galactoside, with cyanidin-3-O-galactoside being recognized as a key phenolic compound associated with elevated antioxidant and radical-scavenging activity [49].

Flavonoids exert protective effects by neutralizing ROS produced under environmental or physiological stress conditions. They also modulate the activity of key ROS-generating enzymes, such as peroxidase, lipoxygenase, and xanthine oxidase [48]. A polyphenol-rich diet has thus been shown to mitigate chronic disease risk by regulating various physiological pathways, including redox homeostasis, enzymatic activity, cell proliferation, and intracellular signaling mechanisms. Despite their demonstrated bioactivity, polyphenols generally exhibit low oral bioavailability. This is primarily due to extensive biotransformation via phase I and phase II metabolic reactions occurring in enterocytes, hepatocytes, and through microbial metabolism in the gut [50]. For example, the bioavailability of the predominant anthocyanins and proanthocyanidins found in *Aronia* is estimated to be below 6% of the ingested dose [51]. Despite their limited bioavailability, polyphenols from *Aronia* remain highly biologically active, presenting what is often referred to as the "low bioavailability/high bioactivity paradox" [52]. Although this paradox remains to be fully elucidated, several studies have reported that polyphenols derived from *Aronia* exert their biological effects in a dose-dependent manner, with lower doses producing more favorable outcomes than higher ones [53].

Black chokeberry anthocyanins are being actively investigated for their anticancer potential, owing to their capacity to modulate oxidative stress and inflammatory pathways [52]. For instance, *Aronia* concentrate has been shown to protect Raw 264.7 macrophage cells from NF-κB pathway activation while suppressing the release of key pro-inflammatory molecules such as tumor necrosis factor-alpha (TNF-α), interleukin 6 (IL-6), and interleukin 8 (IL-8) from human peripheral monocytes. When combined with sodium selenite, it demonstrates a synergistic effect in inhibiting prostaglandin E2 (PGE-2) production, cytokine secretion, and NF-κB signaling [54]. In addition, *Aronia* extract has been shown to suppress ROS formation in macrophages, leading to decreased NF-κB signaling and subsequent inhibition of iNOS-mediated nitric oxide (NO) synthesis [55].

Complementary findings reveal in more detail that black chokeberry polyphenols (BCPs) significantly attenuate nitric oxide (NO) production and reduce the expression of pro-inflammatory mediators, including monocyte chemoattractant protein 1 (MCP-1), interleukin 1β (IL-1β), TNF-α, and IL-6. This anti-inflammatory action is paralleled by a dose-dependent modulation of oxidative stress biomarkers such as GPx, CAT, and malondialdehyde (MDA), ultimately contributing to improved glucose tolerance, reduced systemic inflammation, and mitigation of high-fat diet-induced obesity in animal models [56].

In addition to its rich polyphenolic content, the polysaccharide fraction of *Aronia melanocarpa* (AMP) has demonstrated notable neuroprotective effects by modulating key signaling pathways such as AMP-activated protein kinase (AMPK)/Sirtuin 1 (SIRT 1)/NF-κB and nuclear factor erythroid 2-related factor 2 (Nrf-2)/heme oxygenase 1 (HO-1), which contribute to the reduction of inflammation and oxidative stress in the aging brain. Furthermore, AMP activates the phosphoinositide 3-kinase (PI3K)/mammalian target of rapamycin) mTOR/AKT pathway and regulates apoptosis-related protein families, suggesting a promising role in preventing age-associated neurological decline [57]. Complementing these findings, recent evidence shows that supplementation with *Aronia* also positively influences systemic inflammatory biomarkers by significantly reducing C-reactive protein (CRP), TNF-α, and IL-6 levels while elevating the anti-inflammatory cytokine interleukin 10 (IL-10). This is accompanied by enhanced antioxidant defense mechanisms, as indicated by increased activities of enzymes such as SOD, GPx, and CAT (Figure 1), further supporting its potential in mitigating oxidative stress and inflammation [33]. Taken together, these findings underscore the significant potential of *A. melanocarpa* as a functional food with multifaceted health benefits, particularly in modulating oxidative stress and inflammation, thereby supporting its therapeutic application in age-related and chronic inflammatory conditions [58].

3.3. The Role of Irisin and Myostatin in Overall Muscle State

In recent years, it has been increasingly recognized that muscle contraction triggers the release of peptides and proteins termed myokines, conferring secretory properties to skeletal muscle tissue. Myokines function as important biological mediators with autocrine, paracrine, or endocrine effects, influencing essential processes such as metabolism, angiogenesis, and inflammation at a systemic level [59].

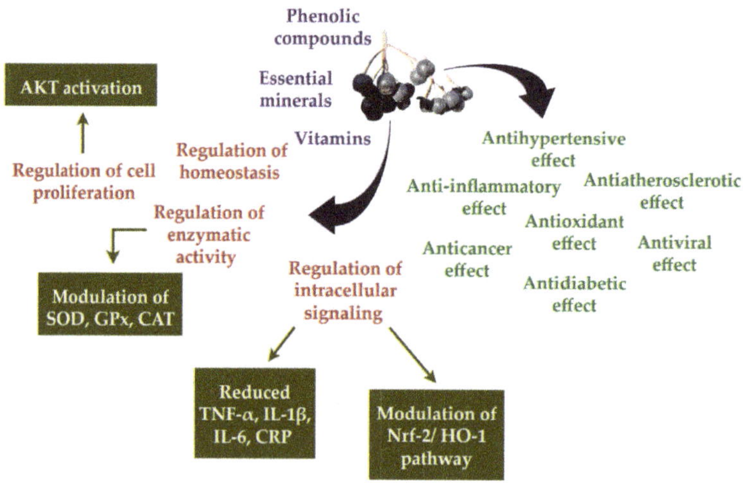

Figure 1. Proposed mechanisms underlying the biological effects of black chokeberry (*Aronia melanocarpa*). The fruit is rich in phenolic compounds, vitamins, and essential minerals, which contribute to the regulation of homeostasis, enzymatic activity, and intracellular signaling. These actions involve AKT activation and modulation of key antioxidant enzymes, such as SOD, GPx, and CAT. As a result, pro-inflammatory mediators, including TNF-α, IL-1β, IL-6, and CRP, are reduced, while the Nrf-2/HO-1 signaling pathway is activated. Collectively, these molecular effects translate into a wide range of physiological benefits, including antihypertensive, anti-inflammatory, anti-atherosclerotic, antioxidant, anticancer, antiviral, and antidiabetic properties. Abbreviations: AKT, protein kinase B; CAT, catalase; CRP, *C*-reactive protein; GPx, glutathione peroxidase; HO-1, heme oxygenase 1; IL-1β, interleukin 1β; IL-6, interleukin 6; Nrf-2, nuclear factor erythroid 2-related factor 2; SOD, superoxide dismutase; TNF-α, tumor necrosis factor α.

One well-studied myokine is myostatin (MSTN), a pro-oxidant that stimulates ROS production in muscle cells. Myostatin, also known as growth differentiation factor 8 (GDF-8) and a member of the transforming growth factor-beta (TGF-β) superfamily, contributes to muscle atrophy by inducing protein degradation [60]. It causes oxidative stress in skeletal muscle cells through activation of TNF-α signaling mediated by NF-κB and NADPH oxidase. Elevated TNF-α levels, in turn, enhance myostatin expression, creating a feedback loop that exacerbates muscle wasting by activating intracellular proteolytic pathways, notably the ubiquitin–proteasome system. Therefore, inhibiting myostatin-induced ROS production represents a promising strategy to minimize muscle loss characteristic of sarcopenia [61].

Another intriguing myokine is irisin, a cleaved form of fibronectin type III domain-containing protein 5 (FNDC5), produced during physical exercise and shown to have multiple health benefits (Figure 2). Both irisin and its precursor FNDC5 are downregulated in conditions of reduced protein synthesis within muscle [62]. Phenotypic studies in mice demonstrate that FNDC5/irisin deficiency in aging individuals leads to aggravated muscle atrophy, including decreased grip strength and reduced muscle mass. Conversely, administration of recombinant irisin intraperitoneally in aged or senescent mice improves sarcopenic symptoms and attenuates age-related adipose tissue expansion [63]. Irisin is also known to modulate glucose metabolism, inflammation, and the immune response, exhibiting notable anti-inflammatory and anti-apoptotic effects. It reduces lipopolysaccharide (LPS)-induced liver injury and inflammatory cytokine production. In vitro, LPS-treated Raw 264.7 macrophage-like cells of animal models (cell line derived from a mouse tumor induced by Abelson murine leukemia virus) show elevated NLRP3 (NOD-, LRR- and pyrin domain-containing protein 3) inflammasome activity, inflammation, and ROS- and NF-κB-mediated apoptosis—effects that can be reversed by irisin treatment [64]. Interestingly, extracts from *A. melanocarpa* demonstrate the ability to activate the AKT signaling pathway, which is directly related to myogenesis and may potentiate the effects of myokines such as irisin while simultaneously reducing the negative impact of myostatin [12].

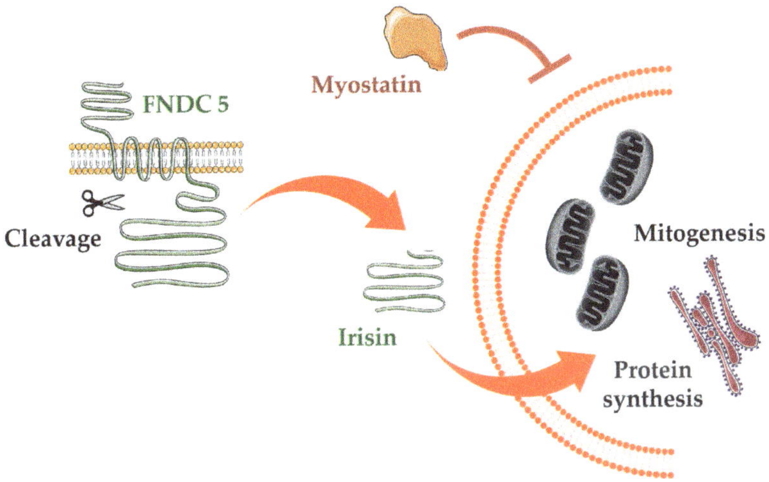

Figure 2. Mechanism of FNDC-5 cleavage and subsequent irisin-mediated effects on muscle cells. FNDC-5, a transmembrane protein, undergoes proteolytic cleavage to release the myokine irisin. Irisin then acts on muscle cells to promote mitochondrial biogenesis (mitogenesis) and enhance protein synthesis, contributing to improved muscle function and metabolic regulation. Myostatin, a negative regulator of muscle growth, inhibits this pathway, counteracting irisin's anabolic effects. This schematic highlights the interplay between FNDC-5-derived irisin signaling and myostatin-mediated inhibition in skeletal muscle physiology. Abbreviations: FNDC-5, fibronectin type III domain-containing protein 5.

3.4. Role of Oxidative Stress and Inflammation in the Development of Sarcopenia

Oxidative stress is a fundamental contributor to cellular aging in general. The uninterrupted progression of regenerative processes is essential for maintaining proper tissue homeostasis and functional integrity [65].

Living organisms are continuously exposed to oxidative stress, which induces oxidative modifications in deoxyribonucleic acid (DNA). One such modification is 8-hydroxy-2′-deoxyguanosine (8-OHdG), a well-established biomarker of oxidative stress and DNA damage detectable both in physiological fluids and cells [66]. Another sign of oxidative stress is MDA, a result of polyunsaturated fatty acid peroxidation within cells. Increased free radical production results in elevated MDA levels [67].

Age-related conditions such as sarcopenia are directly linked to increased oxidative stress in cells [68]. During aging, basal ROS levels rise in muscle fibers and satellite cells, causing oxidation of DNA, proteins, and lipids, disrupting myogenic protein metabolism, and inhibiting skeletal muscle cell differentiation. Specifically, elevated ROS such as hydrogen peroxide (H_2O_2) can suppress phosphorylation of mTOR, AKT, and other downstream signaling molecules, leading to muscle atrophy or sarcopenia due to inhibited protein synthesis [69]. Thus, the pathogenesis of geriatric diseases, including sarcopenia, arises from an imbalance between antioxidant defenses and ROS production, with antioxidant capacity reduced and ROS generation unchanged or increased [70].

The cellular response to ROS production is crucial for preventing further oxidative damage and maintaining cell survival. ROS levels are directly associated with NF-κB-dependent genes, while NF-κB activity is, in turn, modulated by ROS. ROS induce the expression of pro-inflammatory mediators such as IL-1β, TNF-α, interleukin 4 (IL-4), interleukin 12 (IL-12), and IL-6 through NF-κB signaling. NF-κB proteins are transcription factors that play a central role in inflammation and immunity, highlighting the interplay between oxidative stress and inflammation [71,72]. Aerobic cells express varying levels of three key antioxidant enzymes: SOD, CAT, and GPx. These enzymes are essential for cell survival, as their inhibition leads to cell cycle arrest and cell death [73]. Cells also possess transcription factors involved in protective mechanisms. Oxidative stress, defined as an imbalance between ROS production and elimination by defense systems, can lead to chronic inflammation [74]. One such transcription factor is Nrf-2, which supports cellular defenses against oxidative stress and inflammation by inducing the expression of antioxidant genes, including HO-1 and SOD. Nrf-2 deficiency correlates with increased oxidative stress, which promotes NF-κB activity and results in elevated production of pro-inflammatory mediators [75]. Under basal conditions, Nrf2 remains sequestered in the cytoplasm through its association with Keap 1 (Kelch-like ECH associating protein 1), which facilitates its ubiquitin-mediated degradation. However, upon exposure to ROS or electrophilic insults, Nrf2 dissociates from Keap 1 and is stabilized, allowing its translocation into the nucleus where it activates the transcription of antioxidant and cytoprotective genes [76]. Notably, Nrf-2 expression declines with age, leading to dysregulated antioxidant defenses and increased cellular oxidative stress [77].

Evidence suggests that polyphenol-based therapies not only prevent inflammation but also inhibit free radical formation. Furthermore, they activate multiple protective genes such as Nrf-2, AMPK, SOD, CAT, HO-1, SIRT 1, and other key proteins involved in mitochondrial biogenesis [78].

The polyphenols in *A. melanocarpa* have been shown to activate Nrf2-dependent antioxidant defense and suppress NF-κB-mediated inflammation—two key mechanisms in the pathogenesis of sarcopenia [51,79].

3.5. Macrophages as Part of the Balance Between Pro- and Anti-Inflammatory Responses

Macrophages represent a highly heterogeneous and multifunctional group of differentiated mononuclear phagocytes. They are involved in all phases of the immune response, from its initiation, through the development and regulation of the inflammatory process, to the complete restoration of tissues. Macrophages also participate in tissue development, remodeling, and the maintenance of tissue homeostasis [80]. Classically activated macrophages, or M1 macrophages, exhibit a pro-inflammatory phenotype, secreting cytokines such as IL-1β, IL-6, and TNF-α. M1 macrophages are characterized by high expression levels of surface markers, including cluster of differentiation 80 (CD80), cluster of differentiation 86 (CD86), and major histocompatibility complex molecules (MHC class II), relying predominantly on anaerobic glycolysis to meet their energy demands while producing substantial amounts of ROS [81]. Alternatively activated (non-classical) macrophages, or M2 macrophages, are associated with tissue repair and restoration of tissue homeostasis. They secrete anti-inflammatory molecules, including IL-10 and TGF-β, as well as extracellular matrix proteins that support tissue healing. M2 macrophages also express numerous surface markers, such as cluster of differentiation 163 (CD163) and cluster of differentiation 206 (CD206). However, they produce lower levels of ROS, relying primarily on β-oxidation and oxidative phosphorylation to fulfill their energy requirements [82].

The ratio between the two macrophage phenotypes, M1 and M2, can fluctuate over the course of the inflammatory response and depends on microenvironmental factors [83].

An altered balance between M1 and M2 macrophages is considered potentially detrimental, as both prolonged M1 activation and impaired M2 functions may trigger and perpetuate chronic inflammation [84].

It has been observed that the healing process in the musculoskeletal system of elderly individuals is delayed, a phenomenon closely linked to dysregulated inflammatory control [85]. The maintenance of a pro-inflammatory microenvironment during aging leads to the activation of adaptive compensatory mechanisms, which in turn result in delayed tissue recovery [86].

Data from experimental models suggest that biologically active compounds in *A. melanocarpa* may help support the balance between M1 and M2 macrophages, thereby facilitating skeletal muscle regeneration [87].

4. Limitations

Despite the promising findings for *Aronia melanocarpa*'s antioxidant and anti-inflammatory benefits in the context of sarcopenia, some significant limitations must be recognized. First, the majority of current research is based on in vitro and animal models, which may not fully translate to human physiology. Existing clinical trials are limited in number, with small sample sizes, brief intervention periods, and varied groups, limiting the generalizability of findings. Furthermore, several studies use a variety of Aronia-derived products (juices, extracts, powders), making dosage and formulation standardization challenging. Another major issue is the low oral bioavailability of polyphenols, which raises questions about the effective doses required to exert biological effects in skeletal muscle.

5. Conclusions

Sarcopenia is a complex, multifactorial condition in which oxidative stress and chronic inflammation play central roles. These processes accelerate mitochondrial dysfunction, impair anabolic signaling, and limit muscle regenerative capacity, ultimately leading to a decline in functional capacity. Nutritional strategies that target these pathways are therefore of high interest.

Aronia melanocarpa is among the richest dietary sources of polyphenols, with compelling preclinical evidence supporting its ability to activate antioxidant defenses, suppress pro-inflammatory signaling, and enhance muscle metabolism through AKT and mTOR pathways. These mechanisms suggest a plausible role for *Aronia* in protecting vulnerable type II fibers and mitigating age-related muscle atrophy.

Nonetheless, clinical data to date are limited, short-term, and heterogeneous, with small sample sizes and a variety of formulations. Polyphenols have low absorption, which hampers translation into effective therapies. Well-controlled, long-term clinical trials using standardized *Aronia* formulations are required to assess whether the intriguing molecular and preclinical findings transfer into considerable increases in muscle mass, strength, and function in older individuals.

Overall, *Aronia melanocarpa* has promising but preliminary prospects as a safe and accessible dietary component that may help maintain muscular health during aging. Its potential as a nutraceutical candidate should be viewed as speculative and exploratory until more substantial clinical data are obtained.

Author Contributions: K.M. and I.D.: conceptualization, methodology, investigation, resources, and visualization; K.M.: original draft preparation; K.M. and A.B.: review and editing; A.B.: supervision. All authors have read and agreed to the published version of the manuscript.

Funding: The article processing charge (APC) was funded by the Medical University of Plovdiv, project No. HO-14/2025.

Institutional Review Board Statement: Not applicable.

Informed Consent Statement: Not applicable.

Data Availability Statement: The original contributions presented in this study are included in the article. Further inquiries can be directed to the corresponding author.

Acknowledgments: The literature review was conducted within the framework of project No. HO-14/2025 of the Medical University of Plovdiv, entitled "Investigation of oxidative stress and the inflammatory response in skeletal muscles of aged rats following supplementation with *Aronia melanocarpa* juice".

Conflicts of Interest: The authors declare no conflicts of interest.

Abbreviations

The following abbreviations are used in this manuscript:

AKT	Protein kinase B
AMPK	Adenosine monophosphate-activated protein kinase
CAT	Catalase
CD 80	Cluster of differentiation 80
CD 86	Cluster of differentiation 86
CD 163	Cluster of differentiation 163
CD 206	Cluster of differentiation 206
CRP	C-reactive protein
DNA	Deoxyribonucleic acid
FNDC-5	Fibronectin type III domain-containing protein 5
GDF-8	Growth differentiation factor 8
GPx	Glutathione peroxidase
HO-1	Heme oxygenase 1
IL-1β	Interleukin 1β
IL-4	Interleukin 4
IL-6	Interleukin 6
IL-8	Interleukin 8
IL-10	Interleukin 10
IL-12	Interleukin 12
Keap 1	Kelch-like ECH-associating protein 1
LPS	Lipopolysaccharide
MCP-1	Monocyte chemoattractant protein 1
MDA	Malondialdehyde
MHC II	Histocompatibility complex molecules class II
MSTN	Myostatin
mTOR	Mammalian target of rapamycin
NADPH	Nicotinamide adenine dinucleotide phosphate (reduced form)
NF-κB	Nuclear factor kappa B
NLRP-3	NOD-, LRP-, and pyrin domain-containing protein 3
NO	Nitric oxide
Nrf-2	Nuclear factor erythroid 2-related factor 2
8-OHdG	8-hydroxy-2′-deoxyguanosine
PGE-2	Prostaglandin E2
PI3K	Phosphoinositide 3-kinase
Raw 264.7	Cell line derived from a mouse tumor induced by Abelson murine leukemia virus
ROS	Reactive oxygen species
SIRT 1	Sirtuin 1
SOD	Superoxide dismutase

TGF-β	Transforming growth factor-beta
TNF-α	Tumor necrosis factor-alpha

References

1. Dziechciaż, M.; Filip, R. Biological psychological and social determinants of old age: Bio-psycho-social aspects of human aging. *Ann. Agric. Environ. Med.* **2014**, *21*, 835–838. [CrossRef]
2. Henze, H.; Jung, M.; Ahrens, H.E.; Steiner, S.; von Maltzahn, J. Skeletal muscle aging—Stem cells in the spotlight. *Mech. Ageing Dev.* **2020**, *189*, 111283. [CrossRef]
3. Kirkland, J.L.; Tchkonia, T. Cellular senescence: A translational perspective. *eBioMedicine* **2017**, *21*, 21–28. [CrossRef] [PubMed]
4. Birch, J.; Gil, J. Senescence and the SASP: Many therapeutic avenues. *Genes Dev.* **2020**, *34*, 1565–1576. [CrossRef]
5. Rossiello, F.; Jurk, D.; Passos, J.F.; d'Adda di Fagagna, F. Telomere dysfunction in ageing and age-related diseases. *Nat. Cell Biol.* **2022**, *24*, 135–147. [CrossRef] [PubMed]
6. Franceschi, C.; Garagnani, P.; Parini, P.; Giuliani, C.; Santoro, A. Inflammaging: A new immune-metabolic viewpoint for age-related diseases. *Nat. Rev. Endocrinol.* **2018**, *14*, 576–590. [CrossRef] [PubMed]
7. Laviano, A.; Gori, C.; Rianda, S. Sarcopenia and nutrition. *Adv. Food Nutr. Res.* **2014**, *71*, 101–136. [CrossRef]
8. Antuña, E.; Cachán-Vega, C.; Bermejo-Millo, J.C.; Potes, Y.; Caballero, B.; Vega-Naredo, I.; Coto-Montes, A.; Garcia-Gonzalez, C. Inflammaging: Implications in sarcopenia. *Int. J. Mol. Sci.* **2022**, *23*, 15039. [CrossRef]
9. El-Kenawi, A.; Ruffell, B. Inflammation, ROS, and mutagenesis. *Cancer Cell* **2017**, *32*, 727–729. [CrossRef]
10. Fulle, S.; Protasi, F.; Di Tano, G.; Pietrangelo, T.; Beltramin, A.; Boncompagni, S.; Vecchiet, L.; Fanò, G. The contribution of reactive oxygen species to sarcopenia and muscle ageing. *Exp. Gerontol.* **2004**, *39*, 17–24. [CrossRef]
11. Robinson, S.M.; Reginster, J.Y.; Rizzoli, R.; Shaw, S.C.; Kanis, J.A.; Bautmans, I.; Bischoff-Ferrari, H.; Bruyère, O.; Cesari, M.; Dawson-Hughes, B.; et al. Does nutrition play a role in the prevention and management of sarcopenia? *Clin. Nutr.* **2018**, *37*, 1121–1132. [CrossRef] [PubMed]
12. Yun, C.E.; So, H.K.; Vuong, T.A.; Na, M.W.; Anh, S.; Lee, H.K.; Kim, K.H.; Kang, J.S.; Bae, G.U.; Lee, S.J. Aronia upregulates myogenic differentiation and augments muscle mass and function through muscle metabolism. *Front. Nutr.* **2021**, *8*, 753643. [CrossRef] [PubMed]
13. Cruz-Jentoft, A.J.; Sayer, A.A. Sarcopenia. *Lancet* **2019**, *393*, 2636–2646. [CrossRef]
14. Li, C.W.; Yu, K.; Shyh-Chang, N.; Jiang, Z.; Liu, T.; Ma, S.; Luo, L.; Guang, L.; Liang, K.; Ma, W.; et al. Pathogenesis of sarcopenia and the relationship with fat mass: Descriptive review. *J. Cachexia Sarcopenia Muscle* **2022**, *13*, 781–794. [CrossRef]
15. Tournadre, A.; Vial, G.; Capel, F.; Soubrier, M.; Boirie, Y. Sarcopenia. *Jt. Bone Spine* **2019**, *86*, 309–314. [CrossRef]
16. Grosman, Y.; Kalichman, L. The Intersection of Sarcopenia and Musculoskeletal Pain: Addressing Interconnected Challenges in Aging Care. *Int. J. Environ. Res. Public Health* **2025**, *22*, 547. [CrossRef]
17. Abenavoli, L.; Statsenko, M.; Scarlata, G.G.M.; Morano, D.; Myazin, R.; Emelyanov, D. Sarcopenia and Metabolic Dysfunction-Associated Steatotic Liver Disease: A Narrative Review. *Livers* **2024**, *4*, 495–506. [CrossRef]
18. Papadopoulou, S.K. Sarcopenia: A Contemporary Health Problem among Older Adult Populations. *Nutrients* **2020**, *12*, 1293. [CrossRef]
19. Cho, M.R.; Lee, S.; Song, S.K. A review of sarcopenia pathophysiology, diagnosis, treatment and future direction. *J. Korean Med. Sci.* **2022**, *37*, e146. [CrossRef]
20. Yuan, S.; Larsson, S.C. Epidemiology of sarcopenia: Prevalence, risk factors, and consequences. *Metabolism* **2023**, *144*, 155533. [CrossRef] [PubMed]
21. Nasrollahizadeh, A.; Javankiani, S.; Ebrahimi, P.; Sharifi, F.; Soltani, P.; Amiri, M.; Moodi, M.; Khorashadizadeh, M.; Fakhrzadeh, H.; Ramezani, P.; et al. Sarcopenia association with physical and psychological indices in community-dwelling aged population: Birjand Longitudinal Aging Study (BLAS). *Aging Clin. Exp. Res.* **2025**, *37*, 198. [CrossRef] [PubMed]
22. Lauretani, F.; Russo, C.R.; Bandinelli, S.; Bartali, B.; Cavazzini, C.; Di Iorio, A.; Corsi, A.M.; Rantanen, T.; Guralnik, J.M.; Ferrucci, L. Age-associated changes in skeletal muscles and their effect on mobility: An operational diagnosis of sarcopenia. *J. Appl. Physiol.* **2003**, *95*, 1851–1860. [CrossRef]
23. Jung, H.N.; Jung, C.H.; Hwang, Y.C. Sarcopenia in youth. *Metabolism* **2023**, *144*, 155557. [CrossRef]
24. Joseph, A.M.; Adhihetty, P.J.; Buford, T.W.; Wohlgemuth, S.E.; Lees, H.A.; Nguyen, L.M.D.; Aranda, J.M.; Sandesara, B.D.; Pahor, M.; Manini, T.M.; et al. The impact of aging on mitochondrial function and biogenesis pathways in skeletal muscle of sedentary high- and low-functioning elderly individuals. *Aging Cell* **2012**, *11*, 801–809. [CrossRef]
25. Walston, J.D. Sarcopenia in older adults. *Curr. Opin. Rheumatol.* **2012**, *24*, 623–627. [CrossRef] [PubMed]
26. Meng, S.J.; Yu, L.J. Oxidative stress, molecular inflammation and sarcopenia. *Int. J. Mol. Sci.* **2010**, *11*, 1509–1526. [CrossRef]
27. Szentesi, P.; Csernoch, L.; Dux, L.; Keller-Pintér, A. Changes in redox signaling in the skeletal muscle with aging. *Oxid. Med. Cell. Longev.* **2019**, *2019*, 4617801. [CrossRef] [PubMed]

28. Gomes, M.J.; Martinez, P.F.; Pagan, L.U.; Damatto, R.L.; Cezar, M.D.M.; Lima, A.R.R.; Okoshi, K.; Okoshi, M.P. Skeletal muscle aging: Influence of oxidative stress and physical exercise. *Oncotarget* **2017**, *8*, 20428–20440. [CrossRef]
29. Forrester, S.J.; Kikuchi, D.S.; Hernandes, M.S.; Xu, Q.; Griendling, K.K. Reactive oxygen species in metabolic and inflammatory signaling. *Circ. Res.* **2018**, *122*, 877–902. [CrossRef]
30. Hong, Y.; Boiti, A.; Vallone, D.; Foulkes, N.S. Reactive oxygen species signaling and oxidative stress: Transcriptional regulation and evolution. *Antioxidants* **2024**, *13*, 312. [CrossRef]
31. Perandini, L.A.; Chimin, P.; Lutkemeyer, D.D.S.; Câmara, N.O.S. Chronic inflammation in skeletal muscle impairs satellite cell function during regeneration: Can physical exercise restore the satellite cell niche? *FEBS J.* **2018**, *285*, 1973–1984. [CrossRef]
32. Alway, S.E.; Myers, M.J.; Mohamed, J.S. Regulation of satellite cell function in sarcopenia. *Front. Aging Neurosci.* **2014**, *6*, 246. [CrossRef]
33. Sarıkaya, B.; Kolay, E.; Guney-Coskun, M.; Yiğit-Ziolkowski, A.; Aktaç, Ş. The effect of black chokeberry (*Aronia melanocarpa*) on human inflammation biomarkers and antioxidant enzymes: A systematic review of randomized controlled trials. *Nutr. Rev.* **2025**, *83*, 1083–1098. [CrossRef] [PubMed]
34. Dowling, P.; Gargan, S.; Swandulla, D.; Ohlendieck, K. Fiber-type shifting in sarcopenia of old age: Proteomic profiling of the contractile apparatus of skeletal muscles. *Int. J. Mol. Sci.* **2023**, *24*, 2415. [CrossRef]
35. Temple, N.J. A rational definition for functional foods: A perspective. *Front. Nutr.* **2022**, *9*, 957516. [CrossRef]
36. Slavin, J.L.; Lloyd, B. Health benefits of fruits and vegetables. *Adv. Nutr.* **2012**, *3*, 506–516. [CrossRef]
37. Jurikova, T.; Mlcek, J.; Skrovankova, S.; Sumczynski, D.; Sochor, J.; Hlavacova, I.; Snopek, L.; Orsavova, J. Fruits of black chokeberry (*Aronia melanocarpa*) in the prevention of chronic diseases. *Molecules* **2017**, *22*, 944. [CrossRef] [PubMed]
38. Tolić, M.T.; Jurčević, I.L.; Krbavčić, I.P.; Marković, K.; Vahčić, N. Phenolic content, antioxidant capacity and quality of chokeberry (*Aronia melanocarpa*) products. *Food Technol. Biotechnol.* **2015**, *53*, 171–179. [CrossRef]
39. Platonova, E.Y.; Shaposhnikov, M.V.; Lee, H.Y.; Lee, J.H.; Min, K.J.; Moskalev, A. Black chokeberry (*Aronia melanocarpa*) extracts in terms of geroprotector criteria. *Trends Food Sci. Technol.* **2021**, *114*, 570–584. [CrossRef]
40. Ren, Y.; Frank, T.; Meyer, G.; Lei, J.; Grebenc, J.R.; Slaughter, R.; Gao, Y.G.; Kinghorn, A.D. Potential benefits of black chokeberry (*Aronia melanocarpa*) fruits and their constituents in improving human health. *Molecules* **2022**, *27*, 7823. [CrossRef]
41. Sidor, A.; Gramza-Michałowska, A. Black Chokeberry *Aronia melanocarpa* L.—A Qualitative Composition, Phenolic Profile and Antioxidant Potential. *Molecules* **2019**, *24*, 3710. [CrossRef] [PubMed]
42. Zapolska-Downar, D.; Bryk, D.; Małecki, M.; Hajdukiewicz, K.; Sitkiewicz, D. *Aronia melanocarpa* fruit extract exhibits anti-inflammatory activity in human aortic endothelial cells. *Eur. J. Nutr.* **2012**, *51*, 563–572. [CrossRef] [PubMed]
43. Parzonko, A.; Naruszewicz, M. Cardioprotective effects of *Aronia melanocarpa* anthocynanins. From laboratory experiments to clinical practice. *Curr. Pharm. Des.* **2016**, *22*, 174–179. [CrossRef]
44. Park, S.; Kim, J.I.; Lee, I.; Lee, S.; Hwang, M.W.; Bae, J.Y.; Heo, J.; Kim, D.; Han, S.Z.; Park, M.S. *Aronia melanocarpa* and its components demonstrate antiviral activity against influenza viruses. *Biochem. Biophys. Res. Commun.* **2013**, *440*, 14–19. [CrossRef]
45. Dvorska, D.; Mazurakova, A.; Lackova, L.; Sebova, D.; Kajo, K.; Samec, M.; Brany, D.; Svajdlenka, E.; Treml, J.; Mersakova, S.; et al. *Aronia melanocarpa* L. fruit peels show anti-cancer effects in preclinical models of breast carcinoma: The perspectives in the chemoprevention and therapy modulation. *Front. Oncol.* **2024**, *14*, 1463656. [CrossRef]
46. Luzak, B.; Golanski, J.; Rozalski, M.; Krajewska, U.; Olas, B.; Watala, C. Extract from *Aronia melanocarpa* fruits potentiates the inhibition of platelet aggregation in the presence of endothelial cells. *Arch. Med. Sci. AMS* **2010**, *6*, 141–144. [CrossRef]
47. Banjari, I.; Misir, A.; Šavikin, K.; Jokić, S.; Molnar, M.; De Zoysa, H.K.S.; Waisundara, V.Y. Antidiabetic Effects of *Aronia melanocarpa* and Its Other Therapeutic Properties. *Front. Nutr.* **2017**, *4*, 53. [CrossRef]
48. Staszowska-Karkut, M.; Materska, M. Phenolic composition, mineral content, and beneficial bioactivities of leaf extracts from black currant (*Ribes nigrum* L.), raspberry (*Rubus idaeus*), and aronia (*Aronia melanocarpa*). *Nutrients* **2020**, *12*, 463. [CrossRef]
49. Go, M.Y.; Kim, J.; Jeon, C.Y.; Shin, D.W. Functional activities and mechanisms of *Aronia melanocarpa* in human health. *Curr. Issues Mol. Biol.* **2024**, *46*, 8071–8087. [CrossRef] [PubMed]
50. Luca, S.V.; Macovei, I.; Bujor, A.; Miron, A.; Skalicka-Woźniak, K.; Aprotosoaie, A.C.; Trifan, A. Bioactivity of dietary polyphenols: The role of metabolites. *Crit. Rev. Food Sci. Nutr.* **2020**, *60*, 626–659. [CrossRef]
51. Xie, L.; Lee, S.G.; Vance, T.M.; Wang, Y.; Kim, B.; Lee, J.Y.; Chun, O.K.; Bolling, B.W. Bioavailability of anthocyanins and colonic polyphenol metabolites following consumption of aronia berry extract. *Food Chem.* **2016**, *211*, 860–868. [CrossRef] [PubMed]
52. Liu, J.; Zhou, H.; Song, L.; Yang, Z.; Qiu, M.; Wang, J.; Shi, S. Anthocyanins: Promising natural products with diverse pharmacological activities. *Molecules* **2021**, *26*, 3807. [CrossRef] [PubMed]
53. Case, A.J.; Agraz, D.; Ahmad, I.M.; Zimmerman, M.C. Low-dose *Aronia melanocarpa* concentrate attenuates paraquat-induced neurotoxicity. *Oxid. Med. Cell. Longev.* **2016**, *2016*, 5296271. [CrossRef]
54. Appel, K.; Meiser, P.; Millán, E.; Collado, J.A.; Rose, T.; Gras, C.C.; Carle, R.; Muñoz, E. Chokeberry (*Aronia melanocarpa* (Michx.) Elliot) concentrate inhibits NF-κB and synergizes with selenium to inhibit the release of pro-inflammatory mediators in macrophages. *Fitoterapia* **2015**, *105*, 73–82. [CrossRef]

55. Sreedharan, S.; Nair, V.; Bhargava, P.; Cisneros-Zevallos, L. Protective role of polyphenols from aronia berry (*Aronia melanocarpa*) against LPS-induced inflammation in colon cells and macrophages. *Nutrients* **2025**, *17*, 1652. [CrossRef] [PubMed]
56. Zhu, Y.; Cai, P.J.; Dai, H.C.; Xiao, Y.H.; Jia, C.L.; Sun, A.D. Black chokeberry (*Aronia melanocarpa* L.) polyphenols attenuate obesity-induced colonic inflammation by regulating gut microbiota and the TLR4/NF-κB signaling pathway in high fat diet-fed rats. *Food Funct.* **2023**, *14*, 10014–10030. [CrossRef]
57. Zhao, Y.; Liu, X.; Zheng, Y.; Liu, W.; Ding, C. *Aronia melanocarpa* polysaccharide ameliorates inflammation and aging in mice by modulating the AMPK/SIRT1/NF-κB signaling pathway and gut microbiota. *Sci. Rep.* **2021**, *11*, 20558. [CrossRef]
58. Xu, J.; Li, F.; Zheng, M.; Sheng, L.; Shi, D.; Song, K. A comprehensive review of the functional potential and sustainable applications of *Aronia melanocarpa* in the food industry. *Plants* **2024**, *13*, 3557. [CrossRef]
59. Mancinelli, R.; Checcaglini, F.; Coscia, F.; Gigliotti, P.; Fulle, S.; Fanò-Illic, G. Biological aspects of selected myokines in skeletal muscle: Focus on aging. *Int. J. Mol. Sci.* **2021**, *22*, 8520. [CrossRef]
60. Lee, S.J. Targeting the myostatin signaling pathway to treat muscle loss and metabolic dysfunction. *J. Clin. Investig.* **2021**, *131*, e148372. [CrossRef]
61. Sriram, S.; Subramanian, S.; Sathiakumar, D.; Venkatesh, R.; Salerno, M.S.; McFarlane, C.D.; Kambadur, R.; Sharma, M. Modulation of reactive oxygen species in skeletal muscle by myostatin is mediated through NF-κB. *Aging Cell* **2011**, *10*, 931–948. [CrossRef]
62. Waseem, R.; Shamsi, A.; Mohammad, T.; Hassan, M.I.; Kazim, S.N.; Chaudhary, A.A.; Rudayni, H.A.; Al-Zharani, M.; Ahmad, F.; Islam, A. FNDC5/irisin: Physiology and pathophysiology. *Molecules* **2022**, *27*, 1118. [CrossRef] [PubMed]
63. Guo, M.; Yao, J.; Li, J.; Zhang, J.; Wang, D.; Zuo, H.; Zhang, Y.; Xu, B.; Zhong, Y.; Shen, F.; et al. Irisin ameliorates age-associated sarcopenia and metabolic dysfunction. *J. Cachexia Sarcopenia Muscle* **2023**, *14*, 391–405. [CrossRef] [PubMed]
64. Li, Q.; Tan, Y.; Chen, S.; Xiao, X.; Zhang, M.; Wu, Q.; Dong, M. Irisin alleviates LPS-induced liver injury and inflammation through inhibition of NLRP3 inflammasome and NF-κB signaling. *J. Recept. Signal Transduct. Res.* **2021**, *41*, 294–303. [CrossRef]
65. Gerosa, L.; Malvandi, A.M.; Malavolta, M.; Provinciali, M.; Lombardi, G. Exploring cellular senescence in the musculoskeletal system: Any insights for biomarkers discovery? *Ageing Res. Rev.* **2023**, *88*, 101943. [CrossRef] [PubMed]
66. Dąbrowska, N.; Wiczkowski, A. Analytics of oxidative stress markers in the early diagnosis of oxygen DNA damage. *Adv. Clin. Exp. Med.* **2017**, *26*, 155–166. [CrossRef]
67. Gaweł, S.; Wardas, M.; Niedworok, E.; Wardas, P. Malondialdehyde (MDA) as a lipid peroxidation marker. *Wiad. Lek.* **2004**, *57*, 453–455.
68. Mecocci, P.; Boccardi, V.; Cecchetti, R.; Bastiani, P.; Scamosci, M.; Ruggiero, C.; Baroni, M. A long journey into aging, brain aging, and Alzheimer's disease following the oxidative stress tracks. *J. Alzheimer's Dis.* **2018**, *62*, 1319–1335. [CrossRef]
69. Chen, M.; Wang, Y.; Deng, S.; Lian, Z.; Yu, K. Skeletal muscle oxidative stress and inflammation in aging: Focus on antioxidant and anti-inflammatory therapy. *Front. Cell Dev. Biol.* **2022**, *10*, 964130. [CrossRef]
70. Vatner, S.F.; Zhang, J.; Oydanich, M.; Berkman, T.; Naftalovich, R.; Vatner, D.E. Healthful aging mediated by inhibition of oxidative stress. *Ageing Res. Rev.* **2020**, *64*, 101194. [CrossRef]
71. Morgan, M.J.; Liu, Z.G. Crosstalk of reactive oxygen species and NF-κB signaling. *Cell Res.* **2011**, *21*, 103–115. [CrossRef] [PubMed]
72. Thoma, A.; Lightfoot, A.P. NF-kB and Inflammatory Cytokine Signalling: Role in Skeletal Muscle Atrophy. *Adv. Exp. Med. Biol.* **2018**, *1088*, 267–279. [CrossRef]
73. Remacle, J.; Michiels, C.; Raes, M. The importance of antioxidant enzymes in cellular aging and degeneration. *EXS* **1992**, *62*, 99–108. [CrossRef]
74. Hussain, T.; Tan, B.; Yin, Y.; Blachier, F.; Tossou, M.C.; Rahu, N. Oxidative stress and inflammation: What polyphenols can do for us? *Oxid. Med. Cell. Longev.* **2016**, *2016*, 7432797. [CrossRef]
75. Abdelnaser, M.; Alaaeldin, R.; Attya, M.E.; Fathy, M. Modulating Nrf-2/HO-1, apoptosis and oxidative stress signaling pathways by gabapentin ameliorates sepsis-induced acute kidney injury. *Naunyn-Schmiedebergs Arch. Pharmacol.* **2024**, *397*, 947–958. [CrossRef] [PubMed]
76. Kobayashi, M.; Yamamoto, M. Molecular mechanisms activating the Nrf2-Keap1 pathway of antioxidant gene regulation. *Antioxid. Redox Signal.* **2005**, *7*, 385–394. [CrossRef] [PubMed]
77. Hybertson, B.M.; Gao, B.; Bose, S.K.; McCord, J.M. Oxidative stress in health and disease: The therapeutic potential of Nrf2 activation. *Mol. Aspects Med.* **2011**, *32*, 234–246. [CrossRef]
78. Mohib, M.; Afnan, K.; Paran, T.Z.; Khan, S.; Sarker, J.; Hasan, N.; Hasan, I.; Sagor, A.T. Beneficial role of citrus fruit polyphenols against hepatic dysfunctions: A review. *J. Diet. Suppl.* **2018**, *15*, 223–250. [CrossRef]
79. Wang, Z.; Liu, Y.; Zhao, X.; Liu, S.; Liu, Y.; Wang, D. *Aronia melanocarpa* prevents alcohol-induced chronic liver injury via regulation of Nrf2 signaling in C57BL/6 mice. *Oxid. Med. Cell. Longev.* **2020**, *2020*, 4054520. [CrossRef]
80. Strizova, Z.; Benesova, I.; Bartolini, R.; Novysedlak, R.; Cecrdlova, E.; Foley, L.K.; Striz, I. M1/M2 macrophages and their overlaps—Myth or reality? *Clin. Sci.* **2023**, *137*, 1067–1093. [CrossRef]

81. Luo, M.; Zhao, F.; Cheng, H.; Su, M.; Wang, Y. Macrophage polarization: An important role in inflammatory diseases. *Front. Immunol.* **2024**, *15*, 1352946. [CrossRef] [PubMed]
82. Namgaladze, D.; Brüne, B. Fatty acid oxidation is dispensable for human macrophage IL-4-induced polarization. *Biochim. Biophys. Acta* **2014**, *1841*, 1329–1335. [CrossRef] [PubMed]
83. Anders, H.J.; Ryu, M. Renal microenvironments and macrophage phenotypes determine progression or resolution of renal inflammation and fibrosis. *Kidney Int.* **2011**, *80*, 915–925. [CrossRef]
84. Funes, S.C.; Rios, M.; Escobar-Vera, J.; Kalergis, A.M. Implications of macrophage polarization in autoimmunity. *Immunology* **2018**, *154*, 186–195. [CrossRef]
85. Shavlakadze, T.; McGeachie, J.; Grounds, M.D. Delayed but excellent myogenic stem cell response of regenerating geriatric skeletal muscles in mice. *Biogerontology* **2010**, *11*, 363–376. [CrossRef]
86. Duong, L.; Radley, H.G.; Lee, B.; Dye, D.E.; Pixley, F.J.; Grounds, M.D.; Nelson, D.J.; Jackaman, C. Macrophage function in the elderly and impact on injury repair and cancer. *Immun. Ageing* **2021**, *18*, 4. [CrossRef]
87. Cui, Y.; Lin, Y.; Meng, X.; Ma, J.; Deng, H.; Liu, X.; He, X.; Zhao, J. Cyanidin-3-galactoside from *Aronia melanocarpa* ameliorates PM10-induced pulmonary injury by modulating M1/M2 macrophage polarization and NRF2/Sirt1 MAPK signaling. *J. Funct. Foods* **2021**, *78*, 104363. [CrossRef]

nutrients MDPI

Review

Bacopa monnieri: Preclinical and Clinical Evidence of Neuroactive Effects, Safety of Use and the Search for Improved Bioavailability

Anna Gościniak [1], Anna Stasiłowicz-Krzemień [1], Marta Szeląg [2], Jakub Pawlak [2], Izabela Skiera [2], Hanna Kwiatkowska [2], Natasza Nowak [2], Krzysztof Bernady [2], Piotr Trzaskoma [2], Oskar Zimak-Krótkopad [3] and Judyta Cielecka-Piontek [1,3,*]

[1] Department of Pharmacognosy and Biomaterials, Poznan University of Medical Sciences, Rokietnicka 3, 60-806 Poznan, Poland; agosciniak@ump.edu.pl (A.G.); astasilowicz@ump.edu.pl (A.S.-K.)
[2] The Student Scientific Society of Poznan University of Medical Sciences, Department of Pharmacognosy and Biomaterials, Poznan University of Medical Sciences, Rokietnicka 3, 60-806 Poznan, Poland; m.szelag21@wp.pl (M.S.); jpawlak2910@wp.pl (J.P.); izabela.skiera@wp.pl (I.S.); kwiatkowska.han@gmail.com (H.K.); 85251@student.ump.edu.pl (N.N.); 85334@student.ump.edu.pl (K.B.); piotrtrzaskoma242@gmail.com (P.T.)
[3] Department of Pharmacology and Phytochemistry, Institute of Natural Fibres and Medicinal Plants, Wojska Polskiego 71b, 60-630 Poznan, Poland; oskar.zimak-krotkopad@iwnirz.pl
* Correspondence: jpiontek@ump.edu.pl

Abstract: *Bacopa monnieri*, also known as Brahmi or Waterhyssop, is a plant used in Ayurveda for its memory-enhancing properties and control of blood sugar levels. It contains active compounds such as alkaloids, saponins, and cucurbitacins, which have various biological activities. The plant has been studied for its potential in treating Alzheimer's disease, Parkinson's disease, attention deficit hyperactivity disorder (ADHD), and depression. Animal studies have shown promising results in reducing symptoms and protecting against neurodegeneration. Concerning safety, *Bacopa monnieri* has been found to be generally non-toxic, with no serious side effects reported. However, interactions with certain medications and contraindications in conditions like hyperthyroidism should be considered. Further research is needed to determine optimal dosages and ensure safety, especially for pregnant and breastfeeding women.

Keywords: *Bacopa monnieri*; memory enhancement; Alzheimer's disease; neuroprotection

1. Introduction

Bacopa monnieri is a plant that has been used for 5000 years in Ayurveda, the traditional Indian medicine. It belongs to the *Scrophulariaceae* family and grows naturally in the southeastern regions of Asia (India, Australia, Sri Lanka). This plant, characterized by its obovate leaves and small white flowers, is used in traditional medicine to enhance memory. Additionally, it is used to control blood sugar levels. In the book *Charaka Samhita*, which describes Ayurvedic culture, Bacopa is presented as a plant for treating various mental disorders and is referred to as "medhya rasayana", which translates to "rejuvenating (or revitalizing) herbs" that are believed to enhance memory, mental health, and intellect, as well as to promote long life and rejuvenation [1,2]. Therefore, in Ayurveda, Bacopa was used for insomnia, epilepsy and as an anti-anxiety agent. However, this herb has broader applications in various diseases due to the presence of compounds such as alkaloids and saponins, for example, bacosides A, which may be used to support the treatment of gastric ulcers or Alzheimer's disease (Figure 1) [3,4].

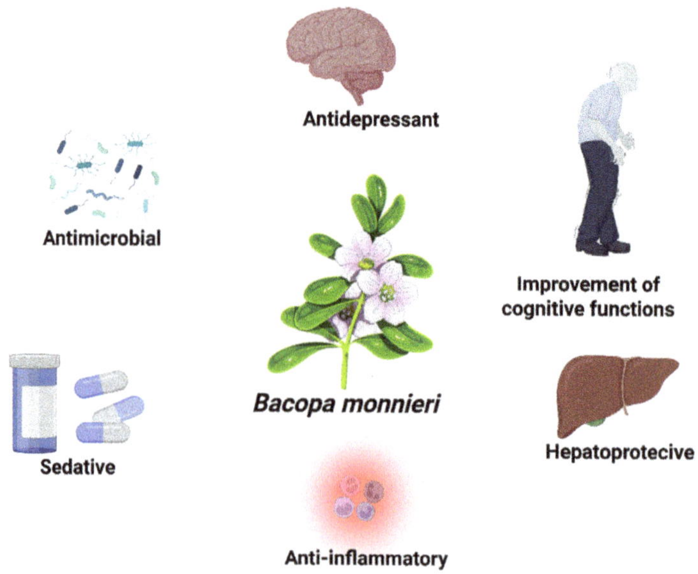

Figure 1. Schematic representation of the main neuropharmacological effects of *Bacopa monnieri.*

Despite human studies showing that *Bacopa monnieri* positively affects learning and word recall, the FDA (Food and Drug Administration) has not approved the medical use of this herb and additionally issued a warning in 2019 to dietary supplement manufacturers producing *Bacopa monnieri* preparations not to make any therapeutic claims regarding this herb [5].

Bacopa monnieri has traditionally been used to enhance memory, and this study aims to review the potential use of the plant in the treatment of Alzheimer's disease, Parkinson's disease, ADHD, and depression. While some modest improvements in memory performance and benefits in conditions like Alzheimer's and depression were observed, the results were inconsistent across tests, indicating the need for more robust, standardized clinical studies [3]. Studies on the activity of plant raw materials are particularly challenging due to the various types of extracts, which differ in composition and concentration of active compounds. The complexity of plant matrices and the diversity of extraction methods further complicate the standardization and reproducibility of results. A review of current research and discussion of safety aspects will help guide future studies in this area.

2. Active Compounds

Bacopa monnieri is rich in secondary metabolites, including a number of alkaloids (herpestine, brahmine), saponins (bacosides, betulic acid, and hersaponin), alcohols, flavonoids, sterol glycosides, sugars, amino acids and cucurbitacins [4,6].

2.1. Saponins

The major chemical compounds from *Bacopa monnieri* are dammarane-type triterpenoid saponins with jujubogenin or pseudojujubogenin moieties as aglycones. These compounds can be found throughout the plant, in the leaves, and in stems [5]. Saponins in the plant include bacosides (Figure 2), Bacopasides, or betulinic acid, which play essential roles in neuronal health and are collectively present at a concentration of up to 6% of the dry weight of the plant [7]. Among these, bacoside A stands out as a major saponin fraction, comprising approximately 38% of the dry mass of standardized methanolic extract [8], and includes four saponin glycosides: Bacopaside II, Bacopaside X, Bacoside A3 and Bacopasaponin C. Bacoside A demonstrated anti-tumor activity in in vitro studies on cell lines as well as in vivo studies conducted on mice [9]. Moreover, Bacoside B (which contains Bacopaside IV, V, N1 and N2 and varies in optical rotation with bacoside A) can be isolated and is considered one of the bioactive marker compounds for this species. A yield of 0.65% (dry weight basis) has been reported for isolated bacoside B [10], which is considered a bioactive marker compound for this species. Bacogenins A1–A5 are the acid-hydrolyzed derivatives of bacosides. The major component is bacogenin A4—ebelin lactone. Bacopasides I-XII interact with sterols and are involved in membrane disruption. Among bacopasaponins, Bacopasaponin C comprises 0.3–0.6% of the ethanolic extracts of *Bacopa monnieri*. Bacopasaponin C is a glycoside of pseudojujubogenin with glucose and rhamnose as sugar units, and it shows anti-dandruff properties. The HPLC-based study quantified individual components of bacoside A in *Bacopa monnieri*. Bacoside A3 ranged from 0.14% to 0.85%, and Bacopaside II from 0.12% to 0.69%. These values reflect regional variation and confirm measurable quantities of bacoside A components in the plant [4,11,12].

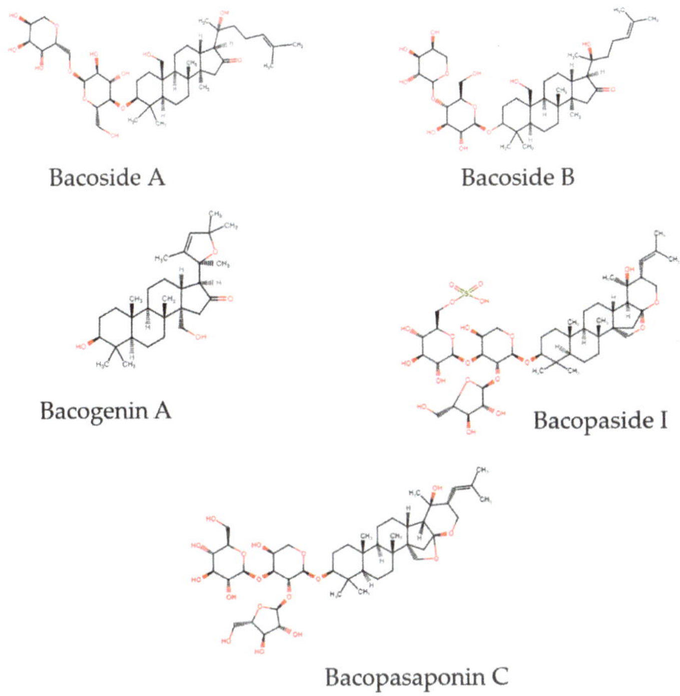

Figure 2. Chemical structures of the major active compounds found in *Bacopa monnieri*.

2.2. Alkaloids

The primary alkaloids found in *Bacopa monnieri* include brahmine, which is believed to contribute to its neuroprotective effects. Brahmine was one of the first alkaloids to be isolated from the plant. Herpestine is another notable alkaloid found in *Bacopa monnieri*. It contains nitrogen atoms and has a complex molecular structure typical of alkaloids. Herpestine may influence neurotransmitter systems, such as serotonin and dopamine, which are crucial for mood regulation and cognitive functions. These constituents have been identified in ethanolic extracts and contribute to the plant's pharmacological profile. Herpestine is of interest for its potential neuromodulatory effects, while monnierin is associated with cognitive-enhancing activity. Their detection underscores the chemical complexity of *Bacopa monnieri* and supports its traditional use in cognitive and neuroprotective therapies [5].

2.3. Cucurbitacins

Cucurbitacins are a class of highly oxygenated tetracyclic triterpenoids known for their bitter taste and pharmacological properties. Cucurbitacins have a tetracyclic triterpenoid core structure consisting of four fused rings derived from cucurbitane. Bacopa contains cucurbitacins such as cucurbitacin B and cucurbitacin E, which contribute to its biological properties. The structure of cucurbitacin B is presented in Figure 3. Cucurbitacin E has recently been reported to possess inhibitory effects on the growth of human colon, breast, lung, and central nervous system cancer cell lines [13,14]. Cucurbitacin B induces cell cycle arrest and inhibits angiogenesis and tumor cell migration, indicating its potential as a promising candidate for anticancer drug development. It is important to note that cucurbitacin B is not a primary bioactive constituent of *Bacopa monnieri*, whose pharmacological effects are mainly attributed to bacosides [11,15].

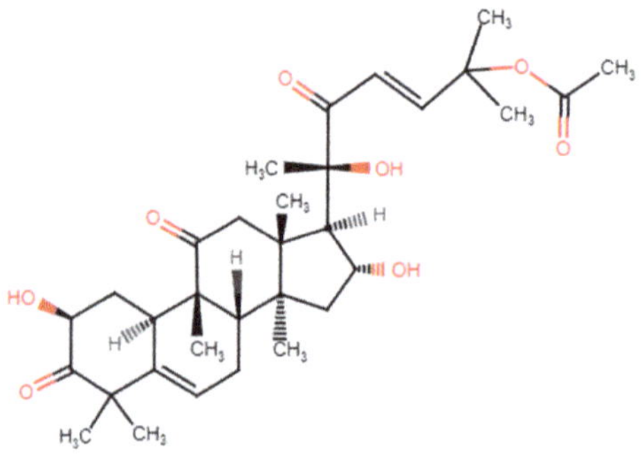

Figure 3. Structure of cucurbitacin B present in *Bacopa monnieri*.

3. Biological Activity

Bacopa monnieri shows great potential for multi-targeted activity, primarily due to its rich profile of bioactive compounds. It is particularly renowned for its impact on the nervous system, as it exhibits neuroprotective effects on multiple levels of neural functioning and across various neurodegenerative pathways. The neuroprotective actions of *Bacopa monnieri* are mediated through a diverse range of mechanisms (Figure 4).

Foremost among them is its potent antioxidant activity, which mitigates oxidative stress by neutralizing reactive oxygen species and inhibiting lipid peroxidation, thereby preserving neuronal integrity [16,17]. The plant also displays anti-amyloidogenic properties, reducing the aggregation and deposition of amyloid-beta peptides—an essential mechanism in the context of Alzheimer's disease [18]. Additionally, Bacopa acts as an acetylcholinesterase inhibitor [19], enhancing cholinergic transmission through increased acetylcholine levels, which contributes to improved memory and cognitive performance. It further influences neuroinflammation and mitochondrial function, reducing neuronal apoptosis and promoting cellular resilience [20]. The above, along with additional mechanisms, are discussed in detail in the following subsections.

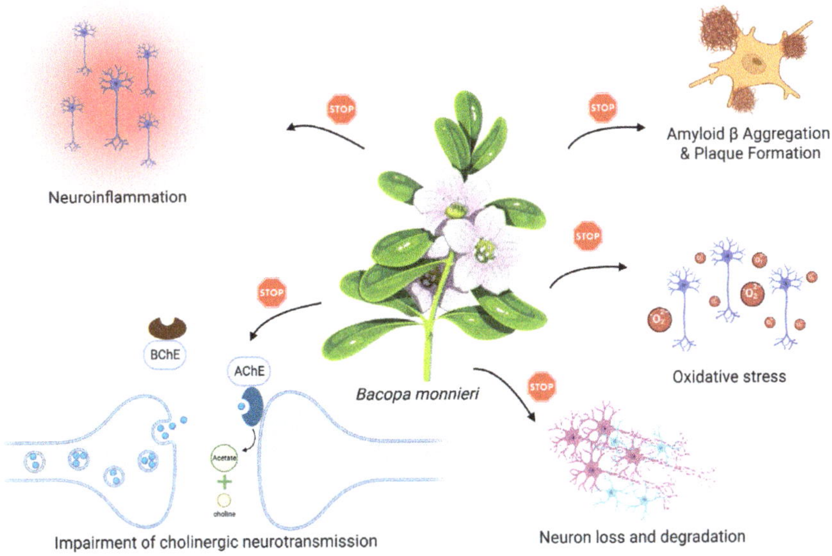

Figure 4. Schematic representation of the neuroprotective mechanisms of *Bacopa monnieri*.

3.1. Alzheimer's Disease

Alzheimer's disease (AD) is a chronic, progressive neurodegenerative disease characterized by irreversible damage to the central nervous system. It leads to cerebral dementia, associated with the loss of many cognitive functions such as memory, speech, and the ability to learn new skills. The source of this disease is not entirely clear, which makes it challenging to find appropriate medications to prevent its rapid progression. Currently, cholinesterase inhibitors and glutamate antagonists are used. In the course of the disease, abnormal deposition of beta-amyloid protein in the brain is observed in the form of plaques and Tau protein. They induce the development of free radicals that impair glucose transport in nerve cells, leading to damage and death of neurons [21]. Death of neurons causes dysfunction of the cholinergic system—deficits in cortical choline acetyltransferase concentrations, reduced choline release, and reduced acetylcholine secretion [22,23].

Treatment of Alzheimer's disease relies on delaying the progression of the disease by potentiating transmission in the cholinergic system. There is no effective causal treatment. Alzheimer's disease is a neurodegenerative disease that affects the elderly and is estimated to account for 60% of all dementia cases in people over the age of 65. The statistics do not indicate improvement, as it is estimated that by 2050, the number of patients may increase two- or threefold. However, the troublesome side effects on the gastrointestinal tract, which lead to damage to the stomach lining and peptic ulcers, often do not allow for long-term pharmacological therapy in Alzheimer's disease [6].

In an in silico study conducted by Roy et al. [24], it was shown that out of 17 compounds found in *Bacopa monnieri*, 2 saponins, Bacopasaponin G and Bacopasaponin N, exhibited inhibitory effects on Caspase-3 and tau-protein kinase, which are factors related to Alzheimer's disease. These findings suggest potential therapeutic activity; however, further in vitro and in vivo studies are necessary to confirm this.

Using methanol extracts has shown the anti-amyloidogenic potential of Brahmi by significantly affecting the dissociation of amyloid protein aggregates [25]. A study on cultured rat cells confirmed these findings, showing a reduction in beta-amyloid deposition in the brain. The neuroprotective effect of *Bacopa monnieri* was likely due to its ability to inhibit acetylcholinesterase activity rather than mitigating glutamate-induced toxicity. Additionally, neurons treated with the extract exhibited lower levels of reactive oxygen species, suggesting a reduction in intracellular oxidative stress and an extension of neuronal lifespan. The extract also demonstrated antioxidant properties and inhibited lipid peroxidation [26].

Following the experiment on 72 mice, it was shown that supplementation with *Bacopa monnieri* (100 mg/kg for 180 days) significantly improved cognitive function. In healthy mice, memory, concentration, and learning ability were enhanced, while in Alzheimer's mice, cognitive performance was restored to near-normal levels. These effects were confirmed by the Morris water maze test, with statistical analysis indicating significant differences between groups (F significant, $p < 0.01$) [27].

In a randomized, double-blind clinical trial, 60 healthy, elderly volunteers taking 300 mg and 600 mg of Brahmi showed reduced acetylcholinesterase activity, which resulted in improved attention and memory. Hence, *Bacopa monnieri* may be useful in the treatment of Alzheimer's disease as well as attention deficit disorder. Moreover, no side effects or toxicity were observed [28].

While *Bacopa monnieri* has demonstrated promising cognitive benefits in clinical studies, its efficacy in Alzheimer's disease (Figure 5) must be evaluated in the context of existing pharmacological treatments. Current drugs for Alzheimer's, such as acetylcholinesterase inhibitors (AChEIs), primarily aim to mitigate cognitive decline by enhancing cholinergic transmission or modulating excitotoxicity. In a 52-week, randomized, double-blind study, Brahmi demonstrated an effect comparable to donepezil, a drug used to treat Alzheimer's disease. The efficacy and safety of *Bacopa monnieri* (300 mg) and synthetic donepezil 10 mg were compared in 48 patients with Alzheimer's disease and mild cognitive impairment. They showed no significant difference between them after 1 year of treatment [29].

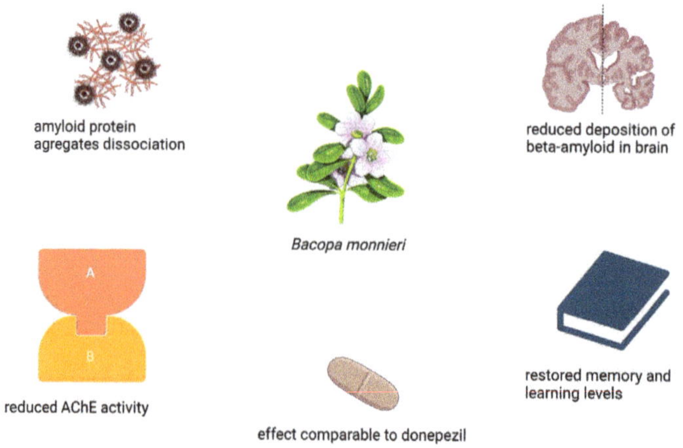

Figure 5. Schematic representation of the effects of *Bacopa monnieri* in patients with Alzheimer's disease.

3.2. *Parkinson's Disease*

Parkinson's disease is a neurodegenerative disorder that consists of selective death of nigral dopaminergic neurons and the presence of Lewy bodies containing α-synuclein. These factors lead to motor symptoms such as tremors and muscle stiffness as well as cognitive impairment. The disease is caused by a combination of numerous factors, including age, genetic liability, brain injuries, and exposure to toxins [30].

Bacopa monnieri has shown promising neuroprotective properties in the context of Parkinson's disease (Figure 6). In silico studies using molecular docking confirmed the potential ability of Bacoside-A to interact with the active site of Parkinson's disease protein 7 (DJ-1) [31] and Bacopaside-XII to inhibit Kelch-like ECH-associated protein 1 (KEAP1) [32]. DJ-1 and KEAP1 play a role in the accumulation of Lewy bodies by causing oxidative stress, and its inhibition may result in improvement of the symptoms.

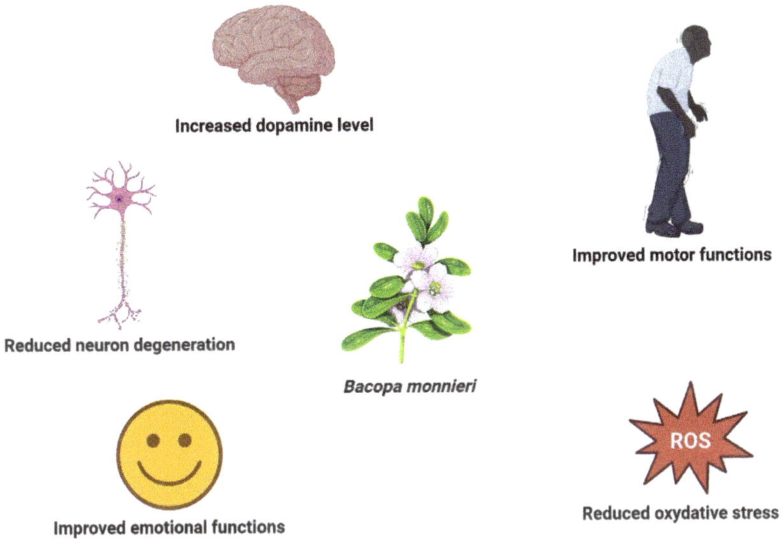

Figure 6. Schematic representation of the effects of *Bacopa monnieri* effects in Parkinson's disease.

Experiments conducted on invertebrates also provided promising results. Transgenic *Caenorhabditis elegans* expressing α-synuclein and *C. elegans* exposed to 25 mM 6-hydroxydopamine were administered a *B. monnieri* tincture (100 g DW/650 mL 96% ethanol) diluted ten times in *E. coli* OP50 liquid culture for 48 h. Transgenic *C. elegans* treated with *Bacopa monnieri* developed significantly reduced accumulation of α-synuclein and lipoperoxidation compared to the control group. Furthermore, *Bacopa monnieri* reduced degeneration of dopaminergic neurons in the group exposed to 6-hydroxydopamine [33].

In other study, transgenic Parkinson's *Drosophila melanogaster* was exposed to 0.25, 0.5, and 1.0 μL/mL *Bacopa monnieri* extract for 24 days. It was observed that *Bacopa monnieri* treatment reduced oxidative stress and delayed motor impairment compared to the untreated control group [34].

In a study on male albino mice conducted by Singh et al. [32], animals received oral administration of *Bacopa monnieri* extract (40 mg/kg) for 30 days. They were injected intraperitoneally with MPTP (1-methyl-4-phenyl-1,2,3,6-tetrahydropyridine) (15 mg/kg) from days 15 to 30 to induce Parkinson's-like neurodegeneration. Mice treated with *Bacopa monnieri* showed improved motor performance and reduced dopaminergic neuron degeneration compared to the MPTP-only group. Brain analysis revealed lower oxidative stress markers and pro-apoptotic proteins, along with increased antioxidant activity and Bcl-2 expression.

Similar results were observed in mice treated with 40 mg/kg *Bacopa monnieri* extract for 3 weeks followed by intraperitoneal injections of 30 mg/kg MPTP from the second to third week and in the group simultaneously exposed to MPTP and *Bacopa monnieri*, which indicates both the neuroprotective and neurorescue potential of *Bacopa monnieri* [32]. An experiment conducted by Shinomol et al. [35] on rats exposed orally to 180 mg/kg *Bacopa monnieri* extract for 80 days and intraperitoneally to 2.5 mg/kg rotenone from the 20th to 80th day also resulted in increased noradrenaline, adrenaline, dopamine, and serotonin and reduced MAO levels in brain tissue.

The double-blind, placebo-controlled, parallel trial conducted by Fuentes dos Santos et al. [36] on 20 volunteers with Parkinson's disease suggests that *Bacopa monnieri* could be useful in PD therapy. Patients were administered 225 or 400 mg of *Bacopa monnieri* extract a day for 90 days. A significant improvement in both motor and emotional function was observed, which resulted in increased quality of life. However, to confirm the potential of *Bacopa monnieri*, more clinical trials are needed.

3.3. *Attention Deficit Hyperactivity Disorder (ADHD)*

Attention deficit hyperactivity disorder (ADHD) is one of the most common neurodevelopmental disorders in children, manifesting itself in problems with inattention, hyperactivity, and impulsivity, which result in learning and social difficulties [37].

Dave et al. [38] conducted a study on 27 children who met the criteria for ADHD. Participants took 225 mg of *Bacopa monnieri* extract a day for 6 months. The symptoms of ADHD, excluding social problems, were significantly reduced after treatment, especially self-control, which increased in 89% of the children. Additionally, levels of restlessness in 85% of participants were reduced. Results clearly confirm that *Bacopa monnieri* has the potential for application in ADHD therapy. That improvement may be caused by the influence on the dopamine level, which decreased in the prefrontal cortex in patients diagnosed with ADHD.

3.4. *Depression*

Major depressive disorder (depression) is a common and significant mental disorder that impacts one's emotions, thoughts, and behaviors in multiple ways. It affects up to 21% of the population. The disorder is characterized by feeling dismal, displaying a lack of enthusiasm for pursuits that were previously engaged in with eagerness, a significant change in sleeping schedule (sleeping too much or too little), and thoughts of death and/or suicide. The symptoms are not identical in every patient, and it requires at least 2 weeks of observation to be clinically diagnosed [39]. Seeking natural remedies might play a vital role since they have fewer side effects [40].

Researchers aimed to evaluate the antidepressant effects of the methanolic extract of *Bacopa monnieri* through various behavioral models designed to demonstrate antidepressant activity, with tests yielding positive results. Swiss albino mice were subjected to various behavioral models, including the forced swimming test, the locomotor activity test, and the tail suspension test [41]. The forced swimming test assessed depressive behavior in mice given either water, methanolic extract, or imipramine [42]. During the test session, the animals were exposed to stressful conditions for 5 min. The study revealed that the methanolic extract of *Bacopa monnieri* significantly decreased the immobility duration in the forced swimming test ($p < 0.001$) [41]. The Open Field Maze test measured locomotion, rearing, and defecation. Mice treated with extract or imipramine showed significant increases in all parameters compared to controls ($p < 0.001$) [43].

A study on Charles Foster rats used a learned helplessness test with shock pretreatment and avoidance training. Rats received *Bacopa monnieri* extract (20 or 40 mg/kg) or imipramine (15 mg/kg). The control group received a carboxymethyl cellulose suspension. Bacopa significantly reduced escape failures and increased avoidance responses after 5 days [8].

3.5. Anxiety

Anxiety is a common reaction to stress, but anxiety disorders go beyond ordinary feelings of nervousness or uneasiness. They are characterized by excessive fear or apprehension. They represent the most prevalent category of mental disorders, impacting nearly 30% of adults during their lifetime. Simple anxiety may go beyond to more severe disorders such as panic disorder [44]. *Bacopa monnieri* has demonstrated multiple beneficial effects in individuals suffering from anxiety (Figure 7). A dose of 150 mg of a standardized extract of *Bacopa monnieri* (Bacognize) administered twice daily for six weeks was tested in a randomized group of people subjected to neuropsychological tests [45]. The results indicated a significant improvement in the Bacopa group compared to the placebo-treated group. Considerable differences were shown in the logical memory test and the reduction in distractibility. The improvement could be a result of the antioxidant effect and action on both calcium channels and acetylcholine, which are Bacopa-dependent.

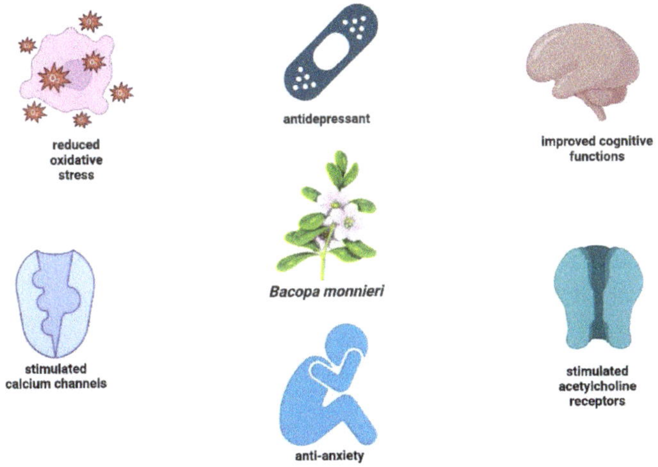

Figure 7. Schematic representation of the anxiolytic effects of *Bacopa monnieri*.

Bacopa monnieri provides a wide range of potential therapeutic effects, as summarized in Table 1, where the collected studies reflect its promising activity demonstrated across different study types and disease models.

Table 1. Summary of study results on various diseases.

Disease	Type of Study	Study Group	Duration of the Study	Dose	Conclusions	Reference
Alzheimer's disease	In silico	-	-	-	Inhibitory effects on the CASP-3 and TPK I	Roy et al. [3]
	In silico	-	-	-	The anti-amyloidogenic effect from dissociation of amyloid protein aggregates	Subramanian et al. [4]
	In vitro	Cortical cell cultures were prepared from 18-day-old rat fetuses	72 h	10–100 μg/μL (extract: 18 kg DW/triple percolation with 95% ethanol, 8 h)	The anti-amyloidogenic effect, limiting deposition beta-amyloid in brain	Limpeanchob et al. [6]
	In vivo	72 healthy and AD mice	180 day	100 mg/kg (methanolic extract)	Memory and learning deficits restored to normal levels;	Kunte and Kuna [27]
	Randomized, double-blind clinical trial	60 healthy volunteers	12 weeks	300 mg, 600 mg (methanolic extract)	memory enhancement and reduction in AChE activity	Peth-Nui et al. [28]
	Randomized, double-blind clinical trial	48 patients with AD and mild cognitive impairment	45 months	300 mg (standardized extract)	Effect comparable to donepezil	Prabhakar et al. [29]
Parkinson's disease	In silico	-	-	-	Interaction of Basocide-A with active site of DJ-1	Chandrasekar et al. [21]
	In silico	-	-	-	Inhibition of KEAP1 by Bacopaside-XII	Singh et al. [32]
	In vivo	*Caenorhabditis elegans*	48 h	*B. monnieri* tincture (100 g DW/650 mL 96% ethanol), diluted ten times in E. coli OP50 liquid culture	Reduction in α-synuclein accumulation, degeneration of dopaminergic neurons, and lipoperoxidation	Jadiya et al. [22]
	In vivo	Transgenic PD *Drosophila melanogaster*	24 days	0.25; 0.5; 1.0 μL/mL (extract: 30 g DW/300 mL acetone)	Delayed motor impairment, reduction in oxidative stress, and brain apoptosis	Siddique et al. [24]
	In vivo	24 male albino mice	30 days	40 mg/kg (extract: 500 g DW/1000 mL ethanol)	Better results in motor tests, reduced lipid peroxidation, conjugated dienes, caspase-3, Bax protein, dopaminergic neuron degeneration, increased Bcl-2 protein, antioxidant activity, nitrate level in nigrostriatal system	Singh et al. [25]
	In vivo	32 Swiss albino mice	3 weeks	40 mg/kg (commercial extract)	Better results in motor tests, reduced lipid peroxidation, increased GSH, dopamine, and nitrate level in the nigrostriatal system	Singh et al. [23]
	In vivo	24 male Wistar rats	80 days	180 mg/kg (ethanolic extract)	Increased noradrenaline, adrenaline, dopamine, serotonin, reduced MAO in brain tissue	Shinomol et al. [26]
	Double-blind placebo-controlled, parallel trial	20 volunteers with Parkinson's disease	90 days	225; 400 mg a day (commercial extract)	Improvement in quality of life, emotional and motor functions	Fuentes dos santos et al. [36]

Table 1. *Cont.*

Disease	Type of Study	Study Group	Duration of the Study	Dose	Conclusions	Reference
ADHD	Open-label trial	27 children meeting the criteria for ADHD	6 months	225 mg a day (commercial extract)	Significant reduction in ADHD symptoms except for social problems	Dave et al. [38]
Anxiety	Double-blind placebo-controlled, parallel trial	60 students aged 19–22 having basic computer literacy	6 weeks	150 mg two times a day (standardized extract, 15.57 of bacopasaponins (%*w*/*w*)	Significant effect on cognitive functions	Kumar et al. [45]
Depression	In vivo	Inbred Charles Foster albino rats	5 days	20 and 40 mg/kg, once a day (methanolic extract)	Decreased escape failures and increased avoidance responses	Sairam et al. [8]
		Swiss albino mice	5 min	50, 100 and 200 mg/kg (sample extract) 30 mg/kg (standard drug)	Confirmed antidepressant-like effect of methanolic extract of *B. monniera*	Mannan et al. [41]

3.6. Other Bioactive Properties

Bacopa monnieri, in addition to its neuroprotective properties, exhibits a range of other health-promoting effects. It is well-known for its adaptogenic properties, helping the body cope with stress and maintain physiological balance [4]. The plant demonstrates anti-inflammatory effects, which may assist in reducing inflammation within the body, as well as antioxidant properties that protect cells from oxidative stress [3]. Furthermore, studies suggest its beneficial impact on the cardiovascular system, including lowering blood pressure and supporting vascular health. *Bacopa monnieri* also exhibits hepatoprotective properties, aiding in liver regeneration and shielding it from toxins. Additionally, some research highlights its potential anticancer effects and its ability to boost immune system function. This wide spectrum of properties makes *Bacopa monnieri* a compelling subject for further investigation into its systemic health benefits [9].

3.7. Limitations of Studies

Despite the promising results obtained in numerous studies on *Bacopa monnieri*, there are a number of important limitations that need to be taken into account when interpreting their results and potential clinical application. Most of the available studies are in silico analyses, in vitro experiments, or animal model studies. Although they point to potential mechanisms of action and beneficial effects of *Bacopa monnieri* on neuroprotective parameters, a systematic assessment of the quality of this evidence is lacking. In many cases, these studies are characterized by small samples, lack of blinding, and short durations, limiting the generalizability of the results to the human population. Translating the results of preclinical studies into clinical effects remains a major challenge. In silico and in vivo studies indicate anti-amyloidogenic and antioxidant effects, among others, but clinical studies confirming these mechanisms in Alzheimer's patients are lacking. Even well-designed human clinical trials, e.g., comparing Brahmi with donepezil, are few and need to be replicated in wider study groups [29]. One key limitation is the considerable variability in the composition of *Bacopa monnieri* extracts. Differences due to the extraction method (ethanolic vs. methanolic), the source of the plant material, the culture conditions, or the type of standardized active compounds used (e.g., bacosides) affect the reproducibility of the results and their comparability. Non-standardized preparations make it difficult to replicate test results and may have varying pharmacological and safety profiles.

4. Safety of Use

Evaluating the safety of plant raw materials is important for many reasons. It allows assessing the impact on both human health and the environment. *Bacopa monnieri*, which is widely known in Ayuverdhist medicine, has also been of scientific interest for its effects on the nervous system. Currently, however, there is still a lack of research on the safe use of the raw materials in pregnant and breastfeeding women, which is important from the point of view of fetal and child development in the early months of life.

4.1. Doses Used

Studies to date do not report strict daily doses to ensure adequate safety, as *Bacopa monnieri* is generally a non-toxic plant. Ethanol extract was most commonly used in the studies. Doses are usually in the range of 300 to 600 mg daily. Based on a clinical study conducted, among others, by Benso et al., doses of 320 mg and 640 mg were shown to have a positive effect on human cognitive function (memorization, eye tracking, etc.). Slightly stronger effects were observed in those who received the 640 mg dose [46]. In a study conducted by Dave et al. [38], a safe dose for children aged 6 to 12 years was developed. The study involved 31 children with ADHD. The children were given a dose of 225 mg per day for 6 months. The dosage has proven not only safe but also effective in eliminating ADHD symptoms in children within a certain age range. Clinical studies have demonstrated that daily doses of 300 to 600 mg of *Bacopa monnieri* extract standardized for the amount of bacosides, equivalent to 5 to 10 g of the dried herb, can enhance cognitive function and alleviate symptoms of anxiety and depression [47]. These effects are typically observed after 12 weeks of consistent supplementation. However, further research is needed to refine these dosage recommendations and to assess the long-term safety and efficacy of Bacopa monnieri across diverse populations.

4.2. Toxicity In Vitro

The purpose of the toxicity study is to provide the necessary information on the safety of the herbal product before evaluating its potential benefits in clinical trials. Sireeratawong et al. conducted a study to assess the chronic and acute toxicity of *Bacopa monnieri* extract in rats. In the acute toxicity study, female rats were divided into two groups. Group I (control) was administered distilled water at 1 mL/kg, and Group II (test) was administered *Bacopa monnieri* extract at 5000 mg/kg. The rats were subjected to close observation for 14 days. Body weight and hematological, biochemical, and histopathological parameters were evaluated. As a result, no significant changes were observed in the aforementioned parameters. In addition, the high dose of 5000 mg/kg did not contribute to the death of rats. Although the control and treatment groups' body weights differed somewhat at the start of the experiment, this difference was not statistically significant. Body weight changed little but significantly only after 14 days. Since it can be the result of variations in food consumption, this little increase in body weight in the treated animals might still be regarded as normal. Rats treated with *B. monnieri* showed no significant histological changes in any of their internal organs, including the kidneys and liver. Doses of 30, 60, 300, and 1500 mg/kg/day of *Bacopa monnieri* extract were used for chronic toxicity testing. The control group was given distilled water, and the test group was given appropriate doses of *Bacopa monnieri* extract for 270 days. In the conducted study, there were no significant changes which would indicate toxicity of the extract [48]. The clinical study, which was conducted on 23 volunteers, showed no alarming changes indicating toxicity of the preparation containing *Bacopa monnieri*. Each participant received a 300 mg tablet and a 450 mg tablet for 30 days. Each dose was consumed for 15 days. Studies that were conducted before and after the use of the product showed no serious side effects. In some cases, gastrointestinal disorders in the form of diarrhea have appeared. Based on studies to date, there are no contraindications to the withdrawal of preparations containing *Bacopa monnieri* extract resulting from the toxicity of the plant material [49].

4.3. Possible Side Effects

At the moment, there are no reports of serious adverse effects. The most common side effects are gastrointestinal disorders. A study by Morgan and Stevens evaluating the effects of *Bacopa monnieri* on the memory of the elderly found that nausea, excessive abdominal cramps, and frequent bowel movements appeared after prolonged use [50].

Singh and Singh conducted a study to assess the effect of *Bacopa monnieri* extract on mouse fecundity. *Bacopa monnieri* was found to have the ability to induce reversible suppression of spermatogenesis and fertility in mice. However, it does not affect libido or cause toxic effects [51].

Administration of a dose of 500 mg/kg to rats resulted in decreased appetite and increased concentrations of albumin, urea, nitrogen, and aspartate aminotransferase, among others. Nevertheless, no notable changes in organ weights were observed at the end of the 90-day study [52].

4.4. Contraindications

Despite the high tolerance and safety of using *Bacopa monnieri* extract, there are also contraindications to using preparations containing this herb. Studies have shown that due to the inhibition of cytochrome isoenzymes (CYP2C9, CYP2C19, CYP1A2, CYP2D6, CYP3A4), interactions occur between the drug and the herb. Such interaction occurs between the extract of *Bacopa monnieri* and amitriptyline (a drug with antidepressant and sedative effects). *Bacopa monnieri*, by inhibiting cytochrome isoenzymes CYP3A and CYP2C responsible for the metabolism of amitriptyline, reduces the first-pass metabolism of this drug and additionally decreases the clearance of the mentioned drug after oral administration. Inhibition of cytochrome isoenzymes by Bacopa may lead to side effects of drugs metabolized by the inhibited isoenzymes. It has been shown that due to the herb–drug interaction, side effects occurred with the simultaneous intake of Bacopa extract and agomelatine—an antidepressant (metabolized by CYP1A2); back pain and excessive sweating were observed. A similar interaction is shown with the combination of *Bacopa monnieri* and Moclobemide—an antidepressant (metabolized by CYP2C19); myocardial infarction was observed as a side effect [53].

Particular caution should be exercised in cases of hyperthyroidism, as an in vivo study on male mice demonstrated that *Bacopa monnieri* leaf extract (200 mg/kg) significantly affects T4 (thyroxine) levels. The concentration of this hormone increased by 41%, which is undesirable in hyperthyroidism, where this hormone is already elevated. Attention should be paid to medications affecting T4 levels when simultaneously using *Bacopa monnieri* to avoid further increasing thyroxine levels [54].

Another study demonstrated that gastrointestinal side effects from using *Bacopa monnieri* extract are caused by the cholinergic action of this plant, leading to cholinergic stimulation of the gastrointestinal system, resulting in effects such as increased tension and peristalsis of the stomach and intestines, abdominal cramps, increased bowel movements, and peptic ulcer disease. On the other hand, *Bacopa monnieri* may also be useful in peptic ulcer disease not only due to its potential stress-relieving effects, which can mitigate the exacerbation of the disease, but also through its influence on the growth of *Helicobacter pylori*. Research indicates that chronic stress can weaken the gastric mucosa, making it more susceptible to *H. pylori* infection, a key factor in the development of peptic ulcers [55]. *Bacopa monnieri* ethanol extract showed antiulcer activity in a mouse model at a dose of 400 mg/kg body weight. At this dose, therapeutic effectiveness comparable to omeprazole, used in the treatment of gastric ulcers, at a dose of 20 mg/kg body weight was observed. The result is associated with increased mucin secretion and reduced desquamation of mucosal cells [56].

The cholinergic action of *Bacopa monnieri* results in increased acetylcholine levels (acetylcholinesterase inhibition), so special attention should be paid when simultaneously administering *Bacopa monnieri* extract and acetylcholinesterase inhibitors (AChE-I) currently used in treating Alzheimer's disease, to avoid a radical increase in acetylcholine levels. Due to its function, high acetylcholine levels may lead to bradycardia, so individuals predisposed to slow heart rates should consult their doctor about whether *Bacopa monnieri* extract supplementation is safe [50]. Early studies suggest that the concomitant use of *Bacopa monnieri* and galantamine may have a synergistic effect on cognitive function. Still, there is a need for further research into the potential risk of side effects and pharmacodynamic interactions [57]. Considering also its acetylcholine-enhancing properties, it can cause stomach ulcers, worsening of asthma, and chronic obstructive pulmonary disease or urogenital tract obstruction, which indicates monitoring of patients at risk [50]. It is also important to monitor patients taking medications for hypothyroidism through the effect of

Bacopa on the release of thyroid hormones to avoid excessive concentrations of the drug in the body, which can cause health risks for patients [54].

4.5. Bacopa Extract in At-Risk and Sensitive Groups

The use of Bacopa extract among vulnerable groups such as children, the elderly, or pregnant women is of particular interest because of their physiological differences. Despite its promising properties for supporting the nervous system, information on its safety of use in the previously mentioned populations is limited.

Among the clinical trials using Bacopa extract in recent years, two studies by the research group Kean et al. conducted on children aged 6–14 years can be found. The study tested the effectiveness of the extract in children diagnosed with ADHD. During the study, only a few cases of gastrointestinal discomfort were reported, which were short-lived and did not result in treatment discontinuation [58,59]. Other studies include two conducted on children aged 4–18 years and 6–12 years. The studies focused on the extract's properties for increasing children's intellectual abilities and reducing symptoms of ADHD. During the study, as in the previously cited ones, several cases of gastrointestinal disturbances were found, including vomiting and upset stomach lasting about three days, after which no further side effects were observed [60,61].

Another vulnerable population is the elderly. A recent study conducted by Best et al. on middle-aged and elderly patients (35–65 years) used a mixture containing *Bacopa monnieri*. Despite the sensitivity of this group to a number of medicinal substances, in this case, no side effects or intolerance to the received preparation were found during the study or during the follow-up phase [62]. Some studies reported the appearance of gastrointestinal disorders, in particular nausea, increased bowel movements and abdominal cramps, or, less frequently, dry mouth. Other side effects included fatigue and "flu-like" symptoms [50,57,63,64].

In the case of the last sensitive population, which is pregnant and lactating women, there is a lack of clinical studies on the safety of *Bacopa monnieri* extract. Only animal studies are available that do not address the aspect of safety during pregnancy and lactation [65,66]. As a result, many researchers note that women should not use Bacopa-containing supplements during this time. Further clinical studies evaluating the potential benefits and risks in this population are needed [67].

5. Bioavailability

Bacoside A is one of the main active compounds found in *Bacopa monnieri*. However, its water insolubility results in low bioavailability when administered orally. Additionally, it has a bitter taste, which is unacceptable for patients when using oral preparations. Research has been conducted to increase the bioavailability of bacoside A and simultaneously remove its bitter taste for more effective action of *Bacopa monnieri* and dose reduction. An inclusion complex with cyclodextrin (β-CD) was utilized to address both drawbacks of bacoside A. Bacoside A/β-CD complexes were created in various molar concentrations (1:1, 1:2, 1:3, 1:4, 1:5) using the co-precipitation method—each sample was tested separately. It was shown that the best solubility was exhibited by the sample with a *Bacopa monnieri*/β-CD ratio of 1:4 (solubility increased threefold). Additionally, the bitter taste of Bacoside A was masked [3].

In vivo studies conducted on mice attempted to enhance the anti-amnesic effect of the *Bacopa monnieri* extract using a new formulation, namely with the use of phospholipids. The study involved mice suffering from amnesia due to the natural aging process. A complex was created using Bacopa extract and L α-phosphatidylcholine to increase absorption in intestinal fluids. Due to their biocompatibility with phytochemical compounds, phospholipids caused the *Bacopa monnieri* preparation in complex form to demonstrate greater anti-amnesic efficacy than the ordinary preparation of this plant at the same dose (40 mg/kg, p.o.). In the Morris water maze test, a significant reduction in escape latency time (ELT), as well as an increase in time spent in the target quadrant (TSTQ), was observed in the phospholipid complex group, indicating improved acquisition and recall of spatial memory. Additionally, the complex caused a much stronger inhibition of AChE activity in the brain compared to the conventional *Bacopa monnieri* extract, suggesting a more effective enhancement of cholinergic transmission, which is crucial for memory processes [68].

The phospholipid complex contained high concentrations of active bacosides (Bacoside-A: 51.92%; Bacopaside-I: 43.2%; Bacopaside-II: 48.6%), which maintained effective concentrations of active compounds for a longer period compared to the conventional extract, indicating formulation stability and efficacy, and suggesting a prolonged half-life (t ½) and slower elimination. Following oral administration, the phospholipid complex showed higher serum concentrations of bacosides (Bacopaside I/BPC complex at 12.21 μg/mL vs. BE at 10.41 μg/mL; Bacopaside II/BPC complex at 12.28 μg/mL vs. BE at 10.38 μg/mL). This represents a 17–18% increase in maximum concentration (Cmax) for the bacosides. The physical intercalation of bacosides into the phospholipid layers enhances their solubility and facilitates transport across lipid-rich biological barriers such as the intestinal membrane and the blood–brain barrier. The presence of L-α-phosphatidylcholine improves molecular compatibility and absorption of phytocompounds in the gastrointestinal tract [4].

6. Modern Methods of Administration

Modern drug delivery methods are becoming increasingly popular in the context of phytotherapy. *Bacopa monnieri*, thanks to its pleiotropic effect, can be administered to patients in a variety of ways, increasing both its effectiveness and bioavailability. Researchers are interested not only in oral administration but also in transdermal or injectable forms. A major role is played by nanotechnology, which has made it possible to develop nanoparticles that make it possible, among other things, to overcome the blood–brain barrier. In addition, scientific reports also inform about other methods of administration of active ingredients such as bilosomes, ethosomes, and polymerosomes. With these innovations, *Bacopa monnieri* is gaining prominence in the context of a holistic approach to health and well-being.

6.1. Bilosomes

Bacopa monnieri extracts must cross the blood–brain barrier in order to work in the central nervous system. For this purpose, an attempt was made to place the extract in nanovesicles, forming liposomes and bilosomes. Two methods were used to obtain these formulations: solvent evaporation and thin-film hydration with phosphatidylcholine. Bilosomes and liposomes were analyzed in detail and characterized by homogeneous particle size and appropriate zeta potential. Bacopa extract at a dose of 200 mg/kg was used in a study on Swiss mice with memory loss. The use of bilosomes resulted in more effective memory improvement compared to liposomes. This is due to better bioavailability and greater stability in simulated gastric and intestinal juice conditions. It is worth noting that 1/10th of the dose considered in the acute toxicity evaluation was used for the study. This is due to the vastly improved bioavailability, which still requires more advanced studies such as radio-labeling [69].

6.2. Ethosomes

Pertaining to skin aging, Brahmi plays a crucial role in maintaining a youthful and healthy appearance due to its antioxidant properties, which protect the skin from free radicals—one of the main contributors to premature aging. Brahmi also contains compounds that stimulate collagen production and improve skin elasticity, reducing the appearance of wrinkles. This effect is attributed to the plant's chemical composition, particularly the presence of bacosides and alkaloids. Studies have been conducted in which *Bacopa monnieri* extract was incorporated into nanolipoidal vesicles, such as ethosomes, to enhance its penetration into the deeper layers of goat skin, aiming to increase collagen production and reduce elastin degradation in the dermal layer. Ethosomes exhibit flexibility and deformability, allowing them to penetrate the disordered stratum corneum and reach deeper skin layers. Through the use of ethosomes, *Bacopa monnieri* extract was able to penetrate up to a depth of 30–40 μm in goat skin. Permeation analysis demonstrated that systems following zero-order kinetics provide continuous substance release over an extended period, enhancing therapeutic effects. Therefore, ethosomes are suitable for transdermal delivery of herbal extracts [70].

6.3. Nanoparticles

Bacoside II, a bioactive compound present in *Bacopa monnieri*, exhibits in vitro cytotoxic effects against various cancer cell lines. It has been shown to induce cell cycle arrest and apoptosis in colorectal cancer cell lines while also inhibiting the migration and tubulogenesis of endothelial cell lines, thereby demonstrating anti-angiogenic properties. Research investigating the effects of PLGA-PEG-encapsulated Bacopaside II nanoparticles (BM1NPs), characterized by prolonged retention time in systemic circulation, on C6 glioma cells have revealed that BM1NP accelerates particle internalization within these cells. This suggests its potential anti-tumor activity through increased ROS levels, inhibition of cell proliferation, and induction of apoptosis in C6 glioma cells [71].

Studies were also conducted in which, similarly to the aforementioned approach, formulated solid lipid nanoparticles (SLNs) were used to facilitate the transport of the bacoside-rich extract across the blood–brain barrier. Swiss albino male mice were utilized in these experiments. The results demonstrated that SLNs exhibited greater efficacy in alleviating neurodegeneration compared to the extract alone, indicating their potential as a delivery system for bacosides across the blood–brain barrier in the treatment of Alzheimer's disease [72].

Similar experiments have been conducted in the context of epilepsy treatment, where the extract was converted into nanoparticles (BM3NP and BM4NP). Following the administration of BM3NP and BM4NP, KA-treated rats exhibited a significant reduction in epileptic spikes, a decrease in sleep latency, and an increase in NREM sleep duration, demonstrating the potential of nanoparticles in neutralizing epileptic seizures [73]. Further clinical studies may provide additional confirmation of the efficacy of herbal extracts in this regard.

6.4. Limitations of Modern Delivery Systems

Although advanced delivery systems show promise in improving the effectiveness of *Bacopa monnieri*, they also have some important limitations. One major issue is the lack of direct comparisons with traditional forms such as oral extracts or tinctures. Many studies report positive results using modern systems, but because they use different methods, doses, and models, it is hard to say which method works best overall. More consistent studies using the same standards are needed to compare their effectiveness. Another challenge is related to regulations and safety. Products that use nanotechnology must go through detailed safety testing, especially because their long-term effects on the body are not yet fully understood [74]. Also, the process of obtaining approval for these products can be complex and varies between countries, making it harder to bring them to market [75]. Advanced drug delivery systems, such as nanoparticles, liposomes, and other nanocarriers, often entail higher production costs due to their complexity and the specialized technologies required for their manufacture. These increased costs can pose significant barriers to large-scale production and widespread adoption [76]. Advanced drug delivery systems can be problematic if they do not take familiar forms that are acceptable to patients. The route and form of administration are key factors influencing patient acceptability. Acceptability is significantly affected by characteristics such as appearance, ease of swallowing, taste (palatability), and handling of the dosage form, particularly in the case of solid oral formulations. Attributes like size, shape, and texture also play an important role in shaping patient preferences, which can impact treatment adherence and overall effectiveness [77]. New or unfamiliar technologies, as well as alternative routes of administration, may cause discomfort, uncertainty, or resistance among users. In summary, while modern delivery systems offer exciting possibilities, more research is needed to compare them fairly, ensure their safety, and make them practical and acceptable for everyday use.

7. Legal Aspects

In the European Union (EU), *Bacopa monnieri* is considered a pharmacopeial plant, and a monograph by the European Medicines Agency (EMA) is currently being developed for this plant. *Bacopa monnieri* can be legally used as an ingredient in dietary supplements; however, it is not classified as a novel food since it was used in dietary supplements in the EU before 15 May 1997, and is therefore not subject to Regulation (EU) 2015/2283. However, applications other than dietary supplements—such as *Bacopa monnieri* in food—may require authorization under the Novel Food Regulation (EU) 2015/2283 before being placed on the EU market. Additionally, general food safety regulations must be considered, including Regulation (EC) No 178/2002, which establishes the general principles and requirements of food law, as well as other regulations that may restrict or regulate the use of the product in specific EU member states [78]. The U.S. Food and Drug Administration (FDA) has not issued specific regulations regarding *Bacopa monnieri* dietary supplements and has not approved this plant as a drug. Therefore, it has not made any official statements regarding its safety or effectiveness. The FDA has issued several general regulations concerning dietary supplements, such as the Dietary Supplement Health and Education Act (DSHEA) and the Current Good Manufacturing Practice (CGMP). DSHEA defines dietary supplements and establishes rules for their labeling and sale, while CGMP sets quality standards for the manufacturing process of dietary supplements. The FDA only intervenes if a supplement is found to be unsafe or is marketed illegally. Therefore, it is recommended that a healthcare professional be consulted before taking any dietary supplement containing *Bacopa monnieri* [79]. Preparations containing *Bacopa monnieri* are regulated in Canada as Natural Health Products (NHPs). They are, therefore, subject to the relevant regulations established by Health Canada, such as the Natural Health Products Regulations and the Natural Health Products Ingredients Database. *Bacopa monnieri* is used in dietary supplements; however, there are restrictions on the maximum dosage, which depend on factors such as age and health status. Additionally, manufacturers and importers must obtain the appropriate license to conduct such activities and comply with quality manufacturing standards [80,81].

8. Conclusions and Perspectives

Bacopa monnieri shows a wide range of neuroprotective effects, including antioxidant, anti-inflammatory, and cholinergic actions, which may help support cognitive and emotional functions. Results from preclinical studies and early clinical trials suggest its potential as a complementary treatment for neurodegenerative and neurodevelopmental disorders. To move forward, research should focus on connecting laboratory findings with real clinical benefits. While comparisons with standard drugs like donepezil are encouraging, they need to be backed by well-designed clinical trials that directly compare treatments and explore how *Bacopa monnieri* works in the human body. Modern delivery methods such as bilosomes and nanoparticles offer promising ways to improve the effectiveness of *Bacopa monnieri* by enhancing its absorption and stability. However, these approaches still need to be carefully tested for safety, patient acceptance, and scalability for wider use. Future studies should aim to confirm how *Bacopa monnieri* works in the human brain, identify who benefits most from its use, and ensure that extracts are consistent in quality and composition. Building a stronger link between lab research and clinical practice will be key to unlocking the full therapeutic potential of this plant.

Author Contributions: Conceptualization, J.C.-P. and A.G.; methodology, J.C.-P. and A.G.; investigation, A.G., M.S., J.P., K.B., N.N., H.K., I.S., P.T. and O.Z.-K.; resources, J.C.-P.; writing—original draft preparation, M.S., J.P., K.B., N.N., H.K., I.S. and P.T.; writing—review and editing, J.C.-P., O.Z.-K., A.S.-K. and A.G.; visualization, M.S; supervision, J.C.-P.; project administration, J.C.-P.; funding acquisition, J.C.-P. All authors have read and agreed to the published version of the manuscript.

Funding: This research was funded in whole by the National Science Centre, Poland, via grant Preludium nr UMO-2021/41/N/NZ7/01125. For the purpose of open access, the author has applied a CC-BY public copyright licence to any Author Accepted Manuscript (AAM) version arising from this submission.

Institutional Review Board Statement: Not applicable.

Informed Consent Statement: Not applicable.

Data Availability Statement: Not applicable.

Acknowledgments: Structures were downloaded from Reaxys. Figures were created with Biorender.com.

Conflicts of Interest: The authors declare no conflicts of interest.

Abbreviations

The following abbreviations are used in this manuscript:

ADHD	Attention deficit hyperactivity disorder
FDA	Food and Drug Administration
AChE-I	Acetylcholinesterase inhibitors
T4	Thyroxine
KEAP1	Kelch-like ECH-associated protein 1
MPTP	1-methyl-4-phenyl-1,2,3,6-tetrahydropyridine
DJ-1	Parkinson disease protein 7
DSHEA	Dietary Supplement Health and Education Act
CGMP	Current Good Manufacturing Practice

References

1. Ghosh, S.; Kumar, V.; Mukherjee, H.; Saini, S.; Gupta, S.; Chauhan, S.; Kushwaha, K.; Lahiri, D.; Sircar, D.; Roy, P. Assessment of the Mechanistic Role of an Indian Traditionally Used Ayurvedic Herb *Bacopa monnieri* (L.) Wettst. for Ameliorating Oxidative Stress in Neuronal Cells. *J. Ethnopharmacol.* **2024**, *328*, 117899. [CrossRef] [PubMed]
2. Dash, V.B.; Kashyap, V.L. *Materia Medica of Ayurveda*; Concept Publishing Company: New Delhi, India, 1980.
3. Brimson, J.M.; Brimson, S.; Prasanth, M.I.; Thitilertdecha, P.; Malar, D.S.; Tencomnao, T. The Effectiveness of *Bacopa monnieri* (Linn.) Wettst. as a Nootropic, Neuroprotective, or Antidepressant Supplement: Analysis of the Available Clinical Data. *Sci. Rep.* **2021**, *11*, 596. [CrossRef] [PubMed]
4. Fatima, U.; Roy, S.; Ahmad, S.; Ali, S.; Elkady, W.M.; Khan, I.; Alsaffar, R.M.; Adnan, M.; Islam, A.; Hassan, M.I. Pharmacological Attributes of *Bacopa monnieri* Extract: Current Updates and Clinical Manifestation. *Front. Nutr.* **2022**, *9*, 972379. [CrossRef]
5. Pandey, A.; Madan, S.; Sandhiya, K.; Sharma, R.; Raturi, A.; Bhatt, A.; Gaurav, N. Comparison of Antioxidant, Phytochemical Profiling of *Bacopa monnieri* (Brahmi). *Scientifictemper* **2022**, *13*, 286–293. [CrossRef]

6. Vo, T.P.; Nguyen, T.H.P.; Nguyen, V.K.; Dang, T.C.T.; Nguyen, L.G.K.; Chung, T.Q.; Vo, T.T.H.; Nguyen, D.Q. Extracting Bioactive Compounds and Proteins from *Bacopa monnieri* Using Natural Deep Eutectic Solvents. *PLoS ONE* **2024**, *19*, e0300969. [CrossRef]
7. Murthy, P.B.S.; Raju, V.R.; Ramakrisana, T.; Chakravarthy, M.S.; Kumar, K.V.; Kannababu, S.; Subbaraju, G.V. Estimation of Twelve Bacopa Saponins in *Bacopa monnieri* Extracts and Formulations by High-Performance Liquid Chromatography. *Chem. Pharm. Bull.* **2006**, *54*, 907–911. [CrossRef] [PubMed]
8. Sairam, K.; Dorababu, M.; Goel, R.K.; Bhattacharya, S.K. Antidepressant Activity of Standardized Extract of *Bacopa monniera* in Experimental Models of Depression in Rats. *Phytomedicine* **2002**, *9*, 207–211. [CrossRef]
9. Prakash, N.S.; Sundaram, R.; Mitra, S.K. In Vitro and In Vivo Anticancer Activity of Bacoside A from Whole Plant of *Bacopa monnieiri* (Linn). *Am. J. Pharmacol. Toxicol.* **2011**, *6*, 11–19. [CrossRef]
10. Dubey, T.; Chinnathambi, S. Brahmi (*Bacopa monnieri*): An Ayurvedic Herb against the Alzheimer's Disease. *Arch. Biochem. Biophys.* **2019**, *676*, 108153. [CrossRef]
11. Bhandari, P.; Kumar, N.; Singh, B.; Kaul, V.K. Cucurbitacins from *Bacopa monnieri*. *Phytochemistry* **2007**, *68*, 1248–1254. [CrossRef]
12. Deepak, M.; Sangli, G.K.; Arun, P.C.; Amit, A. Quantitative Determination of the Major Saponin Mixture Bacoside A in *Bacopa monnieri* by HPLC. *Phytochem. Anal.* **2005**, *16*, 24–29. [CrossRef] [PubMed]
13. Lan, T.; Wang, L.; Xu, Q.; Liu, W.; Jin, H.; Mao, W.; Wang, X.; Wang, X. Growth Inhibitory Effect of Cucurbitacin E on Breast Cancer Cells. *Int. J. Clin. Exp. Pathol.* **2013**, *6*, 1799–1805. [PubMed]
14. Jayaprakasam, B.; Seeram, N.P.; Nair, M.G. Anticancer and Antiinflammatory Activities of Cucurbitacins from *Cucurbita Andreana*. *Cancer Lett.* **2003**, *189*, 11–16. [CrossRef]
15. Martínez-García, M.; Garduño-Solórzano, G.; Lopes, G.; Sanchez, B.A.; Urbatzka, R.; Hentschke, G.S.; Campos, J.E.; Vasconcelos, V.M.O. Antioxidant, Anti-Inflammatory and Anti-Obesity Potential of Extracts Containing Phenols, Chlorophyll and Carotenoids from Mexican Wild Populations of *Bacopa monnieri* (L.) Wettst. *Biology* **2023**, *12*, 620. [CrossRef]
16. Meena, U.K.; Maurya, A.K. *Bacopa monnieri* Extract Diminish Hypoxia-Induced Anxiety by Regulating HIF-1α Signaling and Enhancing the Antioxidant Defense System in Hippocampus. *Neuromolecular Med.* **2025**, *27*, 11. [CrossRef]
17. Russo, A.; Izzo, A.A.; Borrelli, F.; Renis, M.; Vanella, A. Free Radical Scavenging Capacity and Protective Effect of *Bacopa monniera* L. on DNA Damage. *Phytother. Res.* **2003**, *17*, 870–875. [CrossRef] [PubMed]
18. Malishev, R.; Shaham-Niv, S.; Nandi, S.; Kolusheva, S.; Gazit, E.; Jelinek, R. Bacoside-A, an Indian Traditional-Medicine Substance, Inhibits β-Amyloid Cytotoxicity, Fibrillation, and Membrane Interactions. *ACS Chem. Neurosci.* **2017**, *8*, 884–891. [CrossRef]
19. Shoukat, S.; Zia, M.A.; Uzair, M.; Attia, K.A.; Abushady, A.M.; Fiaz, S.; Ali, S.; Yang, S.H.; Ali, G.M. *Bacopa monnieri*: A Promising Herbal Approach for Neurodegenerative Disease Treatment Supported by in Silico and in Vitro Research. *Heliyon* **2023**, *9*, e21161. [CrossRef]
20. Deolankar, S.C.; Najar, M.A.; Ramesh, P.; Kanichery, A.; Kudva, A.K.; Raghu, S.V.; Prasad, T.S.K. Discovery of Molecular Networks of Neuroprotection Conferred by Brahmi Extract in Aβ42-Induced Toxicity Model of Drosophila Melanogaster Using a Quantitative Proteomic Approach. *Mol. Neurobiol.* **2023**, *60*, 303–316. [CrossRef]
21. Tiwari, S.; Atluri, V.; Kaushik, A.; Yndart, A.; Nair, M. Alzheimer's Disease: Pathogenesis, Diagnostics, and Therapeutics. *Int. J. Nanomed.* **2019**, *14*, 5541–5554. [CrossRef]
22. Chen, Z.-R.; Huang, J.-B.; Yang, S.-L.; Hong, F.-F. Role of Cholinergic Signaling in Alzheimer's Disease. *Molecules* **2022**, *27*, 1816. [CrossRef] [PubMed]
23. Canu, N.; Amadoro, G.; Triaca, V.; Latina, V.; Sposato, V.; Corsetti, V.; Severini, C.; Ciotti, M.T.; Calissano, P. The Intersection of NGF/TrkA Signaling and Amyloid Precursor Protein Processing in Alzheimer's Disease Neuropathology. *Int. J. Mol. Sci.* **2017**, *18*, 1319. [CrossRef]
24. Roy, S.; Chakravarty, S.; Talukdar, P.; Soumendra; Talapatra, N. Identification of Bioactive Compounds Present in *Bacopa monnieri* Linn. Against Caspase-3 and Tau Protein Kinase I to Prevent Alzheimer's Disease: An in Silico Study. *Pharma Innov. J.* **2019**, *8*, 855–861.
25. Mathew, M.; Subramanian, S. Evaluation of the anti-amyloidogenic potential of nootropic herbal extracts in vitro. *Int. J. Pharm. Sci. Res.* **2012**, *3*, 4276–4280.
26. Neuroprotective Effect of Bacopa monnieri on Beta-Amyloid-Induced Cell Death in Primary Cortical Culture-PubMed. Available online: https://pubmed.ncbi.nlm.nih.gov/18755259/ (accessed on 5 February 2025).
27. Peera, D.K. Neuroprotective Effect of *Bacopa monniera* on Memory Deficits and ATPase System in Alzheimer's Disease (AD) Induced Mice. *J. Sci. Innov. Res.* **2013**, *2*, 719–735.
28. Peth-Nui, T.; Wattanathorn, J.; Muchimapura, S.; Tong-Un, T.; Piyavhatkul, N.; Rangseekajee, P.; Ingkaninan, K.; Vittaya-Areekul, S. Effects of 12-Week *Bacopa monnieri* Consumption on Attention, Cognitive Processing, Working Memory, and Functions of Both Cholinergic and Monoaminergic Systems in Healthy Elderly Volunteers. *Evid. Based Complement. Altern. Med.* **2012**, *2012*, 606424. [CrossRef]

29. Modi, M.; Prabhakar, S.; Vishnu, V.; Mohanty, M.; Sharma, A.; Medhi, B.; Mittal, B.; Khandelwal, N.; Goyal, M.; Lal, V.; et al. Efficacy of *Bacopa monnieri* (Brahmi) and Donepezil in Alzheimer's Disease and Mild Cognitive Impairment: A Randomized Double-Blind Parallel Phase 2b Study. *Ann. Indian Acad. Neurol.* **2024**, *23*, 767–773. [CrossRef]
30. Vázquez-Vélez, G.E.; Zoghbi, H.Y. Parkinson's Disease Genetics and Pathophysiology. *Annu. Rev. Neurosci.* **2021**, *44*, 87–108. [CrossRef]
31. Chandrasekar, S.; Thangarajan, S.; Loganathan, S.; Sundaram, S.; Kumarasamy, P. Molecular Docking Studies of Bacoside-A, an Active Component of *Bacopa monniera* with DJ1 for Anti-Parkinson's Drug Design. *Biomirror* **2013**, *4*, 67.
32. Singh, B.; Pandey, S.; Rumman, M.; Kumar, S.; Kushwaha, P.P.; Verma, R.; Mahdi, A.A. Neuroprotective and Neurorescue Mode of Action of *Bacopa monnieri* (L.) Wettst in 1-Methyl-4-Phenyl-1,2,3,6-Tetrahydropyridine-Induced Parkinson's Disease: An In Silico and In Vivo Study. *Front. Pharmacol.* **2021**, *12*, 616413. [CrossRef]
33. Jadiya, P.; Khan, A.; Sammi, S.R.; Kaur, S.; Mir, S.S.; Nazir, A. Anti-Parkinsonian Effects of *Bacopa monnieri*: Insights from Transgenic and Pharmacological Caenorhabditis Elegans Models of Parkinson's Disease. *Biochem. Biophys. Res. Commun.* **2011**, *413*, 605–610. [CrossRef] [PubMed]
34. Siddique, Y.H.; Mujtaba, S.F.; Faisal, M.; Jyoti, S.; Naz, F. The Effect of *Bacopa monnieri* Leaf Extract on Dietary Supplementation in Transgenic Drosophila Model of Parkinson's Disease. *Eur. J. Integr. Med.* **2014**, *6*, 571–580. [CrossRef]
35. Swathi, G.; Rajendra, W. Protective role of *Bacopa monnieri* on induced parkinson's disease with particular reference to catecholamine system. *Int. J. Pharm. Pharm. Sci.* **2014**, *6*, 379–382.
36. Santos, A.F.D.; Souza, M.M.Q.; Amaral, E.C.; Albuquerque, E.R.; Bortoloti, D.S.; Gasparotto Junior, A.; Lourenço, E.L.B.; Lovato, E.C.W.; Lívero, F.A.D.R. *Bacopa monnieri* in Patients with Parkinson's Disease: A Pilot Study. *J. Med. Food* **2023**, *26*, 2.
37. Sharma, A.; Couture, J. A Review of the Pathophysiology, Etiology, and Treatment of Attention-Deficit Hyperactivity Disorder (ADHD). *Ann. Pharmacother.* **2014**, *48*, 209–225. [CrossRef] [PubMed]
38. Dave, U.P.; Dingankar, S.R.; Saxena, V.S.; Joseph, J.A.; Bethapudi, B.; Agarwal, A.; Kudiganti, V. An Open-Label Study to Elucidate the Effects of Standardized *Bacopa monnieri* Extract in the Management of Symptoms of Attention-Deficit Hyperactivity Disorder in Children. *Adv. Mind Body Med.* **2014**, *28*, 10–15.
39. Schechter, L.E.; Ring, R.H.; Beyer, C.E.; Hughes, Z.A.; Khawaja, X.; Malberg, J.E.; Rosenzweig-Lipson, S. Innovative Approaches for the Development of Antidepressant Drugs: Current and Future Strategies. *NeuroRx* **2005**, *2*, 590–611. [CrossRef]
40. Chaachouay, N.; Zidane, L. Plant-Derived Natural Products: A Source for Drug Discovery and Development. *Drugs Drug Candidates* **2024**, *3*, 184–207. [CrossRef]
41. Mannan, A.; Abir, A.B.; Rahman, R. Antidepressant-like Effects of Methanolic Extract of *Bacopa monniera* in Mice. *BMC Complement. Altern. Med.* **2015**, *15*, 337. [CrossRef]
42. Yankelevitch-Yahav, R.; Franko, M.; Huly, A.; Doron, R. The Forced Swim Test as a Model of Depressive-like Behavior. *J. Vis. Exp.* **2015**, *97*, e52587. [CrossRef]
43. Seibenhener, M.L.; Wooten, M.C. Use of the Open Field Maze to Measure Locomotor and Anxiety-like Behavior in Mice. *J. Vis. Exp.* **2015**, *96*, e52434. [CrossRef]
44. Psychiatry.Org-What Are Anxiety Disorders? Available online: https://www.psychiatry.org/patients-families/anxiety-disorders/what-are-anxiety-disorders (accessed on 25 June 2024).
45. Kumar, N.; Abichandani, L.G.; Thawani, V.; Gharpure, K.J.; Naidu, M.U.R.; Venkat Ramana, G. Efficacy of Standardized Extract of *Bacopa monnieri* (Bacognize®) on Cognitive Functions of Medical Students: A Six-Week, Randomized Placebo-Controlled Trial. *Evid. Based Complement. Altern. Med.* **2016**, *2016*, 4103423. [CrossRef] [PubMed]
46. Benson, S.; Downey, L.A.; Stough, C.; Wetherell, M.; Zangara, A.; Scholey, A. An Acute, Double-Blind, Placebo-Controlled Cross-over Study of 320 Mg and 640 Mg Doses of *Bacopa monnieri* (CDRI 08) on Multitasking Stress Reactivity and Mood. *Phytother. Res.* **2014**, *28*, 551–559. [CrossRef]
47. *Bacopa monnieri* . In *LiverTox: Clinical and Research Information on Drug-Induced Liver Injury*; National Institute of Diabetes and Digestive and Kidney Diseases: Bethesda, MD, USA, 2012.
48. Sireeratawong, S.; Jaijoy, K.; Khonsung, P.; Lertprasertsuk, N.; Ingkaninan, K. Acute and Chronic Toxicities of *Bacopa monnieri* Extract in Sprague-Dawley Rats. *BMC Complement. Altern. Med.* **2016**, *16*, 249. [CrossRef]
49. Pravina, K.; Ravindra, K.R.; Goudar, K.S.; Vinod, D.R.; Joshua, A.J.; Wasim, P.; Venkateshwarlu, K.; Saxena, V.S.; Amit, A. Safety Evaluation of BacoMind in Healthy Volunteers: A Phase I Study. *Phytomedicine* **2007**, *14*, 301–308. [CrossRef]
50. Morgan, A.; Stevens, J. Does *Bacopa monnieri* Improve Memory Performance in Older Persons? Results of a Randomized, Placebo-Controlled, Double-Blind Trial. *J. Altern. Complement. Med.* **2010**, *16*, 753–759. [CrossRef] [PubMed]
51. Singh, A.; Singh, S.K. Evaluation of Antifertility Potential of Brahmi in Male Mouse. *Contraception* **2009**, *79*, 71–79. [CrossRef]
52. Saraf, M.K.; Prabhakar, S.; Pandhi, P.; Anand, A. *Bacopa monniera* Ameliorates Amnesic Effects of Diazepam Qualifying Behavioral-Molecular Partitioning. *Neuroscience* **2008**, *155*, 476–484. [CrossRef]
53. Siwek, M.; Woroń, J.; Wrzosek, A.; Gupało, J.; Chrobak, A.A. Harder, Better, Faster, Stronger? Retrospective Chart Review of Adverse Events of Interactions between Adaptogens and Antidepressant Drugs. *Front. Pharmacol.* **2023**, *14*, 1271776. [CrossRef]

54. Kar, A.; Panda, S.; Bharti, S. Relative Efficacy of Three Medicinal Plant Extracts in the Alteration of Thyroid Hormone Concentrations in Male Mice. *J. Ethnopharmacol.* **2002**, *81*, 281–285. [CrossRef]
55. Levenstein, S.; Rosenstock, S.; Jacobsen, R.K.; Jorgensen, T. Psychological Stress Increases Risk for Peptic Ulcer, Regardless of Helicobacter Pylori Infection or Use of Nonsteroidal Anti-Inflammatory Drugs. *Clin. Gastroenterol. Hepatol.* **2015**, *13*, 498–506.e1. [CrossRef] [PubMed]
56. Evaluation of Antiulcerogenic Activity of Bacopa monnieri (LINN.) on Ethanol-Induced Gastric Injury in Mice. Available online: https://www.researchgate.net/publication/326032975_Evaluation_of_Antiulcerogenic_Activity_of_Bacopa_Monnieri_LINN_on_Ethanol-Induced_Gastric_Injury_In_Mice (accessed on 5 February 2025).
57. Calabrese, C.; Gregory, W.L.; Leo, M.; Kraemer, D.; Bone, K.; Oken, B. Effects of a Standardized *Bacopa monnieri* Extract on Cognitive Performance, Anxiety, and Depression in the Elderly: A Randomized, Double-Blind, Placebo-Controlled Trial. *J. Altern. Complement. Med.* **2008**, *14*, 707–713. [CrossRef] [PubMed]
58. Kean, J.D.; Downey, L.A.; Sarris, J.; Kaufman, J.; Zangara, A.; Stough, C. Effects of *Bacopa monnieri* (CDRI 08®) in a Population of Males Exhibiting Inattention and Hyperactivity Aged 6 to 14 Years: A Randomized, Double-Blind, Placebo-Controlled Trial. *Phytother. Res.* **2022**, *36*, 996–1012. [CrossRef] [PubMed]
59. Kean, J.D.; Kaufman, J.; Lomas, J.; Goh, A.; White, D.; Simpson, D.; Scholey, A.; Singh, H.; Sarris, J.; Zangara, A.; et al. A Randomized Controlled Trial Investigating the Effects of a Special Extract of *Bacopa monnieri* (CDRI 08) on Hyperactivity and Inattention in Male Children and Adolescents: BACHI Study Protocol (ANZCTRN12612000827831). *Nutrients* **2015**, *7*, 9931–9945. [CrossRef]
60. Usha, P.D.; Wasim, P.; Joshua, J.A.; Geetharani, P.; Murali, B.; Mayachari, A.S.; Venkateshwarlu, K.; Saxena, V.S.; Deepak, M.; Amit, A. BacoMind®: A Cognitive Enhancer in Children Requiring Individual Education Programme. *J. Pharmacol. Toxicol.* **2008**, *3*, 302–310. [CrossRef]
61. Acquarulo, B.; Tandon, P.; Macica, C.M. Suspected cholinergic toxicity due to cevimeline hydrochloride and Bacopa monnieri interaction: A case report. *J. Med. Case Rep.* **2022**, *16*, 253. [CrossRef]
62. Best, T.; Miller, J.; Teo, W.-P. Neurocognitive Effects a Combined Polyphenolic-Rich Herbal Extract in Healthy Middle-Aged Adults-a Randomised, Double-Blind, Placebo-Controlled Study. *Nutr. Neurosci.* **2024**, *27*, 1293–1305. [CrossRef]
63. Roodenrys, S.; Booth, D.; Bulzomi, S.; Phipps, A.; Micallef, C.; Smoker, J. Chronic Effects of Brahmi (*Bacopa monnieri*) on Human Memory. *Neuropsychopharmacology* **2002**, *27*, 279–281. [CrossRef]
64. Stough, C.K.; Pase, M.P.; Cropley, V.; Myers, S.; Nolidin, K.; King, R.; Camfield, D.; Wesnes, K.; Pipingas, A.; Croft, K.; et al. A Randomized Controlled Trial Investigating the Effect of Pycnogenol and Bacopa CDRI08 Herbal Medicines on Cognitive, Cardiovascular, and Biochemical Functioning in Cognitively Healthy Elderly People: The Australian Research Council Longevity Intervention (ARCLI) Study Protocol (ANZCTR12611000487910). *Nutr. J.* **2012**, *11*, 11. [CrossRef]
65. Abhishek, M.; Rubal, S.; Rohit, K.; Rupa, J.; Phulen, S.; Gurjeet, K.; Raj, S.A.; Manisha, P.; Alka, B.; Ramprasad, P.; et al. Neuroprotective Effect of the Standardised Extract of *Bacopa monnieri* (BacoMind) in Valproic Acid Model of Autism Spectrum Disorder in Rats. *J. Ethnopharmacol.* **2022**, *293*, 115199. [CrossRef]
66. Sudhishma; Devadasa Acharya, S.; Ullal, S.D.; Blossom, V.; Parida, A.; Noushida, N. Levetiracetam Exposure during Prenatal and Postnatal Period Induces Cognitive Decline in Rat Offsprings, Not Completely Prevented by *Bacopa monnieri*. *J. Complement. Integr. Med.* **2022**, *19*, 897–903. [CrossRef] [PubMed]
67. Chaudhari, K.S.; Tiwari, N.R.; Tiwari, R.R.; Sharma, R.S. Neurocognitive Effect of Nootropic Drug Brahmi (*Bacopa monnieri*) in Alzheimer's Disease. *Ann. Neurosci.* **2017**, *24*, 111–122. [CrossRef] [PubMed]
68. Habbu, P.; Madagundi, S.; Kulkarni, R.; Jadav, S.; Vanakudri, R.; Kulkarni, V. Preparation and Evaluation of *Bacopa*–Phospholipid Complex for Antiamnesic Activity in Rodents. *Drug Invent. Today* **2013**, *5*, 13–21. [CrossRef]
69. Narayanan, V.A.; Sharma, A.; Rajesh, K.S.; Arunraj, T.R.; Gururaj, M.P.; Parasuraman, S.; John, A. Bilosomes as a Potential Carrier to Enhance Cognitive Effects of *Bacopa monnieri* Extract on Oral Administration. *J. Health Allied Sci. NU* **2023**, *13*, 421–430. [CrossRef]
70. Dwivedi, D.; Nimisha; Mishra, N.; Singh, S.P.; Shukla, A.K. Performance Evaluation of Bacopa monneri-Loaded Ethosomes for Topical Delivery. | EBSCOhost. Available online: https://openurl.ebsco.com/contentitem/doi:10.31018/jans.v16i3.5435?sid=ebsco:plink:crawler&id=ebsco:doi:10.31018/jans.v16i3.5435 (accessed on 17 February 2025).
71. Sekhar, V.C.; Viswanathan, G.; Baby, S. Bacopaside II Nanoparticles Inhibit Proliferation of C6 Glioma Cells. *Phytomedicine Plus* **2021**, *1*, 100040. [CrossRef]
72. Kumar, R.; Garg, R.; Khurana, N. A Comparative in Vivo Evaluation of Anti-Alzheimer Activity of Bacopa Extract and Its Solid Lipid Nanoparticles. *Curr. Bioact. Compd.* **2021**, *17*, 6–16. [CrossRef]
73. Sekhar, V.C.; Gulia, K.K.; Deepti, A.; Chakrapani, P.S.B.; Baby, S.; Viswanathan, G. Protection by Nano-Encapsulated Bacoside A and Bacopaside I in Seizure Alleviation and Improvement in Sleep-In Vitro and In Vivo Evidences. *Mol. Neurobiol.* **2024**, *61*, 3296–3313. [CrossRef]

74. Ma, X.; Tian, Y.; Yang, R.; Wang, H.; Allahou, L.W.; Chang, J.; Williams, G.; Knowles, J.C.; Poma, A. Nanotechnology in Healthcare, and Its Safety and Environmental Risks. *J. Nanobiotechnol.* **2024**, *22*, 715. [CrossRef]
75. Farjadian, F.; Ghasemi, A.; Gohari, O.; Roointan, A.; Karimi, M.; Hamblin, M.R. Nanopharmaceuticals and Nanomedicines Currently on the Market: Challenges and Opportunities. *Nanomedicine* **2019**, *14*, 93–126. [CrossRef]
76. Ezike, T.C.; Okpala, U.S.; Onoja, U.L.; Nwike, C.P.; Ezeako, E.C.; Okpara, O.J.; Okoroafor, C.C.; Eze, S.C.; Kalu, O.L.; Odoh, E.C.; et al. Advances in Drug Delivery Systems, Challenges and Future Directions. *Heliyon* **2023**, *9*, e17488. [CrossRef]
77. Hauber, B.; Hand, M.V.; Hancock, B.C.; Zarrella, J.; Harding, L.; Ogden-Barker, M.; Antipas, A.S.; Watt, S.J. Patient Acceptability and Preferences for Solid Oral Dosage Form Drug Product Attributes: A Scoping Review. *Patient Prefer. Adherence* **2024**, *18*, 1281–1297. [CrossRef] [PubMed]
78. Food and Feed Information Portal Database | FIP. Available online: https://ec.europa.eu/food/food-feed-portal/screen/novel-food-catalogue/search (accessed on 16 February 2025).
79. Center for Food Safety and Applied Nutrition. Peak Nootropics LLC Aka Advanced Nootropics-557887-02/05/2019. Available online: https://www.fda.gov/inspections-compliance-enforcement-and-criminal-investigations/warning-letters/peak-nootropics-llc-aka-advanced-nootropics-557887-02052019 (accessed on 16 February 2025).
80. Health Canada. Natural Health Product Regulation in Canada: Overview. Available online: https://www.canada.ca/en/health-canada/services/drugs-health-products/natural-non-prescription/regulation.html (accessed on 16 February 2025).
81. Branch, L.S. Consolidated Federal Laws of Canada, Natural Health Products Regulations. Available online: https://laws-lois.justice.gc.ca/eng/regulations/sor-2003-196/page-1.html#h-700387 (accessed on 16 February 2025).

nutrients

MDPI

Systematic Review

Effects of Creatine and β-Alanine Co-Supplementation on Exercise Performance and Body Composition: A Systematic Review

Damoon Ashtary-Larky [1,*], Darren G. Candow [2], Scott C. Forbes [3], Leila Hajizadeh [4], Jose Antonio [5] and Katsuhiko Suzuki [6]

[1] Nutrition and Metabolic Diseases Research Center, Ahvaz Jundishapur University of Medical Sciences, Ahvaz 6135715794, Iran
[2] Faculty of Kinesiology and Health Studies, University of Regina, Regina, SK S4S 0A2, Canada; darren.candow@uregina.ca
[3] Department of Physical Education Studies, Brandon University, Brandon, MB R7A 6A9, Canada; forbess@brandonu.ca
[4] Department of Sport Physiology, Marvdasht Branch, Islamic Azad University, Marvdasht 7371113119, Iran; hajizadehleila266@gmail.com
[5] Department of Health and Human Performance, Nova Southeastern University, Davie, FL 33314, USA; jose.antonio@nova.edu
[6] Faculty of Sport Sciences, Waseda University, Tokorozawa 359-1192, Japan; katsu.suzu@waseda.jp
* Correspondence: damoon_ashtary@yahoo.com; Tel.: +98-9366113574

Abstract: Background/Objectives: Creatine and β-alanine are two widely used dietary supplements known to enhance exercise performance and improve body composition; however, less is known regarding the synergistic effects of combining the two supplements. **Methods**: A systematic search was conducted across PubMed/MEDLINE, Scopus, and Web of Science databases for randomized controlled trials (RCTs) published up to March 2025. Eligible studies included adult participants receiving creatine and β-alanine together compared to creatine or β-alanine alone for at least four weeks and assessed measures of exercise performance and/or body composition. Study quality was assessed using the Cochrane Risk of Bias tool. **Results**: A total of 7 randomized controlled trials ($n = 263$ participants; 231 males and 32 females) met the inclusion criteria. Collectively, the combination of creatine and β-alanine supplementation enhanced high-intensity exercise performance, particularly anaerobic power and repeated-bout performance, compared to creatine or β-alanine alone. Co-ingestion of creatine and β-alanine supplementation did not increase measures of maximal strength compared to creatine alone. The effects of creatine and β-alanine supplementation on body composition were equivocal, with one study reporting greater lean mass gains and fat mass reductions compared to creatine and β-alanine supplementation individually, while another found no significant improvements. Additionally, no significant improvements in aerobic endurance capacity (VO_2max, lactate threshold, or time to exhaustion) were observed from creatine and β-alanine supplementation co-ingestion. **Conclusions**: The combination of creatine and β-alanine supplementation may be effective for enhancing high-intensity exercise performance but has no greater effect on maximal strength, body composition, or measures of aerobic capacity compared to creatine or β-alanine alone.

Keywords: creatine; β-alanine; anaerobic power; maximal strength; endurance; body composition

https://doi.org/10.3390/nu17132074

1. Introduction

Creatine and β-alanine are among the most widely utilized ergogenic supplements to enhance exercise performance [1,2]. Creatine supplementation is well-established for its role in increasing intramuscular phosphocreatine stores, thereby enhancing rapid adenosine triphosphate (ATP) resynthesis during high-intensity, short-duration exercise [3]. Further, creatine has been shown to enhance protein kinetics, satellite cells, and myogenic regulatory factors and attenuate myostatin, inflammation, and oxidative stress [4]. These mechanisms contribute to improvements in power output, and chronic creatine supplementation—typically involving a loading phase of approximately 20 g/day for 5–7 days, followed by a maintenance dose of 2–5 g/day—has been associated with greater gains in lean body mass (LBM) and strength during resistance training [5].

β-Alanine, a non-essential amino acid, serves as a precursor to carnosine [6,7], a key intramuscular buffer that helps regulate exercise-induced acidosis [8]. Chronic β-alanine supplementation (typically 3.2–6.4 g/day for 2–10 weeks) increases muscle carnosine content by approximately 10% after 2 weeks and up to 80% following 10 weeks of supplementation [9]. This elevation in intramuscular carnosine enhances the muscle's buffering capacity, potentially delaying the onset of fatigue and improving high-intensity performance lasting between 1 and 4 min [10].

Given their physiological mechanisms, co-supplementation with creatine and β-alanine has been purported to elicit complementary or potentially synergistic ergogenic effects. Preliminary investigations into the combined effects of creatine and β-alanine supplementation have reported promising but mixed results. Zoeller et al. suggested that co-supplementation with creatine and β-alanine may improve ventilatory threshold (VT) and lactate threshold (LT) during incremental cycling exercise in male participants [11]. Additionally, in the context of strength and power performance, Hoffman et al. reported that 10 weeks of creatine and β-alanine supplementation during resistance training conferred "independent and potentially synergistic" benefits in male athletes [12]. However, despite these positive findings, the evidence remains inconclusive, as some studies have failed to observe additive effects of combining these supplements [9]. Given the variability in outcomes, a systematic review of randomized controlled trials (RCTs) is warranted to elucidate the combined effects of creatine and β-alanine supplementation on exercise performance and body composition. Therefore, this review aims to critically assess the evidence from RCTs on co-supplementation with creatine and β-alanine, with a specific focus on key performance outcomes (strength, power, muscular endurance, and aerobic capacity) and body composition changes (lean mass and fat mass). Given the variability in study designs and methodologies, the findings are synthesized qualitatively, without conducting a meta-analysis, to provide a comprehensive and up-to-date evaluation of the potential additive benefits of combined creatine and β-alanine supplementation. This review seeks to determine whether co-supplementation offers superior ergogenic effects compared to either supplement alone, thereby providing evidence-based insights for athletes, coaches, and sports practitioners regarding its efficacy and the certainty of available evidence. Based on previous studies, we hypothesized that co-supplementation with creatine and β-alanine would have beneficial effects on exercise performance and body composition compared to either supplement alone.

2. Materials and Methods

This systematic review was conducted in accordance with the Preferred Reporting Items for Systematic Reviews and Meta-Analyses (PRISMA) guidelines, ensuring transparent and rigorous reporting [13]. A predefined protocol was established to outline the objectives, inclusion criteria, and methodology for evidence synthesis. This systematic review protocol was registered with the International Prospective Register of Systematic Reviews (PROSPERO) under the registration number CRD420251066302.

2.1. Eligibility Criteria

Studies were included if: (1) population: adults (athletes or untrained) of any sex; (2) intervention: combined supplementation with creatine and β-alanine, administered concurrently for at least 4 weeks (or a duration sufficient to load both supplements), alone or in addition to a training program; multi-ingredient interventions were excluded unless the co-interventions were matched between groups and the only difference was the presence or absence of creatine and β-alanine, allowing isolation of its effects; (3) comparators: placebo or single-supplement groups (creatine-only or β-alanine-only) in a randomized design; (4) outcomes: exercise performance measures (strength, power, endurance, aerobic capacity, etc.) and/or body composition (LBM, fat mass, or body fat percentage); (5) study design: randomized controlled trials only.

Studies were excluded if they investigated acute, single-dose supplementation rather than chronic supplementation; utilized non-randomized designs, observational methodologies, or case studies; or examined multi-ingredient supplements where additional ergogenic substances (e.g., citrulline) were co-administered—unless those ingredients were matched across control groups to isolate the effects of creatine and β-alanine. No restrictions were placed on participant training status or the specific training protocols used, provided that all groups within a study followed comparable training conditions.

2.2. Information Sources and Search Strategy

A comprehensive literature search was performed using PubMed/MEDLINE, Scopus, and Web of Science from inception through March 2025. The following keywords and Boolean combinations were used: "creatine AND beta-alanine", "β-alanine AND creatine AND performance", "combined supplementation", "carnosine", "supplementation", "co-supplementation", "strength", "one-repetition maximum", "1RM", "endurance", "body composition", "VO_2max", "weight loss", "lean mass", and "randomized trial". Reference lists of relevant papers, including previous reviews and position stands, were hand-searched for any additional RCTs. No language restrictions were applied, although all identified studies were in English. Database search results were merged, and duplicates were removed using reference management software (EndNote X9 software).

2.3. Study Selection

The titles and abstracts of retrieved studies were screened to determine their relevance. Full-text articles deemed potentially eligible were then assessed against the predefined inclusion criteria. In cases where eligibility was uncertain, careful reconsideration of the inclusion and exclusion criteria was conducted to ensure objective selection.

2.4. Data Extraction

For each included trial, descriptive data were extracted, including sample size, participant characteristics, training status, supplementation protocol (dosing and duration), training program (if applicable), and comparator groups. Outcome measures related to exercise performance (e.g., one-repetition maximum (1RM) strength, Wingate anaerobic power, jump performance, time-to-exhaustion (TTE), and VO_2max) and body composition (e.g., body mass, lean mass, fat mass, and body fat percentage) were recorded. When available, the magnitude and statistical significance of changes in these outcomes were extracted, particularly in the co-supplementation group compared to control or single-supplement groups.

2.5. Risk of Bias Assessment

The risk of bias was evaluated using the Cochrane risk-of-bias assessment tool, which considers multiple methodological domains, including randomization process, allocation concealment, participant and staff blinding, outcome assessor blinding, completeness of outcome data, selective reporting, and other sources of bias. Based on these criteria, studies were categorized into three groups: high risk of bias (≥2 domains rated as high risk), unclear risk of bias (exactly two domains rated as high risk), and low risk of bias (<2 domains rated as high risk).

2.6. Synthesis of Results

Due to the heterogeneity in study designs and outcome measures, a meta-analysis was not conducted. Instead, a qualitative synthesis was performed, organizing findings into distinct outcome domains: strength and power performance, endurance performance, and body composition. Results from individual studies were systematically reported and compared, emphasizing whether co-supplementation with creatine and β-alanine yielded superior improvements relative to placebo or single-supplement conditions. Where relevant, effect directions and statistical significance were documented. The narrative synthesis integrates these findings with the quality of evidence to derive overall conclusions regarding the efficacy of combined supplementation.

3. Results

3.1. Study Characteristics

As illustrated in Figure 1, a total of seven RCTs published between 2003 and 2022 met the inclusion criteria, collectively enrolling 263 participants [9,11,12,14–17]. Study characteristics are summarized in Table 1. Participants were between 20 and 30 years of age. Six studies included male participants only [11,12,14–17], while one study exclusively examined female participants [9]. The supplementation protocols adhered to standard dosing strategies for creatine and β-alanine. For creatine, most studies implemented a loading phase (~20 g/day or 0.3 g/kg/day, divided into multiple doses over 5–7 days), followed by a maintenance dose (~5–10 g/day) or a body mass-adjusted dose (e.g., 0.1 g/kg/day) [9,11,15,17]. However, some studies employed only a loading phase [14] or a maintenance protocol without an initial loading phase [12], or, in one case, a reversed approach where a maintenance dose was administered before the loading phase [16]. β-Alanine dosing ranged from 3.2 g/day to 6.4 g/day [9,11,12,14–17], typically divided into multiple daily doses to enhance tolerance and minimize paresthesia. The duration of combined supplementation varied between 4 and 10 weeks.

All studies included at least one single-supplement comparison group (creatine-only and/or β-alanine-only) to assess the potential additive effects of co-supplementation. Additionally, all trials except one study [14] incorporated a placebo control group (e.g., dextrose) alongside at least one combined creatine plus β-alanine group.

3.2. Results of Quality Assessment

The quality assessment of included studies, presented in Figure 2, reveals variability in the risk of bias across different methodological aspects. While most studies demonstrated a low risk of bias in key domains such as participant blinding, outcome assessor blinding, and allocation concealment, some exhibited unclear or high risk in specific categories.

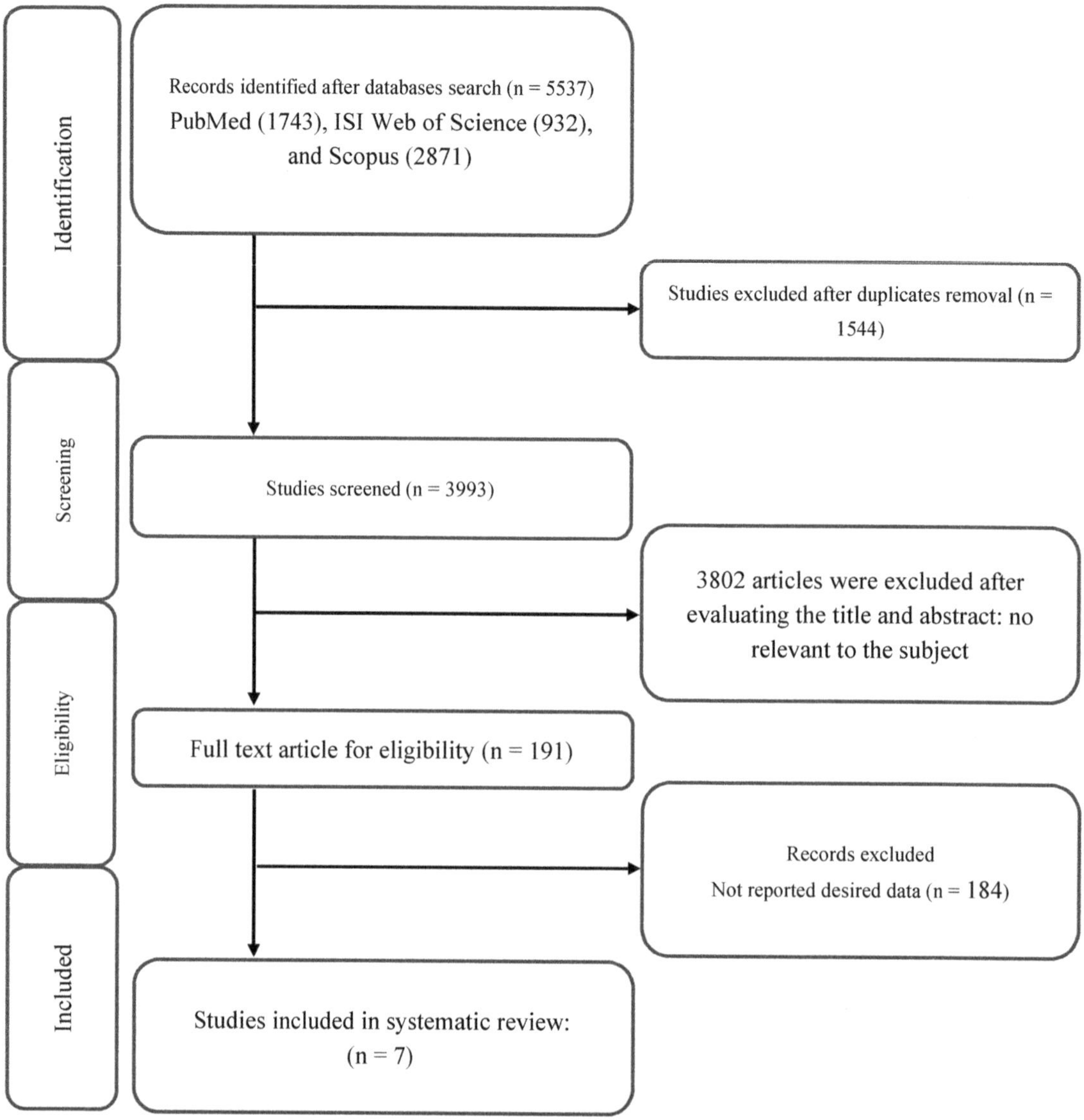

Figure 1. Flow chart of study selection for inclusion trials in the systematic review.

Notably, Harris et al. [17], Zoeller et al. [11], and Okudan et al. [16] had an unclear risk of bias in random sequence generation, indicating potential limitations in randomization procedures. Additionally, selective reporting and incomplete outcome data emerged as the most frequent sources of high risk of bias, particularly in Stout et al. [15] and Samadi et al. [14].

Table 1. Characteristics of included studies in meta-analysis.

Author (Year)	Country	Study Design	Participants	Intervention & Sample Size	Duration (Week)	Mean Age	Cr + βA Dosage & Administration	Training Type	Tests	Placebo	Impact of Cr + BA Compared to Cr or BA Alone
Harris et al. (2003) [17]	USA	P, R, PC, DB	28 Healthy men	βA + Cr: 10 Plac + Cr: 9 Plac + Plac: 9	5	24–30 yrs	βA: 4 × 800 mg/d for 5 wks Cr: 4 × 5 g/d in 5th wk	None	Isometric endurance at 50% MVC, and PO4max test	ND	Body composition: ND Anaerobic performance: ↑ Aerobic performance: ND
Hoffman et al. (2006) [12]	USA	P, R, PC, DB	33 Male strength power athletes	βA + Cr: 11 Cr: 11 Plac: 11	10	NR	Cr: 10.5 g/day; βA: 3.2 g/day	RT	BC (DEXA), 1 RM for squat and bench press, Wingate anaerobic power test and 20 jump power test	Dextrose (10.5 g/day)	Body composition: ↑ Anaerobic performance: ↑ Aerobic performance: ND
Stout et al. (2006) [15]	USA	P, R, PC, DB	51 Untrained healthy men	βA + Cr: 14 βA: 12 Cr: 12 Plac: 13	4	24.5	Day 1–6: βA: 4 × 1.6 g/d Cr: 4 × 5.25 g/d Day 7–28: βA: 2 × 1.6 g/d Cr: 2 × 5.25 g/d	None	Cycle ergometry test, PWC_{FT}	Dextrose (34 g/dose)	Body composition: ND Anaerobic performance: ND Aerobic performance: ↔
Zoeller et al. (2007) [11]	USA	P, R, PC, DB	55 Untrained healthy men	βA + Cr: 16 βA: 14 Cr: 12 Plac: 13	4	24.5	Day 1–6: βA: 4 × 1.6 g/d Cr: 4 × 5.25 g/d Day 7–28: βA: 2 × 1.6 g/d Cr: 2 × 5.25 g/d	None	Graded exercise test to determine VO_2peak, VT and LT	Dextrose (34 g/dose)	Body composition: ND Anaerobic performance: ND Aerobic performance: ↔
Kresta et al. (2014) [9]	USA	P, R, PC, DB	32 Recreation-ally active females	βA + Cr: 9 βA: 8 Cr: 8 Plac: 7	4	21.5	βA: 0.1 g/kg/day Cr: 0.3 g/kg/day (1 week), then 0.1 g/kg/day	None	BC (DEXA), Wingate tests to determine PP, MP & FI, Graded exercise test to determine VO_2peak, VT and LT	Maltodextrin (0.1 g/kg/day for 4 week) + dextrose (0.3 g/kg/day for 1 week)	Body composition: ↔ Anaerobic performance: ↔ Aerobic performance: ↔
Okudan et al. (2015) [16]	Turkey	P, R, PC	44 Untrained healthy men	βA + Cr: 11 βA: 11 Cr: 11 Plac: 11	4	20–22	Day 1–22: βA: 2 × 1.6 g/d Cr: 2 × 5 g/d Day 23–28: βA: 4 × 1.6 g/d Cr: 4 × 5 g/d	None	Wingate Test to determine PP, MP & FI, Graded exercise test to determine VO_2peak, VT and LT	Maltodextrin (20 g/day for day 1–22 and 40 g/day for day 23–28)	Body composition: ND Anaerobic performance: ↑ Aerobic performance: ND
Samadi et al. (2022) [14]	Iran	P, R, PC	20 Active male military personnel	βA + Cr: 10 βA: 10	4	21.5	βA: 6.4 g/day for 28 days; Cr: 0.3 g/kg/day for 7-day loading phase	Military training	RAST, 1RM for bench press and leg press, Vertical Jump Test, and SCET	Equal grams of rice flour	Body composition: ND Anaerobic performance: ↑ Aerobic performance: ND

P = parallel; R = randomized; PC = placebo control; DB = double blind; Cr = creatine; βA = β-alanine; Plac = placebo; MVC = Maximum Voluntary Contraction; PO4max = power output during a 4 min all-out maximal ergometer exercise; ND = not determined; RT = resistance training, BC = body composition, DEXA = dual energy X-ray absorptiometry; 1RM = 1-repetition maximum; PWC_{FT} = physical working capacity at neuromuscular fatigue threshold; VT = ventilatory threshold; LT = lactate threshold; PP = peak power; MP = mean power; FI = fatigue index; RAST = running anaerobic sprint test; SCET = Simulated Casualty Evacuation Test; ↑ = improvement; ↔ = no significant change.

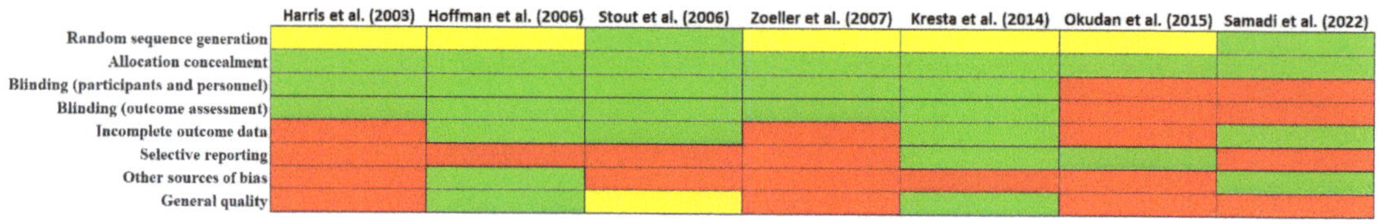

Figure 2. Quality assessment of included studies. Studies with more than two high-risk domains were classified as high risk of bias (red), while those with exactly two high-risk factors were categorized under unclear risk (yellow). Studies exhibiting less than two high-risk domains were considered low risk of bias (green) [9,11,12,14–17].

Overall, based on the Cochrane scoring system, studies with more than two high-risk domains were classified as high risk of bias, while those with exactly two high-risk factors were categorized under unclear risk. Studies exhibiting less than two high-risk domains were considered low risk of bias. These findings emphasize the need for greater methodological rigor in future research to enhance the reliability and validity of reported outcomes.

3.3. *Outcomes Measured*

The primary outcomes assessed across studies included maximal strength (1RM in bench press and squat), anaerobic power (Wingate test outputs, vertical jump), high-intensity exercise capacity (repeated sprint performance, TTE at a fixed intensity), aerobic capacity (VO_2max or VO_2peak), and body composition (fat mass and lean mass). Findings are reported sequentially, beginning with strength and power performance, followed by endurance/aerobic performance, and concluding with body composition outcomes.

3.3.1. Strength and Power Performance

Five trials evaluated muscular strength adaptations (primarily 1RM in resistance exercises) and anaerobic power output following co-supplementation with creatine and β-alanine [9,12,14,16,17]. Findings related to maximal strength are summarized first, followed by studies examining anaerobic power and high-intensity performance.

Maximal Strength

The longest-duration study investigating the effects of creatine and β-alanine co-supplementation was conducted by Hoffman et al., who examined collegiate male football players undergoing 10 weeks of heavy resistance training while receiving either a placebo, creatine alone, or creatine + β-alanine [12]. As expected, the creatine-supplemented group exhibited significantly greater gains in 1RM strength (bench press and squat) compared to the placebo group over the training period. Notably, the combined creatine + β-alanine group demonstrated similar strength improvements to the creatine-only group, with both supplement conditions significantly outperforming the placebo in 1RM gains. However, there was no statistically significant difference in strength gains between the combination group and creatine-only group, suggesting that β-alanine did not provide additional benefits for maximal strength beyond the established ergogenic effects of creatine. These findings indicate that, in the context of resistance-trained male athletes, creatine is the primary contributor to maximal strength improvements, while β-alanine does not further enhance 1RM performance when training and diet are controlled.

A more recent study by Samadi et al. investigated β-alanine as the primary intervention, followed by a short-term creatine loading phase. In this 4-week trial, male military personnel initially supplemented β-alanine (6.4 g/day) for three weeks before being randomized to either continue β-alanine alone or add high-dose creatine (~0.3 g/kg/day) during the final week [14]. The creatine + β-alanine group exhibited significant improvements in vertical jump performance, a key indicator of lower-body power, whereas no such improvement was observed in the β-alanine-only group. The authors also reported trends toward greater muscular strength gains in the creatine + β-alanine group, aligning with previous findings that creatine is a potent enhancer of strength and power. However, the addition of creatine did not result in significant improvements in peak power, average power, minimum power, leg press, or chest press compared to β-alanine alone. These results collectively suggest that while co-supplementation enhances maximal strength compared to no supplementation, this effect is primarily attributable to creatine, with β-alanine providing no additional advantage for 1RM strength gains beyond those achieved with creatine and resistance training alone.

Anaerobic Power and High-Intensity Performance

Harris et al. conducted the first study examining the co-ingestion of creatine and β-alanine [17]. Their findings revealed that power output during a 4-min cycling test was greater in the creatine + β-alanine group than in the creatine-only group, demonstrating that β-alanine supplementation enhanced high-intensity exercise performance beyond creatine alone. Specifically, participants receiving β-alanine exhibited a significant increase in maximal power output during the 4-min all-out ergometer test, with most of the performance gains occurring within the first minute of exercise, prior to full cardiovascular adjustment. This improvement is likely attributed to an increased hydrogen ion (H^+) buffering capacity, facilitated by elevated muscle carnosine levels. However, β-alanine supplementation did not significantly affect isometric endurance or overall force output compared to control groups. These findings suggest that co-supplementation with creatine and β-alanine primarily enhances short-duration, high-intensity performance, whereas its effects on endurance-related strength parameters remain limited compared to creatine alone.

In contrast, Hoffman et al. assessed anaerobic power using a 30-s Wingate test and a 20-repetition jump test in their 10-week study. Neither the creatine group nor the creatine + β-alanine group demonstrated significant improvements in Wingate anaerobic power or the 20-repetition jump test [12]. However, both supplement groups exhibited significant gains in 1RM squat strength, 1RM bench press strength, and average weekly training intensity (% 1RM squat) compared to the placebo, with no significant differences between the creatine-only and creatine + β-alanine groups. The only exception was average weekly training intensity, where the co-supplementation group improved significantly compared to the placebo, suggesting a potential benefit of β-alanine in sustaining training intensity over time.

Further evidence comes from Okudan et al., who conducted a 28-day RCT in untrained young men, specifically investigating repeated Wingate sprint performance across four groups: placebo, creatine-only, β-alanine-only, and combined β-alanine + creatine [16]. Participants completed three consecutive 30-s Wingate tests (separated by brief rest periods) before and after the supplementation period to simulate repeated supramaximal efforts. As expected, the placebo group experienced performance decrements across sprints in both pre- and post-supplementation tests, indicating fatigue accumulation. In contrast, the creatine-only group exhibited significant improvements in peak power output during the second and third sprints, suggesting better maintenance of anaerobic power over repeated efforts. However, the β-alanine + creatine group showed an additional advantage, as they significantly increased mean power output across all three sprints—an improvement not observed in placebo or β-alanine-only conditions. Furthermore, the fatigue index (rate of power decline across sprints) remained stable in groups receiving β-alanine, indicating reduced fatigue accumulation. These findings suggest that while creatine improves peak power, β-alanine contributes to sustained power output and mitigates fatigue in repeated high-intensity efforts.

A study by Kresta et al. in recreationally active women further examined repeated-sprint performance following a 4-week supplementation period with β-alanine, creatine, a combination of both, or a placebo [9]. Participants performed multiple Wingate anaerobic capacity tests before, during, and after supplementation. Unlike previous findings in men, the co-supplementation group did not exhibit significant advantages over the single-supplement groups in any performance measure. The authors concluded that co-supplementation did not provide additive benefits for anaerobic performance in female participants. Additionally, all groups, including the placebo group, experienced some performance improvements with training, further reinforcing the lack of significant differences between supplementation conditions.

3.3.2. Endurance and Aerobic Performance

In this review, the term "endurance" refers to aerobic or high-intensity exercise capacity, including VO_2max, VT, LT, and TTE during sustained exercise. The potential synergistic effects of co-supplementation with creatine and β-alanine on aerobic capacity and endurance performance have been examined in several studies, which are presented below.

Aerobic Power (VO_2max/VO_2peak)

The impact of creatine and β-alanine co-supplementation on maximal aerobic capacity (VO_2max or VO_2peak) has been explored in a limited number of trials. Zoeller et al. conducted an RCT with 55 male participants, examining 4 weeks of supplementation with placebo, creatine, β-alanine, or a combination of both [11]. The study assessed VO_2peak using a graded exercise test on a cycle ergometer, along with VT, LT, and TTE at VO_2peak. The results indicated no significant differences between groups for any of the primary endurance-related outcomes—neither creatine, β-alanine, nor their combination produced statistically significant improvements in VO_2peak or TTE compared to the placebo over 4 weeks. However, the co-supplementation group exhibited the most consistent within-group improvements, showing significant pre-post increases in five of the eight endurance parameters measured (e.g., a trend toward increased VO_2peak and delayed fatigue onset), whereas the single-supplement groups demonstrated improvements in fewer parameters (one in the β-alanine group and two in the creatine group). As the placebo group also showed minor improvements—likely due to training adaptation or test familiarization—the between-group differences did not reach statistical significance. The authors cautiously suggested that co-supplementation "may potentially enhance endurance performance", though the evidence for a true additive effect was weak. From a practical standpoint, any enhancement in VO_2max by these supplements appears to be minimal.

Similarly, Kresta et al., in a study of female participants, found no significant benefit of creatine + β-alanine co-supplementation on VO_2peak [9]. Following 4 weeks of supplementation combined with endurance and cycle training, changes in VO_2peak did not significantly differ between the β-alanine, creatine, combined, or placebo groups. Notably, β-alanine supplementation alone did not outperform the placebo for aerobic capacity, aligning with previous research in male subjects that also failed to demonstrate a significant impact of β-alanine on VO_2max. Although creatine alone showed a non-significant trend toward improved TTE at VO_2peak in the female cohort, the effect was minor. Overall, co-supplementation failed to improve maximal aerobic fitness beyond the effects of training alone, with the authors concluding that their findings support prior literature indicating that creatine has, at best, a modest and inconsistent impact on aerobic capacity.

Submaximal Endurance and Fatigue Thresholds

Several studies have explored whether co-supplementation with creatine and β-alanine influences the onset of fatigue during incremental exercise. As previously noted, Zoeller et al. assessed ventilatory and LT and found no significant group differences, although the combined supplementation group exhibited the largest numerical improvements [11].

A separate study by Stout et al. focused on neuromuscular fatigue thresholds, using a metric known as physical working capacity at the fatigue threshold (PWCFT), derived from electromyographic signals during incremental cycling [15]. In this 28-day trial in untrained men, participants were assigned to one of four groups: placebo, creatine, β-alanine, or creatine + β-alanine. The β-alanine-only and co-supplementation groups both exhibited significant improvements in fatigue threshold compared to the placebo, whereas creatine alone did not. Importantly, the increase in fatigue threshold in the co-supplementation group was not significantly greater than in the β-alanine-only group, indicating that adding creatine did not provide additional benefits for neuromuscular fatigue resistance beyond those conferred by β-alanine alone. The authors concluded that β-alanine was effective in delaying neuromuscular fatigue, while creatine did not contribute meaningfully to this endurance-related outcome. These findings reinforce the notion that β-alanine's buffering capacity plays a crucial role in sustaining high-intensity effort, whereas creatine's role in endurance-type performance is minimal.

Time-to-Exhaustion and Thresholds

Several studies have examined the effects of co-supplementation on TTE at submaximal intensities and related endurance measures. As mentioned, Zoeller et al. found no significant group differences in TTE, though the co-supplementation group exhibited the largest numerical increase [11]. Similarly, Kresta et al. found no significant improvements in TTE or LT across groups [9].

In Kresta's female cohort, β-alanine supplementation for 4 weeks did not significantly increase the LT, though a trend toward improved lactate dynamics was observed after one week in the β-alanine groups. Additionally, Kresta et al. reported a notable finding regarding peak blood lactate levels during the VO_2max test—the β-alanine-only group exhibited significantly higher peak blood lactate than the co-supplementation and placebo groups post-supplementation. This observation suggests a potential enhancement in anaerobic glycolytic capacity in the β-alanine-alone group, though it remains unclear why the co-supplementation group did not exhibit the same response. The lack of significant differences in VT across groups further supports the conclusion that neither creatine nor β-alanine meaningfully enhances endurance-related parameters in the context of aerobic capacity.

3.3.3. Body Composition Outcomes

Data on the effects of co-supplementation with creatine and β-alanine on body composition are limited, as only two studies have investigated this topic. The findings from these two RCTs are presented below.

Lean Body Mass Gains

The most notable finding regarding LBM enhancement comes from the 10-week RCT by Hoffman et al., which examined resistance-trained men undergoing supplementation with creatine, β-alanine, a combination of both, or the placebo [12]. Body composition was assessed using dual-energy X-ray absorptiometry (DEXA). The results demonstrated that the combined creatine + β-alanine group experienced significantly greater gains in LBM compared to both the creatine-only and placebo groups. On average, the co-supplementation group accumulated more LBM than the creatine-alone group, suggesting a potential synergistic effect on muscle hypertrophy or lean tissue retention. Furthermore, the combined group also exhibited a greater reduction in body fat percentage, indicating a possible repartitioning effect, where increases in muscle mass were accompanied by a reduction in fat mass. The authors acknowledged that creatine alone was effective in increasing LBM relative to the placebo, as expected, but the addition of β-alanine appeared to further augment lean mass accrual.

Conversely, a similarly designed study in female participants failed to replicate these findings. Kresta et al. assessed body composition using DXA in college-aged women following 4 weeks of supplementation combined with concurrent training [9]. Their results revealed no significant differences between the creatine + β-alanine group and any other group in terms of changes in LBM or fat mass. All groups, including the placebo, exhibited modest improvements in body composition, likely due to the effects of training adaptation (i.e., slight increases in lean mass and decreases in fat mass). However, none of the supplementation conditions significantly enhanced body composition beyond the effects of training alone in women.

Fat Mass, Body Fat Percentage, and Body Mass

Changes in fat mass were less frequently reported across studies, though they generally followed an inverse relationship to lean mass changes. In Hoffman et al.'s study, the creatine + β-alanine group not only exhibited greater increases in LBM but also demonstrated a significantly greater reduction in body fat percentage compared to the creatine-only and placebo groups [12]. Over 10 weeks of resistance training, the combined supplementation group maintained stable body mass yet experienced a more pronounced decline in absolute fat mass and body fat percentage. This effect may be attributed to the greater increase in lean mass, which lowered the percentage of body fat, or alternatively, an increase in training volume and energy expenditure due to the ergogenic benefits of supplementation. By contrast, Kresta et al. reported no significant differences in fat mass, body fat percentage, or total body mass between groups in their 4-week trial in female participants [9].

4. Discussion

This systematic review aimed to evaluate whether co-supplementation with creatine and β-alanine provides greater improvements in exercise performance and body composition compared to either supplement alone. The findings from RCTs suggest that co-supplementation may be an effective strategy for enhancing certain performance outcomes, particularly strength and high-intensity power output. However, these benefits appear to be primarily driven by the well-established ergogenic effects of creatine. True synergistic effects—where the combination of creatine and β-alanine leads to performance enhancements beyond what either supplement achieves alone—were observed more frequently in anaerobic power and high-intensity performance, with a lower probability of additive effects in maximal strength and body composition. Current evidence regarding the effects of creatine and β-alanine co-supplementation on body composition is both limited and inconsistent. While one study reported greater improvements in lean mass and fat mass reduction compared to individual supplementation, another found no significant changes. Furthermore, co-supplementation did not result in meaningful improvements in aerobic endurance measures, including VO_2max, lactate threshold, or TTE.

4.1. Anaerobic Performance

It is well established that creatine supplementation enhances strength and power [18,19], and all RCTs reviewed in this study confirmed that groups receiving creatine (either alone or in combination) exhibited substantial improvements in strength and anaerobic power relative to the placebo [12,14]. These findings are consistent with decades of research demonstrating that creatine is one of the most effective supplements for increasing muscular strength, primarily by enhancing training capacity, phosphocreatine resynthesis, and neuromuscular function [20–23].

One of the primary mechanisms by which β-alanine is hypothesized to enhance strength and power performance is through its buffering effect on intramuscular acidity [24,25]. The accumulation of H^+ during high-intensity exercise has been shown to impair phosphocreatine resynthesis [26], inhibit glycolytic metabolism [27], and negatively affect muscle contractile function. Thus, it is theoretically plausible that combining creatine with β-alanine could provide additional benefits by simultaneously supporting ATP production (creatine) and buffering metabolic acidosis (β-alanine). However, the question remains whether this combination meaningfully enhances strength and power outcomes beyond what creatine alone achieves.

The evidence from RCTs suggests that any additional benefit of β-alanine in maximal strength gains is minimal. Hoffman et al. found no significant differences in 1RM strength gains (bench press and squat) between the creatine-only and creatine + β-alanine groups, indicating that β-alanine did not further enhance maximal strength beyond the effects of creatine [12]. Other studies that assessed strength outcomes similarly reported that creatine alone was superior to the placebo but did not specifically compare creatine-only vs. creatine + β-alanine for 1RM gains. These results suggest that creatine's mechanism (increasing phosphocreatine availability) is already sufficient to maximize strength adaptations in a resistance training context and that additional buffering from β-alanine does not provide a substantial advantage for maximal strength performance.

In contrast, β-alanine may offer greater benefits in scenarios where repeated maximal efforts are required, such as high-intensity interval training (HIIT), sprinting, or repeated sets of resistance exercise. This is evident in studies where muscle acidosis is a key limiting factor. For example, Okudan et al. examined repeated Wingate sprint performance in untrained men and found that while creatine improved peak power, only the groups receiving β-alanine (β-alanine alone or β-alanine + creatine) were able to sustain power output across multiple sprints and resist fatigue [16]. This suggests that β-alanine's buffering effect translated into reduced performance decrements over successive high-intensity efforts, whereas creatine alone was primarily effective for increasing peak power output. The physiological basis for this synergy is logical: Creatine supplementation enhances ATP-PCr system efficiency, providing energy for short-duration, high-intensity efforts. β-Alanine, via its role in carnosine synthesis, buffers H^+ accumulation, mitigating the decline in pH associated with anaerobic glycolysis and thereby delaying fatigue in subsequent efforts. This complementary interaction likely explains why β-alanine's effects are more apparent in repeated-bout performance rather than in single maximal lifts (e.g., 1RM strength testing).

A recent study by Li et al. in competitive male basketball players provides further insights into the potential benefits of co-supplementation for explosive performance. This 4-week RCT included the placebo, creatine-only, β-alanine-only, L-citrulline-only, or a combination of all three supplements, alongside a sprint interval training program [28]. The study reported that all supplement groups outperformed the placebo in physical performance tests (e.g., vertical jump, 20-m sprint, and change-of-direction speed) and that the combination of multiple supplements provided the broadest performance enhancements. However, because the co-supplementation group in this study included L-citrulline, these results were not included in the current systematic review due to the predefined inclusion criteria.

Despite this limitation, the findings reinforce that creatine and β-alanine—either alone or in combination—are beneficial for power-related outcomes. Additionally, no negative interactions were observed between multiple supplements, suggesting that co-supplementation strategies may provide broad ergogenic benefits without interference.

It is important to note that not all studies demonstrated a clear differentiation in the roles of creatine and β-alanine. For instance, in Kresta et al.'s study on female participants, even repeated Wingate tests did not reveal a distinct advantage of co-supplementation over single-supplement conditions [9]. Several factors may contribute to these findings. One potential explanation is the influence of training status and sex-related differences. The female participants in Kresta's study, despite being recreationally active, likely had lower baseline power outputs and muscle mass compared to male athletes. Consequently, the absolute physiological stress and accumulation of metabolic byproducts (e.g., hydrogen ions) during repeated sprints may have been lower, reducing the potential ergogenic effects of β-alanine. Additionally, the dosing strategy (relative to body weight) and the supplementation duration (4 weeks) may have been insufficient for smaller female participants to achieve a meaningful increase in muscle carnosine levels, thereby limiting the impact of β-alanine on performance.

Another relevant consideration is that creatine's effects on lean mass and power output in women are often less pronounced than in men, potentially due to hormonal differences, muscle fiber composition, or lower total muscle creatine stores [9]. Moreover, Kresta et al. incorporated concurrent endurance training across all study groups, which may have attenuated strength and power adaptations and masked potential supplement effects. This contrasts with Okudan et al.'s study in untrained men, which specifically targeted anaerobic performance (Wingate sprint tests) without endurance training [16]. The differences in training modality and population characteristics suggest that the presence of synergy between creatine and β-alanine may be more evident in anaerobic-focused interventions (e.g., Okudan et al.) but less pronounced in endurance-based or mixed-training contexts (e.g., Kresta et al.).

Another possible reason for inconsistent findings is the presence of ceiling effects [29]. In highly trained populations, such as Hoffman et al.'s collegiate football players, substantial improvements in strength and power are already achieved through training and creatine supplementation alone. In such cases, β-alanine's ability to further enhance performance may be limited, particularly over a relatively short intervention period (e.g., 10 weeks), where creatine and structured training have already maximized neuromuscular adaptations. Conversely, in less-trained individuals, the potential for improvement may be greater, and a supplement that allows for even marginal increases in training capacity (e.g., an additional repetition or a slight delay in fatigue) could lead to measurable performance differences. This may explain why β-alanine's effects were more evident in studies involving untrained participants engaging in repeated high-intensity efforts but less pronounced in well-trained athletes undergoing structured resistance training.

The cumulative evidence from RCTs indicates that co-supplementation with creatine and β-alanine enhances strength and power performance relative to the placebo, particularly when combined with structured training programs. However, these improvements are primarily attributed to creatine's well-established effects on muscular strength and power output. In settings where creatine alone already optimizes neuromuscular performance, β-alanine does not appear to provide additional benefits for maximal strength (e.g., 1RM gains). However, β-alanine may offer advantages in high-intensity, repeated-effort scenarios, where it can delay fatigue and sustain power output over successive efforts.

From a practical standpoint, athletes engaged in strength and power training can expect substantial performance enhancements from creatine alone. Adding β-alanine may be beneficial in scenarios requiring sustained power output over multiple sets or repeated bouts of high-intensity exercise, but its contribution to absolute strength gains appears to be minimal. Future research should explore the long-term effects of co-supplementation across different training populations, with a particular focus on sex-based differences, training status, and sport-specific demands.

4.2. Aerobic Performance

The findings of this review provide limited evidence supporting the efficacy of co-supplementation with creatine and β-alanine in enhancing traditional endurance performance metrics, such as VO_2max or prolonged aerobic exercise capacity, beyond the effects of training alone. This outcome is expected, as creatine supplementation does not inherently improve oxidative metabolism and may even be detrimental to endurance performance if it leads to rapid weight gain without direct benefits to aerobic energy production [30,31]. Conversely, β-alanine's primary ergogenic role is observed in high-intensity exercise lasting approximately 1–4 min, such as an 800–1500 m run or a 1000 m rowing effort, rather than in prolonged endurance events such as marathons [32]. The current body of evidence confirms that VO_2max remains unaffected by β-alanine or creatine supplementation [9,11]. However, for efforts occurring at the metabolic "crossover" between anaerobic and aerobic energy systems, there may be a modest indication of benefit. Stout et al. reported that β-alanine supplementation increased the PWCFT, suggesting an improvement in fatigue resistance [15]. However, the addition of creatine did not further amplify this effect, indicating that β-alanine alone was responsible for the observed improvements. Similarly, Zoeller et al. reported modest improvements in TTE at high intensity in the combined supplementation group, though these improvements were not significantly greater than those observed with β-alanine alone [11]. These findings suggest that β-alanine may provide a slight advantage in events involving sustained high-intensity efforts, such as 2–3-min maximal exertion bouts or sports requiring repeated bursts of high-intensity activity (e.g., boxing rounds, middle-distance track races, or 100–200 m swimming sprints). However, direct evidence from studies specifically targeting such performance scenarios remains lacking.

The findings from Li et al. in competitive basketball players further support the limited impact of co-supplementation on aerobic endurance [28]. In this 4-week study, athletes received creatine, β-alanine, a combination of both, or an additional L-citrulline supplementation regimen alongside their training program. Aerobic fitness was assessed (likely via a shuttle run or VO_2max test), and while all groups improved due to training, the supplemented groups (including the combined group) outperformed the placebo group in general. However, the co-supplementation group did not demonstrate a clear advantage over the single-supplement groups for aerobic performance, suggesting that creatine and β-alanine do not synergistically enhance aerobic endurance when combined.

Another intriguing finding comes from Samadi et al., who observed improved cognitive performance (measured via mathematical processing tasks) in participants receiving β-alanine + creatine supplementation [14]. Given that creatine is well-documented to support cognitive function, particularly in sleep-deprived or hypoxic conditions, and that β-alanine may mitigate central fatigue contributors, the combined supplementation may offer benefits for maintaining cognitive performance under conditions of physical and mental stress. This finding has potential practical applications for military personnel, endurance athletes, and individuals performing high-cognitive-demand tasks under fatigue, warranting further investigation into the neuromuscular and cognitive effects of co-supplementation.

Overall, the current RCT evidence does not strongly support a meaningful synergistic effect of combined creatine and β-alanine on traditional endurance performance. While β-alanine has demonstrated efficacy in delaying fatigue by improving work at the fatigue threshold and extending TTE, co-supplementation with creatine has not consistently yielded additive benefits in VO_2max, lactate threshold, or exercise duration to fatigue beyond what β-alanine or endurance training alone can achieve. Creatine supplementation, on its own, has minimal direct impact on classical endurance metrics and does not appear to synergize with β-alanine for these outcomes. There is some evidence that combined supplementation may slightly improve high-intensity endurance thresholds and capacity, but such effects have been inconsistent across studies and generally not statistically superior to single-supplement interventions.

From a practical standpoint, endurance athletes are unlikely to derive substantial additional benefits from creatine and β-alanine co-supplementation beyond those obtained through structured endurance training alone. However, individuals engaged in mixed metabolic events (e.g., HIIT, combat sports, middle-distance races, or team sports requiring repeated sprint efforts) may experience minor improvements in high-intensity endurance capacity with β-alanine alone, although the contribution of creatine in this context remains limited. Future research should explore the effects of co-supplementation in sport-specific endurance applications, particularly in hybrid aerobic-anaerobic sports where sustained high-intensity efforts play a critical role in performance outcomes.

4.3. Body Composition

Creatine supplementation is well established for its role in increasing LBM, primarily through enhanced intracellular water retention, improved strength, and greater progressive overload during resistance training [4,33]. In contrast, β-alanine's potential effects on body composition are more indirect, hypothesized to occur through increased training volume and higher-intensity efforts, leading to greater hypertrophic adaptation. The proposed synergy between these two supplements is that creatine enhances maximal strength, while β-alanine delays fatigue, allowing for a higher training volume—thereby providing both a heavier and a slightly prolonged training stimulus.

Limited evidence from this review suggests that co-supplementation with creatine and β-alanine may potentially improve body composition adaptations; this effect was observed only in Hoffman et al.'s 10-week study, where the creatine + β-alanine group gained approximately 1 kg more lean mass than the creatine-only group and also experienced greater reductions in body fat [12]. These results suggest a potential recomposition effect, where greater muscle mass is accrued without additional fat gain. For athletes, this could imply an improved lean mass-to-fat ratio over a training cycle, thereby optimizing performance and body composition simultaneously.

The underlying mechanism by which β-alanine might contribute to these improvements remains speculative. One hypothesis is that β-alanine's buffering effect on muscle acidosis allows athletes to sustain higher training volumes or intensities over time, resulting in greater hypertrophic stimulus and potentially increased caloric expenditure [34]. If an athlete can perform additional repetitions before muscular failure or execute high-intensity intervals at a slightly higher power output, these incremental training improvements may accumulate over several weeks, contributing to enhanced lean mass gains and fat loss. Supporting this theory, previous studies have reported that β-alanine supplementation improved training volume in resistance exercise and promoted lean mass gains when combined with HIIT.

Notably, Hoffman et al. observed higher weekly training volume in the squat exercise in the creatine + β-alanine group, potentially explaining the higher lean mass gains in this cohort. However, it is important to acknowledge that not all studies have observed this effect, as some research has failed to find a significant impact of β-alanine on training volume [35,36]. Furthermore, Hoffman et al.'s study design did not include a β-alanine–only group, making it difficult to determine whether the observed benefits were due to a true synergistic effect or simply a larger effect of creatine alone.

Not all studies have demonstrated a significant benefit of co-supplementation with creatine and β-alanine on body composition. A particularly notable finding is the null results reported by Kresta et al., who found that the combination of creatine and β-alanine was not superior to either supplement alone in terms of lean mass or fat mass changes [9]. Several factors may explain these findings, including shorter study duration, lower relative dosage per body weight, and potential sex-specific differences in physiological responses.

Kresta et al. noted that females generally experience smaller increases in lean mass following creatine supplementation compared to males, a trend that was evident in their study, where the creatine-only group exhibited smaller lean mass gains than those typically observed in male-based studies. When juxtaposed with Hoffman et al.'s findings in male participants, it appears plausible that creatine primarily supports muscle energetics, while β-alanine may facilitate greater training volume and quality, potentially maximizing hypertrophic adaptations over time. However, given that Hoffman et al. is the only study to report a significant synergistic effect of co-supplementation on lean mass, these findings should be interpreted with caution.

Some studies suggest that women do not gain as much muscle mass or retain as much water from creatine supplementation as men, potentially due to lower absolute muscle mass, greater baseline intramuscular creatine stores, or hormonal differences. For example, a meta-analysis by Pashayee-Khamene et al. reported that men gained more than twice the amount of lean mass compared to women following creatine supplementation (1.2 kg vs. 0.54 kg) [5].

Additionally, study duration may have influenced the observed outcomes. While Hoffman et al. conducted a 10-week trial, which allowed for more cumulative training adaptations, Kresta et al.'s study lasted only 4 weeks, which may have been insufficient to detect meaningful differences in body composition.

Another important factor is statistical power. Hoffman et al. included 33 participants, and even with this sample size, the between-group differences were only barely significant ($p < 0.05$). In contrast, Kresta et al. divided 32 participants across four groups (~8 per group), significantly reducing statistical power. As a result, the study may have been underpowered to detect modest but potentially meaningful effects of supplementation.

A meta-analysis of 20 RCTs by Ashtary-Larky et al. concluded that, regardless of exercise program, supplementation dose, or study duration, β-alanine supplementation does not significantly increase lean mass or reduce fat mass [37]. This suggests that β-alanine does not have a direct impact on muscle hypertrophy and that the hypertrophic effects observed in creatine + β-alanine co-supplementation studies are primarily attributable to creatine.

Thus, existing evidence does not strongly support the hypothesis that β-alanine enhances the body composition benefits of creatine supplementation. The observed improvements in lean mass in some studies may simply reflect creatine's well-established role in improving muscle energetics and increasing training capacity, rather than a true synergistic effect with β-alanine.

The current body of evidence regarding the benefits of co-supplementation with creatine and β-alanine for body composition remains limited and inconclusive. Given that previous research has not demonstrated a significant effect of β-alanine on lean mass or fat loss, it is unlikely that β-alanine enhances the body composition benefits of creatine supplementation.

Future studies should focus on longer-duration trials with larger sample sizes to determine whether β-alanine contributes to hypertrophic adaptations when combined with creatine. Additionally, research should explore sex-specific responses and variations in training protocols, as current findings suggest that the potential benefits of co-supplementation may be population-dependent.

In practical terms, athletes seeking to optimize muscle hypertrophy and body composition should prioritize creatine supplementation, as its effects on lean mass and strength are well established. While β-alanine may provide ergogenic benefits for sustained high-intensity efforts, its direct role in body composition improvements remains uncertain. Future research is necessary to clarify whether co-supplementation provides advantages over creatine alone, particularly in specific athletic populations or training contexts.

4.4. Dosing Strategies and Interindividual Variability

An important consideration in interpreting the findings of this review is the variation in dosage, duration, and participant characteristics across included studies. For creatine, supplementation protocols included a loading phase (~20 g/day or 0.3 g/kg/day, divided into multiple doses over 5–7 days) followed by a maintenance dose (~5–10 g/day), or in some cases, either a loading-only or maintenance-only protocol. For β-alanine, daily dosages ranged from 3.2 to 6.4 g. Supplementation durations varied between 4 and 10 weeks. Additionally, heterogeneity in participant characteristics—including training status (e.g., trained, recreational, and untrained individuals), sex, and baseline nutritional status—may have influenced the observed outcomes. These variations limit the ability to identify optimal protocols for co-supplementation, highlighting the need for future studies to clarify "how much, how often, and in whom" these supplements are most effective.

Furthermore, individual variability in supplement response—often categorized as "responders" and "non-responders"—is another important factor that may have affected the outcomes assessed in this review. Factors such as genetics [38], muscle fiber composition [39], and baseline dietary creatine [39] or carnosine levels [40] may influence the magnitude of response [39]. For example, Syrotuik and Bell explored responders and non-responders to creatine supplementation [39]. They found that baseline muscle cross-sectional area, a greater proportion of type II muscle fibers, and lower intramuscular creatine stores had greater performance improvements following creatine supplementation and were described as responders. Similarly, beta-alanine responders are more likely to have lower baseline muscle carnosine levels, a greater proportion of Type II muscle fibers, be less well-trained, and follow a vegetarian diet [40]. Importantly, the included RCTs in our systematic review did not stratify or report data based on these variables, which may contribute to the inconsistency and heterogeneity observed across individual studies. Future trials should address this gap by including analyses stratified by response status to better inform individualized recommendations.

4.5. Limitations

This systematic review has several limitations that should be acknowledged. First, the total number of included studies (n = 7) is relatively small, limiting the ability to draw definitive conclusions regarding the effects of creatine and β-alanine co-supplementation. Additionally, for some key performance and body composition outcomes, only a few studies were available, reducing the reliability and generalizability of the findings. The limited number of studies also precludes the possibility of conducting a meta-analysis, which would have provided a more robust quantitative assessment of the combined effects of these supplements.

Second, another main limitation of this review is the considerable methodological heterogeneity among the included studies. Participant populations varied in terms of training status, sex, and baseline fitness level, and dosing protocols for creatine and β-alanine supplementation were not standardized. These differences limit the ability to draw definitive conclusions and hinder the applicability of findings across all populations.

Third, the duration of most included studies was relatively short, with intervention periods typically ranging from 4 to 5 weeks, except for one longer trial lasting 10 weeks. Given that muscle hypertrophy, body recomposition, and chronic adaptations to training require extended periods, the short intervention durations may have limited the ability to detect meaningful long-term effects of creatine and β-alanine co-supplementation. Future research should focus on longer-duration trials to determine whether the potential synergistic effects of these supplements become more pronounced over time.

Despite these limitations, this review provides valuable insights into the effects of creatine and β-alanine co-supplementation on strength, power, endurance, and body composition. However, future studies with larger sample sizes, longer intervention periods, and more standardized outcome measures are needed to further clarify the efficacy and applicability of co-supplementation in different athletic populations.

5. Conclusions

In summary, co-supplementation with creatine and β-alanine may be an effective strategy for enhancing strength, power, and body composition compared to a placebo. However, when comparing creatine and β-alanine combined to either alone, the most consistent benefits tend to enhance high-intensity exercise performance, particularly in activities requiring repeated maximal efforts or sustained anaerobic power output. Although some evidence suggests potential benefits for maximal strength and body composition, the current data remain inconsistent and inconclusive, limiting the ability to draw definitive conclusions regarding a synergistic effect between these supplements. Based on the existing body of research, athletes may potentially benefit from this combination when their primary goal is to enhance high-intensity performance, such as in sprint-based sports, resistance training, or repeated explosive efforts. Conversely, no consistent improvements in aerobic endurance capacity have been observed with creatine and β-alanine co-supplementation, reinforcing the currently limited role of these supplements in oxidative metabolism. Future long-term, well-controlled studies are necessary to further clarify the effects of co-supplementation on different athletic populations and training modalities, ensuring that recommendations are based on reliable and robust evidence. Further, there are large individual responses to creatine and β-alanine supplementation, which may be associated with genetic or baseline differences such as diet, training status, and muscle fiber composition that warrant future considerations.

Author Contributions: Conceptualization, D.A.-L.; methodology, D.A.-L. and L.H.; formal analysis, D.A.-L.; writing—original draft preparation, D.A.-L.; writing—review and editing, S.C.F., D.G.C., J.A. and K.S. All authors have read and agreed to the published version of the manuscript.

Funding: This research received no specific grant from any funding agency in the public, commercial, or not-for-profit sectors.

Conflicts of Interest: D.A.-L. is professionally involved in the health and nutrition industry, including activities related to dietary products and supplementation. No commercial interest influenced the design, analysis, or interpretation of this manuscript. S.C.F. has served as a scientific advisor for a company that sells creatine products and is a scientific advisor of Bear Balanced. SCF has received creatine donations from Creapure for research purposes. J.A. is the CEO and co-founder of the International Society of Sports Nutrition (ISSN), an academic non-profit. The ISSN may be sponsored by companies that manufacture, market, and sell β-alanine and creatine-containing supplements, including Creapure, Bear Balanced, and Create. D.G.C. has received research grants and performed industry-sponsored research involving creatine supplementation, received creatine donation for scientific studies, and travel support for presentations involving creatine supplementation at scientific conferences. In addition, D.G.C. serves on the Scientific Advisory Board for Alzchem and Create (companies that manufacture creatine) and the editorial review board for the Journal of the International Society of Sports Nutrition. D.G.C. is also a sports science advisor to the International Society of Sports Nutrition and serves as an expert witness/consultant in legal cases involving creatine supplementation. All other authors declare no conflicts of interest. K.S. is a board member of the International Society of Exercise Immunology (ISEI), an academic non-profit organization, and has received research grants and performed industry-sponsored research not involving creatine and β-alanine supplements.

Abbreviations

The following abbreviations are used in this manuscript:

RCT	Randomized controlled trials
ATP	Adenosine triphosphate
VT	Ventilatory threshold
LT	Lactate threshold
PRISMA	Preferred Reporting Items for Systematic Reviews and Meta-Analyses
PROSPERO	International Prospective Register of Systematic Reviews
1RM	One-repetition maximum
TTE	Time to exhaustion
PWCFT	physical working capacity at the fatigue threshold
DEXA	dual-energy X-ray absorptiometry
H^+	Hydrogen ions
HIIT	High-intensity interval training
LBM	Lean body mass

References

1. Doherty, M.; Smith, P.M.; Davison, R.R.; Hughes, M.G. Caffeine is ergogenic after supplementation of oral creatine monohydrate. *Med. Sci. Sports Exerc.* **2002**, *34*, 1785–1792. [CrossRef] [PubMed]
2. Hoffman, J.R.; Emerson, N.S.; Stout, J.R. β-alanine supplementation. *Curr. Sports Med. Rep.* **2012**, *11*, 189–195. [CrossRef] [PubMed]
3. Luo, D.; Edwards, S.; Smeuninx, B.; McKendry, J.; Nishimura, Y.; Perkins, M.; Philp, A.; Joanisse, S.; Breen, L. Immobilization leads to alterations in intracellular phosphagen and creatine transporter content in human skeletal muscle. *Am. J. Physiol.-Cell Physiol.* **2020**, *319*, C34–C44. [CrossRef] [PubMed]
4. Farshidfar, F.; Pinder, M.A.; Myrie, S.B. Creatine supplementation and skeletal muscle metabolism for building muscle mass—Review of the potential mechanisms of action. *Curr. Protein Pept. Sci.* **2017**, *18*, 1273–1287. [CrossRef] [PubMed]
5. Pashayee-Khamene, F.; Heidari, Z.; Asbaghi, O.; Ashtary-Larky, D.; Goudarzi, K.; Forbes, S.C.; Candow, D.G.; Bagheri, R.; Ghanavati, M.; Dutheil, F. Creatine supplementation protocols with or without training interventions on body composition: A GRADE-assessed systematic review and dose-response meta-analysis. *J. Int. Soc. Sports Nutr.* **2024**, *21*, 2380058. [CrossRef]
6. Matthews, J.J.; Artioli, G.G.; Turner, M.D.; Sale, C. The physiological roles of carnosine and β-alanine in exercising human skeletal muscle. *Med. Sci. Sports Exerc.* **2019**, *51*, 2098–2108. [CrossRef]
7. Culbertson, J.Y.; Kreider, R.B.; Greenwood, M.; Cooke, M. Effects of beta-alanine on muscle carnosine and exercise performance: A review of the current literature. *Nutrients* **2010**, *2*, 75–98. [CrossRef]
8. Derave, W.; Everaert, I.; Beeckman, S.; Baguet, A. Muscle carnosine metabolism and β-alanine supplementation in relation to exercise and training. *Sports Med.* **2010**, *40*, 247–263. [CrossRef]
9. Kresta, J.Y.; Oliver, J.M.; Jagim, A.R.; Fluckey, J.; Riechman, S.; Kelly, K.; Meininger, C.; Mertens-Talcott, S.U.; Rasmussen, C.; Kreider, R.B. Effects of 28 days of beta-alanine and creatine supplementation on muscle carnosine, body composition and exercise performance in recreationally active females. *J. Int. Soc. Sports Nutr.* **2014**, *11*, 55. [CrossRef]

10. Hobson, R.M.; Saunders, B.; Ball, G.; Harris, R.; Sale, C. Effects of β-alanine supplementation on exercise performance: A meta-analysis. *Amino Acids* **2012**, *43*, 25–37. [CrossRef]
11. Zoeller, R.; Stout, J.; O'kroy, J.; Torok, D.; Mielke, M. Effects of 28 days of beta-alanine and creatine monohydrate supplementation on aerobic power, ventilatory and lactate thresholds, and time to exhaustion. *Amino Acids* **2007**, *33*, 505–510. [CrossRef] [PubMed]
12. Hoffman, J.; Ratamess, N.; Kang, J.; Mangine, G.; Faigenbaum, A.; Stout, J. Effect of creatine and ß-alanine supplementation on performance and endocrine responses in strength/power athletes. *Int. J. Sport Nutr. Exerc. Metab.* **2006**, *16*, 430–446. [CrossRef] [PubMed]
13. Page, M.J.; McKenzie, J.E.; Bossuyt, P.M.; Boutron, I.; Hoffmann, T.C.; Mulrow, C.D.; Shamseer, L.; Tetzlaff, J.M.; Akl, E.A.; Brennan, S.E. The PRISMA 2020 statement: An updated guideline for reporting systematic reviews. *BMJ* **2021**, *372*, 71. [CrossRef]
14. Samadi, M.; Askarian, A.; Shirvani, H.; Shamsoddini, A.; Shakibaee, A.; Forbes, S.C.; Kaviani, M. Effects of four weeks of beta-alanine supplementation combined with one week of creatine loading on physical and cognitive performance in military personnel. *Int. J. Environ. Res. Public Health* **2022**, *19*, 7992. [CrossRef]
15. Stout, J.R.; Cramer, J.T.; Mielke, M.; O'Kroy, J.; Torok, D.J.; Zoeller, R.F. Effects of twenty-eight days of beta-alanine and creatine monohydrate supplementation on the physical working capacity at neuromuscular fatigue threshold. *J. Strength Cond. Res.* **2006**, *20*, 928–931. [PubMed]
16. Okudan, N.; Belviranli, M.; Pepe, H.; Gökbel, H. The effects of beta alanine plus creatine administration on performance during repeated bouts of supramaximal exercise in sedentary men. *J. Sports Med. Phys. Fit.* **2015**, *55*, 1322–1328.
17. Harris, R.C.; Hill, C.; Wise, J.A. Effect of combined beta-alanine and creatine monohydrate supplementation on exercise performance. *Med. Sci. Sports Exerc.* **2003**, *35*, S218. [CrossRef]
18. Rawson, E.S.; Volek, J.S. Effects of creatine supplementation and resistance training on muscle strength and weightlifting performance. *J. Strength Cond. Res.* **2003**, *17*, 822–831.
19. Volek, J.S.; Kraemer, W.J.; Bush, J.A.; Boetes, M.; Incledon, T.; Clark, K.L.; Lynch, J.M. Creatine supplementation enhances muscular performance during high-intensity resistance exercise. *J. Am. Diet. Assoc.* **1997**, *97*, 765–770. [CrossRef]
20. Becque, M.D.; Lochmann, J.D.; Melrose, D.R. Effects of oral creatine supplementation on muscular strength and body composition. *Med. Sci. Sports Exerc.* **2000**, *32*, 654–658. [CrossRef]
21. Kendall, K.L.; Smith, A.E.; Graef, J.L.; Fukuda, D.H.; Moon, J.R.; Beck, T.W.; Cramer, J.T.; Stout, J.R. Effects of four weeks of high-intensity interval training and creatine supplementation on critical power and anaerobic working capacity in college-aged men. *J. Strength Cond. Res.* **2009**, *23*, 1663–1669. [CrossRef] [PubMed]
22. Greenhaff, P.; Bodin, K.; Soderlund, K.; Hultman, E. Effect of oral creatine supplementation on skeletal muscle phosphocreatine resynthesis. *Am. J. Physiol. -Endocrinol. Metab.* **1994**, *266*, E725–E730. [CrossRef] [PubMed]
23. Cramer, J.T.; Stout, J.R.; Culbertson, J.Y.; Egan, A.D. Effects of creatine supplementation and three days of resistance training on muscle strength, power output, and neuromuscular function. *J. Strength Cond. Res.* **2007**, *21*, 668–677. [PubMed]
24. Black, M.I.; Jones, A.M.; Morgan, P.T.; Bailey, S.J.; Fulford, J.; Vanhatalo, A. The effects of β-alanine supplementation on muscle pH and the power-duration relationship during high-intensity exercise. *Front. Physiol.* **2018**, *9*, 111. [CrossRef]
25. Sale, C.; Saunders, B.; Harris, R.C. Effect of beta-alanine supplementation on muscle carnosine concentrations and exercise performance. *Amino Acids* **2010**, *39*, 321–333. [CrossRef]
26. McMahon, S.; Jenkins, D. Factors affecting the rate of phosphocreatine resynthesis following intense exercise. *Sports Med.* **2002**, *32*, 761–784. [CrossRef]
27. Jubrias, S.A.; Crowther, G.J.; Shankland, E.G.; Gronka, R.K.; Conley, K.E. Acidosis inhibits oxidative phosphorylation in contracting human skeletal muscle in vivo. *J. Physiol.* **2003**, *553*, 589–599. [CrossRef]
28. Li, M.; Sheykhlouvand, M. Effects of Combined Versus Single Supplementation of Creatine, Beta-Alanine, and L-Citrulline During Short Sprint Interval Training on Basketball Players' Performance: A Double-Blind Randomized Placebo-Controlled Trial. *Int. J. Sports Physiol. Perform.* **2025**, *20*, 559–567. [CrossRef]
29. Latella, C.; Teo, W.-P.; Spathis, J.; van den Hoek, D. Long-term strength adaptation: A 15-year analysis of powerlifting athletes. *J. Strength Cond. Res.* **2020**, *34*, 2412–2418. [CrossRef]
30. Fernández-Landa, J.; Santibañez-Gutierrez, A.; Todorovic, N.; Stajer, V.; Ostojic, S.M. Effects of creatine monohydrate on endurance performance in a trained population: A systematic review and meta-analysis. *Sports Med.* **2023**, *53*, 1017–1027. [CrossRef]
31. Gras, D.; Lanhers, C.; Bagheri, R.; Ugbolue, U.C.; Coudeyre, E.; Pereira, B.; Zak, M.; Bouillon-Minois, J.-B.; Dutheil, F. Creatine supplementation and VO_2max: A systematic review and meta-analysis. *Crit. Rev. Food Sci. Nutr.* **2023**, *63*, 4855–4866. [CrossRef] [PubMed]
32. Wilson, J.M.; Wilson, G.J.; Zourdos, M.C.; Smith, A.E.; Stout, J.R. Beta-alanine supplementation improves aerobic and anaerobic indices of performance. *Strength Cond. J.* **2010**, *32*, 71–78. [CrossRef]
33. Pinto, C.L.; Botelho, P.B.; Carneiro, J.A.; Mota, J.F. Impact of creatine supplementation in combination with resistance training on lean mass in the elderly. *J. Cachexia Sarcopenia Muscle* **2016**, *7*, 413–421. [CrossRef]

34. Sooneste, H.; Tanimoto, M.; Kakigi, R.; Saga, N.; Katamoto, S. Effects of training volume on strength and hypertrophy in young men. *J. Strength Cond. Res.* **2013**, *27*, 8–13. [CrossRef] [PubMed]
35. de Camargo, J.B.B.; Brigatto, F.; Zaroni, R.; Germano, M.; Souza, D.; Bacurau, R.; Marchetti, P.; Braz, T.; Aoki, M.; Lopes, C. Does beta-alanine supplementation enhance adaptations to resistance training? A randomized, placebo-controlled, double-blind study. *Biol. Sport* **2023**, *40*, 217–224. [CrossRef]
36. Bassinello, D.; de Salles Painelli, V.; Dolan, E.; Lixandrão, M.; Cajueiro, M.; de Capitani, M.; Saunders, B.; Sale, C.; Artioli, G.G.; Gualano, B. Beta-alanine supplementation improves isometric, but not isotonic or isokinetic strength endurance in recreationally strength-trained young men. *Amino Acids* **2019**, *51*, 27–37. [CrossRef]
37. Ashtary-Larky, D.; Bagheri, R.; Ghanavati, M.; Asbaghi, O.; Wong, A.; Stout, J.R.; Suzuki, K. Effects of beta-alanine supplementation on body composition: A GRADE-assessed systematic review and meta-analysis. *J. Int. Soc. Sports Nutr.* **2022**, *19*, 196–218. [CrossRef]
38. Mattos, D.; Santos, C.G.M.; Forbes, S.C.; Candow, D.G.; Rosa, D.; Busnardo, R.G.; Ribeiro, M.D.; Paulucio, D.; Chester, C.; Machado, M. Individual responses to creatine supplementation on muscular power is modulated by gene polymorphisms in military recruits. *J. Sci. Sport Exerc.* **2023**, *5*, 70–76. [CrossRef]
39. Syrotuik, D.G.; Bell, G.J. Acute creatine monohydrate supplementation: A descriptive physiological profile of responders vs. nonresponders. *J. Strength Cond. Res.* **2004**, *18*, 610–617.
40. Trexler, E.T.; Smith-Ryan, A.E.; Stout, J.R.; Hoffman, J.R.; Wilborn, C.D.; Sale, C.; Kreider, R.B.; Jäger, R.; Earnest, C.P.; Bannock, L. International society of sports nutrition position stand: Beta-Alanine. *J. Int. Soc. Sports Nutr.* **2015**, *12*, 30. [CrossRef]

MDPI AG
Grosspeteranlage 5
4052 Basel
Switzerland
Tel.: +41 61 683 77 34

Nutrients Editorial Office
E-mail: nutrients@mdpi.com
www.mdpi.com/journal/nutrients

www.ingramcontent.com/pod-product-compliance
Lightning Source LLC
Chambersburg PA
CBHW061449210926
51850CB00008B/1662